AN ARAMAIC BIBLIOGRAPHY
PART I

Publications of *The Comprehensive Aramaic Lexicon* Project

An Aramaic Bibliography, Part I
Old, Official, and Biblical Aramaic

AN ARAMAIC BIBLIOGRAPHY
PART I

Old, Official, and Biblical Aramaic

Joseph A. Fitzmyer, S.J., and Stephen A. Kaufman
With the collaboration of Stephan F. Bennett and Edward M. Cook

The Johns Hopkins University Press
Baltimore and London

Publication of this work was made possible in part by a grant from
the National Endowment for the Humanities, a Federal agency.

The Johns Hopkins University Press
701 West 40th Street
Baltimore, Maryland 21211-2190
The Johns Hopkins Press Ltd., London

The paper used in this book meets the minimum requirements of
American National Standard for Information Sciences—Permanence
of Paper for Printed Library Materials, ANSI Z39.48-1984.

Library of Congress Cataloging-in-Publication Data

Fitzmyer, Joseph A.
   An Aramaic bibliography / Joseph A. Fitzmyer and Stephen A. Kaufman, with
the collaboration of Stephan F. Bennett and Edward M. Cook.
      p.   cm.
   At head of title: Publications of The Aramaic Lexicon Project.
   Includes bibliographical references.
   Contents: pt. 1. Old, official, and Biblical Aramaic
   ISBN 0-8018-4312-X (pt. 1)
   1. Aramaic philology—Bibliography.   I. Kaufman, Stephen A.   II. Comprehensive
Aramaic Lexicon (Project)   III. Title.
Z7053.F57   1991
[PJ5201]   91-21491
016.492′29—dc20   CIP

CONTENTS

ABBREVIATIONS

AaGDeg	*Altaramäische Grammatik der Inschriften des 10.–8. Jh. v. Chr.* (R. Degen 1969)
AaGSeg	*Altaramäische Grammatik* (S. Segert 1975)
AAL	Afroasiatic Linguistics (Malibu, CA: Undena)
AANL	*Atti della Accademia nazionale dei Lincei,* Classe di scienze morali storiche e filologiche (Rome: Accad. naz. dei Lincei)
AAO	*Album d' antiquités orientales: Recueil de monuments inédits ou peu connus* (C. Clermont-Ganneau 1897)
AASOR	Annual of the American Schools of Oriental Research
AASyr	*Les annales archéologiques arabes syriennes* (Damascus)
ABC	*Assyrian and Babylonian Contracts with Aramaic Reference Notes* (J. H. Stevenson 1902)
AbhKGWG	*Abhandlungen der Königlichen Gesellschaft der Wissenschaften zu Göttingen*
AC	*Aramäische Chrestomathie* (J. J. Koopmans 1962)
AAASH	Acta Antiqua Academiae Scientiarum Hungaricae (Budapest)
AcOr	*Acta Orientalia* (Copenhagen)
AD	*Aramaic Documents of the Fifth Century B.C.* (G. R. Driver 1954)
ADAJ	Annual of the Department of Antiquities of Jordan (Amman)
ADD	*Assyrian Deeds and Documents* (C. H. W. Johns 1901)
AECT	*Aramaic Epigraphs on Clay Tablets of the Neo-Assyrian Period* (F. M. Fales 1986)
Aeg	*Aegyptus*
AF	*Altorientalische Forschungen* (Leipzig: Pfeiffer)
AfO	*Archiv für Orientforschung*
AH	*An Aramaic Handbook* (F. Rosenthal 1967)
AION	*Annali dell' Istituto Orientale di Napoli* (Naples)
AJA	*American Journal of Archaeology* (Princeton)
AJBA	*Australian Journal of Biblical Archaeology*
AJSL	*American Journal of Semitic Languages and Literatures* (Chicago)
AJT	*American Journal of Theology*
AMI	Archäologische Mitteilungen aus Iran
AnBib	Analecta Biblica. Investigationes scientificae in res biblicas (Rome)
ANEP	*The Ancient Near East in Pictures Relating to the Old Testament.* Ed. J. B. Pritchard. Princeton: Princeton Univ. Press 1954. 2nd ed., with supplement, 1969.
ANESTP	*The Ancient Near East.* Supplementary Texts and Pictures Relating to the Old Testament. Ed. J. B. Pritchard. Princeton: Princeton Univ. Press, 1969.
ANET	*Ancient Near Eastern Texts Relating to the Old Testament.* Ed. J. B. Pritchard. Princeton: Princeton Univ. Press 1950. 2nd. ed., 1955; 3rd. ed., with supplement, 1969.

AnOr	Analecta Orientalia
AO	*Aula Orientalis*
AOAT	Alter Orient und Altes Testament (Neukirchen-Vluyn: Neukirchener)
AÖAWW	*Anzeiger der Österreichischen Akademie der Wissenschaften in Wien, phil.-hist. Kl.*
AOS	American Oriental Series (American Oriental Society)
AP	*Aramaic Papyri of the Fifth Century* B.C. (A. Cowley 1923)
APA	*Aramaic Papyri Discovered at Assuan* (A. H. Sayce and A. Cowley 1906)
APE	*Aramäische Papyrus aus Elephantine* (A. Ungnad 1911)
APO	*Aramäische Papyrus und Ostraka aus einer jüdischen Militärkolonie zu Elephantine* (E. Sachau 1911)
ArOr	*Archiv orientální*
As	*Altsyrien* (H. T. Bossert 1951)
ASAE	*Annales du Service des Antiquités de l'Égypte*
ATAT	*Altorientalische Texte zum Alten Testament* (H. Gressmann et al. 1926)
Aug	*Augustinianum*
AUSS	*Andrews University Seminary Studies*
BA	*Biblical Archaeologist*
BARev	*Biblical Archaeology Review*
BASOR	*Bulletin of the American Schools of Oriental Research*
BAT	*Biblical Archaeology Today*, ed. J. Amitai (Jerusalem: Israel Exploration Society, 1985)
BeO	*Bibbia e oriente*
Bib	*Biblica*
BibOr	Biblica et Orientalia (Rome)
BIE	*Bulletin de l'Institut de l'Egypte*
BIFAO	*Bulletin de l'Institut français d'archéologie orientale*
BJPES	*Bulletin of the Jewish Palestine Exploration Society*
BJRL	*Bulletin of the John Rylands (University) Library (of Manchester)*
BLE	*Bulletin de littérature ecclésiastique*
BM	*Beth Mikra* (Jerusalem)
BMAP	*The Brooklyn Museum Aramaic Papyri* (E. G. Kraeling 1953)
BMB	*Bulletin du Musée de Beyrouth*
BN	*Biblische Notizen*
BO	*Bibliotheca Orientalis*
BSOAS	*Bulletin of the School of Oriental and African Studies* (University of London)
BTDAR	*The Balaam Text from Deir 'Alla Re-Evaluated*, ed. J. Hoftijzer and G. van der Kooij. Proceedings of the International Symposium held at Leiden 21–24 August 1989 (Leiden: Brill, 1991).
BW	*The Biblical World*
BZ	*Biblische Zeitschrift*
BZAW	Beihefte zur *ZAW*
CBQ	*Catholic Biblical Quarterly*
CdE	*Chronique d'Egypte*
CIS	*Corpus Inscriptionum Semiticarum, pars secunda: Inscriptiones aramaicae* (Academia Inscriptionum et Litterarum Humaniorum 1888, 1893)

CRAIBL	*Comptes rendus de l'Académie des inscriptions et belles-lettres*
CT	*Cuneiform Texts from Babylonian Tablets in the British Museum*
DAE	*Documents araméens d'Égypte* (P. Grelot 1972)
DOTT	*Documents from Old Testament Times* (D. Winton Thomas 1958)
DTT	*Dansk Teologisk Tidsskrift*
EA	*Épigraphes araméens* (L. Delaporte 1912)
EAS	*Les états araméens de Syrie depuis leur fondation jusqu'à leur transformation en provinces assyriennes* (H. Sader 1987)
EAW	*East and West*
EI	*Eretz-Israel* (Jerusalem: Israel Exploration Society)
EM	*Encyclopedia Miqrait*
EncBib	*Enciclopedia de la Biblia*, ed. A. Díez Macho and S. Bartina, 6 vols. (Barcelona: Garriga)
ERS	*Études sur les religions sémitiques* 2d ed. (M.-J. Lagrange 1905)
EstBib	*Estudios bíblicos*
ESE	*Ephemeris für semitische Epigraphik* (M. Lidzbarski 1902–15)
ETL	*Ephemerides theologicae lovanienses*
ETR	*Etudes theologiques et religieuses*
EVO	*Egitto e Vicino Oriente*
EvT	*Evangelische Theologie*
ExpTim	*Expository Times*
FuB	*Forschungen und Berichte der Staatlichen Museen* (Berlin)
GGA	*Göttingische gelehrte Anzeigen*
GLECS	*Comptes rendus du Groupe Linguistique d'Études Chamito-Sémitiques*
HNE	*Handbuch der nordsemitischen Epigraphik* (M. Lidzbarski 1898)
HomAD-S	*Hommages à André Dupont-Sommer*, ed. A. Caquot and M. Philonenko (Paris: Maisonneuve, 1971)
HSM	Harvard Semitic Monographs
HTR	*Harvard Theological Review*
HUCA	*Hebrew Union College Annual*
ICC	International Critical Commentary
IDB	*Interpreter's Dictionary of the Bible* (Nashville: Abingdon)
IEJ	*Israel Exploration Journal*
IOS	*Israel Oriental Studies*
IR	*Inscriptions Reveal: Documents from the Time of the Bible, the Mishna and the Talmud* (R. Hestrin et al. 1973)
ITQ	*Irish Theological Quarterly*
JA	*Journal asiatique*
JANES	*Journal of the Ancient Near Eastern Society* (formerly of Columbia University)
JAOS	*Journal of the American Oriental Society*
JARCE	*Journal of the American Research Center in Egypt*
JBL	*Journal of Biblical Literature*
JBR	*Journal of Bible and Religion*
JCS	*Journal of Cuneiform Studies*
JEA	*Journal of Egyptian Archaeology*

JEAS	*Jews of Elephantine and Arameans of Syene (Fifth Century B.C.E.)* (B. Porten and J. C. Greenfield 1974)
JEOL	*Jaarbericht van het Vooraziatisch-Egyptisch Genootschap: Ex Oriente Lux*
JESHO	*Journal of the Economic and Social History of the Orient*
JfKF	*Jahrbuch für kleinasiatische Forschung*
JHS	*Journal of Hellenic Studies*
JJLG	*Jahrbuch der Jüdisch-Literarischen Gesellschaft*
JJS	*Journal of Jewish Studies*
JNES	*Journal of Near Eastern Studies*
JNSL	*Journal of Northwest Semitic Languages*
JPOS	*Journal of the Palestine Oriental Society*
JQR	*Jewish Quarterly Review*
JRAS	*Journal of the Royal Asiatic Society*
JSJ	*Journal for the Study of Judaism in the Persian, Hellenistic, and Roman Period*
JSOT	*Journal for the Study of the Old Testament*
JSS	*Journal of Semitic Studies*
JTS	*Journal of Theological Studies*
JZ	*Jüdische Zeitschrift*
KAI	*Kanaanäische und aramäische Inschriften* (H. Donner and W. Röllig 1962, 1964)
KIT	Kleine Texte für Vorlesungen und Übungen
LA	*Les Araméens* (A. Dupont-Sommer 1949)
Leš	*Lešonenu*
MAOG	Mitteilungen der Altorientalischen Gesellschaft, Berlin
MDB	*Le monde de la Bible*
MDOG	Mitteilungen der Deutschen Orient-Gesellschaft zu Berlin
MGWJ	*Monatsschrift für Geschichte und Wissenschaft des Judentums*
MIO	Mitteilungen des Instituts für Orientforschung (Berlin)
MNRAS	*Monthly Notices of the Royal Astronomical Society*
MPAIBL	Mémoires présentés à l'Académie des Inscriptions et Belles-Lettres
MUSJ	*Mélanges de l'Université Saint Joseph*
MVAG	Mitteilungen der Vorderasiatisch-ägyptischen Gesellschaft
NedTT	*Nederlands theologisch Tijdschrift*
NERTOT	*Near Eastern Religious Texts Relating to the Old Testament* (W. Beyerlin 1978)
NESE	*Neue Ephemeris für semitische Epigraphik* (R. Degen et al. 1972, 1974, 1978)
NovT	*Novum Testamentum*
NRV	*Neubabylonische Rechts- und Verwaltungstexte* (O. Krückmann 1933)
NSI	*A Text-Book of North-Semitic Inscriptions* (G. A. Cooke 1903)
NSR	*Nordsyrisch-südanatolische Reliefs* (H. Genge 1979)
NTCS	*Newsletter for Targumic and Cognate Studies*
NTS	*New Testament Studies*
NC	*Numismatic Chronicle*
OIP	Oriental Institute Publications

OLP	Orientalia lovaniensia periodica
OLZ	*Orientalistische Literaturzeitung*
Or	*Orientalia*
OrAnt	*Oriens antiquus*
OrLovAn	Orientalia Lovaniensia Analecta
OS	*Orientalia Suecana*
OTS	*Oudtestamentische Studiën*
PalSb	*Palestinskii Sbornik*
ParPass	*Parola del Passato* (Naples)
PEFQS	*Palestine Exploration Fund: Quarterly Statement*
PEQ	*Palestine Exploration Quarterly*
PSBA	*Proceedings of the Society of Biblical Archaeology*
RA	*Revue d'assyriologie et d'archéologie orientale*
RAO	*Recueil d'archéologie orientale* (C. Clermont-Ganneau 1885–1924)
RArch	*Revue archéologique*
RB	*Revue biblique*
REG	*Revue des études grecques*
REJ	*Revue des études juives*
RES	*Répertoire d'épigraphie sémitique* (Commission du *CIS* 1900–5, 1907–14)
RevQ	*Revue de Qumran*
RevSém	*Revue sémitique*
RIDA	*Revue internationale des droits de l'antiquité* (Brussels)
RivB	*Rivista biblica*
RGG	*Die Religion in Geschichte und Gegenwart: Handwörterbuch für Theologie und Religionswissenschaft*
RHR	*Revue de l'histoire des religions*
RlA	*Reallexikon der Assyriologie*, ed. E. Ebeling, B. Meissner et al.
RQ	*Römische Quartalschrift für christliche Altertumskunde und Kirchengeschichte*
RSO	*Revista degli studi orientali*
RSPT	*Revue des sciences philosophiques et théologiques*
RTAT	*Religionsgeschichtliches Textbuch zum Alten Testament* (W. Beyerlin 1975)
RTP	*Revue de théologie et de philosophie*
SAAB	*State Archives of Assyria Bulletin* (Padua)
SBAW	*Sitzungsberichte der Bayerischen Akademie der Wissenschaft*
SBFLA	*Studii biblici franciscani: Liber Annuus*
SBL	Society of Biblical Literature
Sem	*Semitica*
Shnaton	*Shnaton - Annual for the Biblical and Ancient Near Eastern Society*
SKAWW	*Sitzungsberichte der Kaiserlichen Akademie der Wissenschaften Wien*, Phil.-Hist. Kl.
SPAW	*Sitzungsberichte der Preussischen Akademie der Wissenschaften zu Berlin* Phil.-hist. Kl.
SPB	Studia Post-Biblica
SW	*Semitic Writing* (G. R. Driver 1948)
TAD	*Textbook of Aramaic Documents from Ancient Egypt Newly Copied, Edited and Translated into Hebrew and English* (B. Porten and A. Yardeni 1986 –)

	Vol. 1(=**A**): Letters (1986); Vol. 2(=**B**): Contracts (1989); Vol. 3(=**C**): Lists, Literary and Historical Texts (1991)
TAE	*Textes araméens d'Egypte* (N. Aimé-Giron 1931)
TC	Textes cunéiformes du Louvre
ThGl	*Theologie und Glaube*
TLZ	*Theologische Literaturzeitung*
TQ	*Theologische Quartalschrift*
TRu	*Theologische Rundschau*
TSSI	*Textbook of Syrian Semitic Inscriptions* Volume II. (J. C. L. Gibson 1975)
TUAT	Texte aus der Umwelt des Alten Testaments. Vol. 1. (O. Kaiser 1982–85)
TZ	*Theologische Zeitschrift*
UF	*Ugarit Forschungen*
Vat.	F. Vattioni. 1970–71. Epigrafia aramaica. *Aug* 10:493–532, 11:18–190
VD	*Verbum domini*
VDI	*Vestnik drevnej istorii* (Moscow)
VO	*Vicino oriente* (Rome)
VT	*Vetus Testamentum* (Leiden)
VTSup	Supplements to *Vetus Testamentum* (Leiden)
WO	*Die Welt des Orients* (Göttingen)
WZKM	*Wiener Zeitschrift für die Kunde des Morgenlandes* (Vienna)
ZA	*Zeitschrift für Assyriologie* (Berlin)
ZÄS	*Zeitschrift für ägyptische Sprache und Altertumskunde* (Berlin)
ZAW	*Zeitschrift für die alttestamentliche Wissenschaft*
ZDMG	*Zeitschrift der Deutschen Morgenländische Gesellschaft*
ZDMGSup	Supplements to *ZDMG*
ZDPV	*Zeitschrift des Deutschen Palästina-Vereins*
ZS	*Zeitschrift für Semitistik und verwandte Gebiete*
ZVO	*Zapiski Vostochnogo otdeleniya Rysskogo arkheologicheskogo obshchestva*
ZVR	*Zeitschrift für vergleichende Rechtswissenschaft*

PREFACE

Origins

The origins of this volume go back to 1964, when Fitzmyer spent a sabbatical year using the resources of the libraries of the Princeton Theological Seminary and Princeton University. At that time he began to collect a file with a master card listing the *editio princeps* of every Aramaic inscription, text, or writing from the emergence of the language down to the Syriac period. Many references to secondary literature on the various texts were also collected. That file has been kept up over the years and forms the basis for the bibliography.

In the beginning and along the way, secondary lists found in standard surveys of the Aramaic language and bibliographies of different sorts were utilized. As in all such works, many of the references contained errors and required diligent checking. Moreover, entries to the secondary literature were originally added only as they were encountered, not through any systematic combing of the literature. In spite of these shortcomings, when, at the outset of the *Comprehensive Aramaic Lexicon* (*CAL*) project, the editors agreed that a systematic listing of the corpus of texts to be covered and the current bibliography thereto was a *sine qua non*, Fitzmyer's extensive files seemed a natural starting point for such an endeavor.

Checking of the original entries and entering them into a computer data file took place under the direction of Fitzmyer and Bennett at JHU. Bennett was also entrusted with much of the work of font design and related matters. Subsequently, responsibility for the comprehensiveness of the collection and the design of the finished reference work was assumed by Kaufman, with Cook working at his direction and supervising assistants at HUC.

Some of Fitzmyer's bibliographical file has already been published in earlier forms. Two such installments deserve mention here: Part of his article, "The Contribution of Qumran Aramaic to the Study of the New Testament" (*NTS* 20 [1973–74]:382–407; reprinted with slight revision in Fitzmyer 1979, 85–113) included two charts, one listing Palestinian Aramaic texts and the other, Qumran Aramaic texts. Another bibliographical listing became part of his "Some Notes on Aramaic Epistolography" (1974).

Contents

The present bibliography is meant to be as comprehensive as possible. We have attempted to include every known text, no matter how small or fragmentary, and all substantive secondary discussions of such texts. (Those texts whose status as Aramaic is uncertain are listed in Appendix A.) Naturally, there will be those who will disagree with our determination as to what is or is not Aramaic, as well as whether every offhand mention of an Aramaic text or word merits inclusion in the list of secondary literature. It is also inevitable in a work of such pioneer scope and proportion that users will discover real errors and omissions, despite our best efforts to eliminate them. We shall be grateful to all who spot such oversights and bring them to our attention.

The bibliography is to appear in several parts, the first two of which are based on Fitzmyer's files. This volume, Part I, covers Old Aramaic (from 900 B.C.E. to 700 B.C.E. [or perhaps to 613 B.C.E., the fall of Nineveh]), Standard or Official Aramaic – the so-called Reichsaramäisch (to 200 B.C.E.), and Biblical Aramaic. Part II will include texts from the Middle Period of Aramaic (200 B.C.E. to 300 C.E.). For the sake of completeness, we have chosen to include the dialects of ancient Sam'al and Deir 'Alla in this bibliography, even though it has not yet been decided whether the lexical materials from these dialects will be included in the *CAL*. In the case of Biblical Aramaic, we have not included the innumerable commentaries on the books of Daniel or Ezra, except for those whose relevance to matters Aramaic is noteworthy, but we have included monographs and articles dealing specifically with the contents of the Aramaic chapters in those books.

Structure

Some comments here to guide the user: The work is structured in two major parts. Inasmuch as a large percentage of bibliographic entries, both *editiones principes* and secondary treatments, deal with multiple texts and topics, in order to avoid endless duplicate citations, complete bibliographical information on all such references has been collected in Part II. Appropriate reference to these entries is made in Part I using an author–date style of citation (with the exception of the references in I.A.1, which have been given in complete form in order to aid in the identification of the frequently used abbreviations in the "Easy Access" sections of Part I.B). Book reviews have been cited where known, but no effort has been made to be all-inclusive in this regard. Reviews are cited at three different levels: Brief notices are listed in full under the book reviewed. Those containing substantive additions and corrections are given as complete bibliographic entries and are also cross referenced under the reviewed book, but are not referred to in Part I. Those that make a signficant scholarly contribution in their own right are treated like the previous case but also have cross references to them in Part I like any other entry. To those who may be offended by our decisions in some of these cases we apologize in advance.

Part I is further subdivided into three main chapters: In Chapter I.A are collected references to general topics in Aramaic studies, as they relate to the historical period here under review. Chapter I.C deals with Biblical Aramaic. Chapter I.B, entitled TEXTS, requires some commentary. Most entries contain the following information: a sequential, identifying alphanumeric key (used in collational tables in Appendix B), a brief descriptive title followed by the provenance of the text and its approximate date, and, in the right margin, the siglum to be used in the *CAL* to refer to this text or group of related texts. Where known, a physical description of the text and its current location are given. There follows, only in the case of relatively brief inscriptions (particularly so for those not included in the standard text collections), the text of the inscription as currently read in the *CAL* files. The general intent of this inclusion is to aid the user in evaluating the relevance of various minor inscriptions for specific needs, though on occasion we have ventured to posit a reading at odds with that currently accepted. After a listing of the *editio princeps* (marked "*Ed. Pr.*"), we list (under the rubric "Easy Access") commonly available collections of text editions, translations, and/or illustrations wherein treatment of this material can be found. Lastly, come the cross references to the collected references in Part II (under the heading "Literature"). In the case of large corpora of related materials, such as dockets and seals, a tabular format has sometimes been chosen as being more useful.

The texts are ordered by general geographical origin and date. Additional access points may be found by consulting the several tables in Appendix B. The identification of the *editio princeps* of a given text is not always an easy matter. We have tried to list the first serious treatment of each text rather than mere mention or even a citation; we recognize that not all will agree with our interpretation of the facts.

Entries have been checked using the resources of, above all, the libraries of Woodstock College (now the Woodstock Theological Center Library, housed at Georgetown University), the Catholic University of America, the Johns Hopkins University, Hebrew Union College — Jewish Institute of Religion (Cincinnati), and the Library of Congress. The resources of the libraries of Harvard University, Harvard Divinity School, the Biblical Institute (Rome), the Bodleian and Oriental Institute (Oxford), and the Faculty of Theology of the Katholiek Universitet te Leuven have also been consulted. To the patient reference librarians of all of these fine institutions go our deepest thanks.

Finally, it is our pleasant duty to thank various persons who have helped or have collaborated with us in the production of this bibliography. First of all, the other editor of the *CAL*, Prof. Delbert R. Hillers of the Johns Hopkins University. Second, Naicong Li, programmer for the *CAL* project from 1986 through 1988. Third, various graduate students and research associates who have contributed time to entry checking and data entry: Eleonora Cussini, Doris Gottschalk, Carolyn Higginbotham, Ed Hostetter, Jonathan Lewis, Mark Meehl, Kathy Slanski, Ed Smith, and Jan Verbruggen at JHU, and, at HUC, Dr. Jerome Lund, Dr. Deirdre Dempsey, and Steven Boyd. We are particularly grateful to Dr. Lund for his devoted efforts to bring order out of the chaos of the corpus of seals and to Ms. Cussini for her work on the Babylonian tablets in European collections. Fourth, the scholars around the world who have cooperated with us in seeing that our materials are as complete and up-to-date as possible, among them professors K. Beyer, P. Bordreuil, F. M. Cross, P. E. Dion, F. M. Fales, J. C. Greenfield, D. Gropp, A. Lemaire, B. Levine, E. Lipiński, A. Millard, T. Muraoka, J. Naveh, B. Porten, F. Rosenthal, M. Sokoloff, and J. M. Wesselius. B. Porten also provided us with the sigla to be used in his essential *TAD* volumes long in advance of their publication. Lastly, our thanks to Ms. Jacqueline Wehmueller, acquisitions editor of the Johns Hopkins University Press, for her patience and help in seeing this volume through the press.

1

PART ONE

A. ARAMAIC STUDIES — GENERAL

A.1   COLLECTIONS — Texts, Translations, Illustrations

Academia Inscriptionum et Litterarum Humaniorum. 1888, 1893. *Corpus Inscriptionum Semiticarum, pars 2: Inscriptiones aramaicae.* Ed. C. J. de Vogüé. 2 vols. Paris: Imprimerie Nationale [Librairie C. Klincksieck]. [= *CIS*]

Aimé-Giron, N. 1931. *Textes araméens d'Egypte.* Service des antiquités de l'Egypte. Cairo: Imprimerie de l'Institut Français. [= *TAE*]

———. 1939–40. Adversaria semitica. *BIFAO* 38:1–63; *ASAE* 39:339–63; *ASAE* 40:433–66.

Bossert, H. T., in collaboration with R. Naumann. 1951. *Altsyrien: Kunst und Handwerk in Cypern, Syrien, Palästina, Transjordanien und Arabien von den Anfängen bis zum völligen Aufgehen in der griechisch-römischen Kultur.* Die Ältesten Kulturen des Mittelmeerkreises, vol. 3. Tübingen: E. Wasmuth. [= *As*]

Clermont-Ganneau, C. 1885–1924. *Recueil d'archéologie orientale.* 8 vols. Paris: E. Leroux. [= *RAO*]

———. 1897. *Album d'antiquités orientales: Recueil de monuments inédits ou peu connus.* Paris: E. Leroux. [= *AAO*]

Commission du *CIS* 1900–5, 1907–14. *Répertoire d'épigraphie sémitique.* 8 vols. Ed. C. J. de Vogüé. Paris: Imprimerie Nationale [Librairie C. Klincksieck]. [= *RES*]

Cooke, G. A. 1903. *A Text-Book of North-Semitic Inscriptions: Moabite, Hebrew, Phoenician, Aramaic, Nabataean, Palmyrene, Jewish.* Oxford: Clarendon. [= *NSI*]

Cowley, A. 1919. *Jewish Documents of the Time of Ezra: Translated from the Aramaic.* London: Society for Promoting Christian Knowledge.

———. 1923. *Aramaic Papyri of the Fifth Century B. C: Edited with Translations and Notes.* Oxford: Clarendon. Reprint. Osnabrück: Zeller, 1967. [= *AP*]

Degen, R. 1969. *Altaramäische Grammatik der Inschriften des 10.–8. Jh. v. Chr.* Abh. f. d. Kunde d. Morgenlandes 38/3. Wiesbaden: F. Steiner. [= *AaGDeg*]

Degen, R., W. W. Müller, and W. Röllig, eds. 1972, 1974, 1978. *Neue Ephemeris für semitische Epigraphik.* 3 vols. Wiesbaden: Harrassowitz. [= *NESE*]

Delaporte, L. 1912. *Épigraphes araméens: Étude des textes araméens gravés ou écrits sur des tablettes cunéiformes.* Paris: P. Geuthner. [= *EA*]

Donner, H., and W. Röllig. 1962, 1964. *Kanaanäische und aramäische Inschriften (Mit einem Beitrag von O. Rössler): Band I, Texte; Band II, Kommentar; Band III, Glossar und Indizes.* Wiesbaden: Harrassowitz. 3rd rev. edition, 1971–73. [= *KAI*]

Driver, G. R. 1948. *Semitic Writing.* The Schweich Lectures of the British Academy. 3rd rev. edition. London: Oxford University Press. [= *SW*]

————. 1954. *Aramaic Documents of the Fifth Century* B.C., *Transcribed and Edited with Translation and Notes*. Oxford: Clarendon. Abridged and Revised Edition, 1957. [= *AD*]

Dupont-Sommer, A. 1949. *Les Araméens*. L'orient ancien illustré. Paris: Maisonneuve. [= *LA*]

Fales, F. M. 1986. *Aramaic Epigraphs on Clay Tablets of the Neo-Assyrian Period*. Dipartimento di Studi Orientali. Studi Semitici n.s. 2. Rome: Università degli studi "La Sapienza". [= *AECT*]

Genge, H. 1979. *Nordsyrisch-südanatolische Reliefs*. Eine archäologisch–historische Untersuchung: Datierung und Bestimmung. 2 vols. Det Kongelige Danske Videnskabernes Selskab: Hist.-filos. meddelelser 49. Copenhagen: Munksgaard. [= *NSR*]

Gibson, J. C. L. 1975. *Textbook of Syrian Semitic Inscriptions: Volume II, Aramaic Inscriptions Including Inscriptions in the Dialect of Zenjirli*. Oxford: Clarendon. [= *TSSI*]

Ginsberg, H. L. 1969. Aramaic Papyri from Elephantine. In *ANESTP*, 112–13 = *ANET*^{3}, 548–49.

Grelot, P. 1972. *Documents araméens d'Égypte*. Littératures anciennes du Proche-Orient. Paris: Cerf. [= *DAE*]

Gressmann, H., et al., eds. 1926. *Altorientalische Texte zum Alten Testament*. Altorientalische Texte und Bilder zum Alten Testament. Berlin/Leipzig: De Gruyter. 2d edition. [= *ATAT*]

Hestrin, R., et al., eds. 1973. *Inscriptions Reveal: Documents from the Time of the Bible, the Mishna and the Talmud*. Jerusalem: Israel Museum. 2d ed. [= *IR*]

Hug, V. forthcoming. *Altaramäische Grammatik der Texte des 7. und 6. Jr.s v. Chr.* Heidelberger Studien zum Alten Orient 4. Heidelberg: Heidelberger Orientverlag.

Johns, C. H. W. 1901. *Assyrian Deeds and Documents: Cuneiform Texts, Introduction, Officials, Metrology*. 2 vols. Cambridge: Deighton Bell and Co. [= *ADD*]

Kaiser, O., ed. 1982–85. *Rechts- und Wirtschaftsurkunden; Historisch-chronologische Texte*. Texte aus der Umwelt des Alten Testaments. Gütersloh: G. Mohn. [= *TUAT*].

Koopmans, J. J. 1962. *Aramäische Chrestomathie: Ausgewählte Texte (Inschriften Ostraka und Papyri) bis zum 3. Jahrhundert n. Chr. für das Studium der aramäischen Sprache gesammelt*. 2 vols. Leiden: Nederlands Institut voor het Nabije Oosten. [= *AC*]

Kraeling, E. G. 1953. *The Brooklyn Museum Aramaic Papyri: New Documents of the Fifth Century B.C. from the Jewish Colony at Elephantine*. New Haven, Conn.: Yale Univ. Press. Reprint. New York: Arno, 1969. [= *BMAP*]

Krückmann, O. 1933. *Neubabylonische Rechts- und Verwaltungstexte*. Texte und Materialien der Frau Prof. Hilprecht Collection of Babylonian Antiquities 2–3. Leipzig: J. C. Hinrichs. [= *NRV*]

Lagrange, M.-J. 1905. *Études sur les religions sémitiques*. 2d ed. Paris: Lecoffre. [= *ERS*]

Lidzbarski, M. 1898. *Handbuch der nordsemitischen Epigraphik nebst ausgewählten Inschriften.* 2 vols. Weimar: E. Felber. Reprint. Hildesheim: Olms, 1962. [= *HNE*]

———. 1902, 1908, 1915. *Ephemeris für semitische Epigraphik.* 3 vols. Giessen: J. Ricker. [= *ESE*]

Lipiński, E. 1988. Nouveaux recueils de textes araméens et phénico-puniques. *BO* 45:510–17.

Porten, B. in collaboration with J. C. Greenfield. 1974. *Jews of Elephantine and Arameans of Syene (Fifth Century B.C.E.): Fifty Aramaic Texts with Hebrew and English Translations.* Jerusalem: Academon. [= *JEAS*]

Porten, B., and A. Yardeni. 1986 –. *Textbook of Aramaic Documents from Ancient Egypt Newly Copied, Edited and Translated into Hebrew and English.* Vol. 1: Letters (1986); Vol. 2: Contracts (1989); Vol. 3: Lists, Literary and Historical Texts (forthcoming). Texts and Studies for Students. Jerusalem: Hebrew University, Dept. of History of the Jewish People. Distributed by Eisenbraun's. [= *TADA, TADB, TADC*]

Rosenthal, F. 1955. Canaanite and Aramaic Inscriptions. *ANET*, 499–505.

Rosenthal, F., ed. 1967. *An Aramaic Handbook.* 4 vols. Porta Linguarum Orientalium. Wiesbaden: Harrassowitz. [= *AH*]

Rosenthal, F. 1969. Canaanite and Aramaic Inscriptions. *ANESTP*, 217–26 = *ANET*^{3}, 653–62.

Sachau, E. 1907. *Drei aramäische Papyrusurkunden aus Elephantine.* APAW phil.-hist. Kl. Berlin: Königl. Akademie der Wissenschaften.

———. 1911. *Aramäische Papyrus und Ostraka aus einer jüdischen Militärkolonie zu Elephantine: Altorientalische Sprachdenkmäler des 5. Jahrhunderts vor Christus.* 2 vols. Leipzig: Hinrichs. [= *APO*]

Sader, H. 1987. *Les états araméens de Syrie depuis leur fondation jusqu'à leur transformation en provinces assyriennes.* Beiruter Texte und Studien 36. Beirut: Orient-Institut der Deutschen Morgenländischen Gesellschaft. [= *EAS*]

Sayce, A. H. 1906. *Aramaic Papyri Discovered at Assuan.* Ed. A. E. Cowley, W. Spiegelberg, and S. de Ricci. London: A. Moring. [= *APA*]

Segal, J. B. 1983. *Aramaic Texts from North Saqqara with Some Fragments in Phoenician.* Excavations at North Saqqara, Documentary series, Memoir 6. London: Egypt Exploration Society.

Segert, S. 1975. *Altaramäische Grammatik: Mit Bibliographie, Chrestomathie und Glossar.* Leipzig: VEB Verlag Enzyklopädie. [= *AaGSeg*]

Sprengling, M. 1917–18. The Aramaic Papyri of Elephantine in English. *AJT* 21:411–52; 22:349–75.

Staerk, W. 1907. *Die jüdisch-aramäischen Papyri von Assuan sprachlich und sachlich erklärt.* KIT 22–23. Bonn: Marcus & Weber.

———. 1908. *Aramäische Urkunden zur Geschichte des Judentums im VI. und V. Jahrhundert vor Chr. sprachlich und sachlich erklärt.* KIT 32. Bonn: Marcus & Weber.

————. 1912. *Alte und neue aramäische Papyri übersetzt und erklärt.* KIT 94. Bonn: Marcus & Weber.

Stevenson, J. H. 1902. *Assyrian and Babylonian Contracts with Aramaic Reference Notes.* The Vanderbilt Oriental Series. New York, Cincinnati, Chicago: American Book Co. [= *ABC*]

Ungnad, A. 1911. *Aramäische Papyrus aus Elephantine: Kleine Ausgabe unter Zugrundelegung von Eduard Sachaus Erstausgabe.* Leipzig: Hinrichs. [= *APE]*

Vattioni, F. 1970–71. Epigrafia aramaica. *Aug* 10:493–532; 11:18–190. [= **Vat.**]

————. 1970–71. I sigilli, le monete e gli avori aramaici. *Aug* 11:47–87.

de Vogüé, C. J. 1868–77. *Syrie centrale: Inscriptions sémitiques.* Paris: J. Baudry.

Winton Thomas, D., ed. 1958. *Documents from Old Testament Times, Translated with Introductions and Notes by Members of the Society for Old Testament Study.* London: Nelson; New York: Harper. [= *DOTT*]

A.2 BIBLIOGRAPHIES AND SURVEYS

M. Lidzbarski 1898, esp. vol. 1, pp. 4–83 • S. de Ricci 1906 • F. Rosenthal 1939 •
J. J. Koopmans 1957 • F. Vattioni 1969a • E. Y. Kutscher 1970 • H. J. W. Drijvers
1973 • F. Vattioni 1978, esp. pp. 487–93 • M. Bar-Asher 1978 • F. Rosenthal
1978a • F. Vattioni 1979, esp. pp. 662–67 • F. Vattioni 1980, esp. pp. 693–99 • F.
Vattioni 1981a, esp. pp. 675–80 • F. Vattioni 1982, esp. pp. 654–62 • F. Vattioni
1983, esp. pp. 693–99 • F. Vattioni 1984a, esp. pp. 675–80 • F. Vattioni 1985,
esp. pp. 710–21 • W. E. Aufrecht 1985 • A. Lemaire 1986 • R. Contini 1986 • F.
Vattioni 1986a, esp. pp. 603–15 • F. Vattioni 1987 • F. Vattioni 1988, esp. pp.
314–25 • S. P. Brock 1989.

A.3 THE ARAMEANS — History

T. Nöldeke 1871 • E. Sachau 1892 • J. Halévy 1893–94, esp. pp. 324–36; 25–53
• J. F. McCurdy 1908 • S. Schiffer 1911 • E. Kraeling 1918 • K. Galling 1938 •
F. Rosenthal 1939 • K. Elliger 1947 • R. T. O'Callaghan 1948 • N. Schneider
1949 • A. Malamat 1949–50a • A. Dupont-Sommer 1949a • F. Spadafora 1951 •
H. T. Bossert 1951 • P. K. Hitti 1951 • S. Moscati 1951a • A. Dupont-Sommer
1954 • A. Pohl 1954 • M. McNamara 1957 • M. Unger 1957 • A. Malamat 1958
• B. Zahdi 1958–59 • P. Sacchi 1959 • S. Moscati 1959 • P. Sacchi 1960–61 • H.
Tadmor 1961 • J. C. L. Gibson 1961 • B. Mazar 1962 • D. O. Edzard 1964 • G.
Buccellati 1967 • J. A. Fitzmyer 1967a • D. Diringer and R. Regensburger 1968,
esp. p. 1.196–98 • M. Dietrich 1970 • E. Lipiński 1971b • A. Malamat 1973 • J.
Teixidor 1973, esp. p. 404 • J. Mudarres 1974 • J. Teixidor 1974, esp. p. 314 • H.
Tadmor 1975 • W. Helck 1975 • J. A. Brinkman 1977 • M. Elat 1977 • R. Zadok
1977 • D. J. Wiseman 1978 • I. Eph'al 1978 • E. Lipiński 1978c • M. 1979 • E.
Lipiński 1979a • A. R. Millard 1980 • M. J. Mulder 1980 • A. Lemaire 1981 • E.
Akurgal 1981 • M. Heltzer 1981 • H. Tadmor 1982a • J. C. Greenfield 1982a • A.
R. Millard 1983 • B. Porten 1983d • B. Porten 1984 • R. Zadok 1984 • R. Zadok
1984a • A. Lemaire 1984e • E. Bresciani 1985 • C. Cannuyer 1985 • D. C. Snell
1985 • R. A. Stucky 1985 • R. Zadok 1985 • R. Zadok 1985a • A. Lemaire 1985f
• J. C. Greenfield 1986a • B. Mazar 1986 • N. Mendecki 1986 • E. Lipiński 1987
• H. Sader 1987 • J. C. Greenfield 1987 • N. Mendecki 1987 • W. T. Pitard 1987
• J. C. Greenfield 1987a • A. Lemaire 1988a • J. D. Ray 1988 • M. Dandamaev
and V. G. Lukonin 1989 • J. F. Healey 1989 • G. M. Schwartz 1989 • H. Tadmor
1989 • E. Lipiński 1989a • A. R. Millard 1989b • A. R. Millard 1989c • A. R.
Millard 1990.

A.4 THE ARAMAIC LANGUAGE — General Discussions

J. F. McCurdy 1908 • J.-B. Chabot 1910 • O. G. von Wesedonk 1932 • H. L.
Ginsberg 1933–34 • G. Messina 1934 • H. L. Ginsberg 1935–36 • F. Rosenthal
1939 • H. L. Ginsberg 1942 • E. Y. Kutscher 1942–3 • K. Galling 1948 • R. A.
Bowman 1948 • J.-P. Audet 1950 • C. Brockelmann 1954 • F. Rosenthal 1955a •
S. Moscati 1956a • S. Moscati 1956b • W. F. Stinespring 1958 • E. Y. Kutscher
1960 • K. Beyer 1962 • R. Stiehl 1964 • A. Díez Macho 1965 • E. Y. Kutscher

1965 • S. Segert 1965 • J. C. Greenfield 1967–68 • J. A. Fitzmyer 1967a • E. Y. Kutscher 1970 • H. L. Ginsberg 1970 • E. Y. Kutscher 1970a • R. Macuch 1971 • S. A. Kaufman 1974, esp. pp. 152–70 • J. A. Delaunay 1974a • J. C. Greenfield 1974a • J. C. Greenfield 1976b • K. Beyer 1977 • J. C. Greenfield 1978b • J. A. Fitzmyer 1979 • J. A. Fitzmyer 1979a • J. Fellman 1980 • S. A. Kaufman 1980 • F. Rundgren 1981 • J. C. Greenfield 1981a • J. C. Greenfield 1983a • S. A. Kaufman 1983 • K. Beyer 1984 • D. I. Block 1984 • A. Caquot 1984 • S. A. Kaufman 1984 • J. Naveh and J. C. Greenfield 1984 • F. Vattioni 1984 • P. Fronzaroli 1985 • J. C. Greenfield 1985b • H. Marblestone 1985 • K. Beyer 1986 • E. Lipiński 1987 • R. M. Voigt 1987 • G. Garbini 1988 • A. R. Millard 1989 • E. Lipiński 1990 • E. Lipiński 1990a.

A.5 GRAMMARS

K. Marti 1896 • H. L. Strack 1921 • W. B. Stevenson 1924 • H. Bauer and P. Leander 1927 • P. Leander 1928 • H. Bauer and P. Leander 1929 • J. A. Montgomery 1940–41 • L. Palacios 1953 • G. Garbini 1956a • J. J. Koopmans 1957a • F. Rosenthal 1961 • A. F. Johns 1963 • N. H. Richardson 1965 • R. Degen 1969 • J. Teixidor 1971, esp. p. 457 • E. Y. Kutscher 1972 • P.-E. Dion 1974 • S. Segert 1975 • V. Hug forthcoming.

A.6 GRAMMATICAL STUDIES

J. Barth 1901 • E. König 1901a • A. J. Wensinck 1909 • I. Eitan 1927–30 • P. Joüon 1930–31 • J. Cantineau 1931a • A. J. Wensinck 1931, esp. pp. 12, 14 • H. Yalon 1931, esp. pp. 100–102 • J. Cantineau 1932 • P. Joüon 1934 • H. Yalon 1935 • H. H. Schaeder 1938 • C. Brockelmann 1939 • P. Mouterde 1939 • C. Brockelmann 1940 • E. Y. Kutscher 1950 • Z. Ben-Ḥayyim 1951 • S. Moscati 1954 • G. Garbini 1956 • S. Moscati 1956 • J. A. Fitzmyer 1957 • J. Friedrich 1957b • G. Garbini 1957 • S. Segert 1958b • K. Aartun 1959 • G. Garbini 1959 • I. as-Samarra'i 1959 • G. Garbini 1960a • H. B. Rosen 1961 • S. Morag 1962 • S. Moscati 1962 • W. F. Stinespring 1962 • R. Macuch 1965, esp. pp. xlvii–liv • J. A. Soggin 1965 • A. Spitaler 1968 • F. Pennacchietti 1968, esp. pp. 11–35 • R. Degen 1969a • G. Garbini 1969 • G. Garbini 1969a • J. C. Greenfield 1969 • M. Kaddari 1969 • E. Y. Kutscher 1969 • J. Blau 1970 • T. O. Lambdin 1971 • J. L. Malone 1971 • H. Tawil 1972 • D. Boyarin 1972–73 • K. Aartun 1973 • S. A. Kaufman 1974, esp. pp. 116–52 • S. A. Ryder 1974 • G. Janssens 1975–76 • T. Muraoka 1976 • M. M. Bravmann 1977 • E. Clarke 1977 • S. A. Kaufman 1977a • P. Coxon 1977 • P. Grelot 1977 • P. Coxon 1978 • E. Lipiński 1978 • J. D. Whitehead 1978 • D. Pardee 1978a • A. M. R. Aristar 1979 • R. Contini 1979 • R. I. Vasholz 1979–81a • J. Margain 1979–84 • J. Blau 1980 • G. Bonfante 1980 • S. Segert 1980 • R. C. Steiner 1980 • K. Tsereteli 1980 • J. W. Wesselius 1980 • D. Boyarin 1981 • A. Vivian 1981 • E. Qimron 1981–82 • Y. Lerner 1981–82 • J. L. Boyd III 1982 • R. Contini 1982 • W. Diem 1982 • M. Kaddari 1983 • S. A. Kaufman 1983 • S. F. Bennett 1984 • S. A. Kaufman 1984 • R. Macuch 1984–86 • W. R. Garr 1985 • R. D. Hoberman 1985 • T. O. Lambdin 1985 • D. Testen 1985 • J. Blau 1985–86 • W. Diem 1986 • A. Gai 1986 • H.-P. Müller 1986 • A.

M. R. Aristar 1987 • R. Buth 1987 • B. Kienast 1987 • D. M. Stec 1987 • R. C. Steiner 1987 • J. Huehnergard 1987a • E. Qimron 1987–88 • W. Eilers 1988 • A. Faber 1988 • P. Swiggers 1988 • A. Dodi 1989 • S. A. Kaufman 1989 • W. von Soden 1989 • W. R. Garr 1990 • V. Brugnatelli forthcoming.

A.7   PALEOGRAPHY

D. Diringer 1937 • S. A. Birnbaum 1954–57, 1971 • S. Segert 1963 • B. L. Haines 1967 • S. J. Lieberman 1968 • D. Diringer and R. Regensburger 1968, esp. p. 1.198–202 • J. Naveh 1970 • J. Teixidor 1970a, esp. p. 357 • J. Naveh 1971c • J. Naveh 1973 • J. Oelsner 1976 • A. R. Millard 1976b • J. Rosenbaum 1978 • F. M. Fales 1978b • J. Naveh 1982 • P. Swiggers 1983 • A. R. Millard 1984 • E. Attardo 1984 • P. T. Daniels 1984 • M. G. Amadasi Guzzo 1985 • W. Sundermann 1985 • S. A. Kaufman 1986 • E. Puech 1986a • E. A. Knauf 1987 • A. Lemaire 1989.

See also Part B, s.vv., in particular: Fakh, DA.

A.8   ORTHOGRAPHY

G. R. Driver 1948 • F. M. Cross and D. N. Freedman 1952 • A. Spitaler 1952–54 • F. Rosenthal 1953 • M. E. Sherman 1966 • G. Garbini 1969a • L. A. Bange 1971 • S. Segert 1978 • R. Zadok 1979, esp. p. 68 • S. A. Kaufman 1982 • D. N. Freedman and F. I. Andersen 1989 • F. I. Andersen and D. N. Freedman 1989 • E. M. Cook 1990 • R. Macuch 1990.

A.9   LEXICOGRAPHY

W. Gesenius 1833 • B. Davidson 1848 • I. Löw 1881 • S. A. Cook 1898 • I. Löw 1906 • F. Brown, S. R. Driver, and C. A. Briggs 1907, esp. pp. 1078–1118 • P. Leander 1927 • F. Rundgren 1953, esp. pp. 304–14 • W. Baumgartner 1953 • S. B. Sperry 1955 • H. Petschow 1956, esp. pp. 52–54 • P. Grelot 1956 • I. N. Vinnikov 1958–65 • R. Stiehl 1959–62 • S. Segert 1960 • J. C. Greenfield 1962 • M. Ellenbogen 1962 • S. Segert 1962 • C.-F. Jean and J. Hoftijzer 1965 • R. Frankena 1965, esp. pp. 134–36 • W. von Soden 1966–77 • S. Segert 1967 • R. Degen 1968–69 • E. Vogt 1971 • H. Donner 1973 • J. Teixidor 1973, esp. pp. 432–33 • R. Brauner 1974 • S. A. Kaufman 1974 • J. Teixidor 1975, esp. p. 264 • R. Degen 1975 • W. E. Aufrecht and J. C. Hurd 1975 • J. Teixidor 1976, esp. p. 310, 335 • R. Brauner 1977 • J. C. Greenfield 1978c • K. Beyer 1979 • P. Reymond 1980 • L. A. Mitchell 1984, esp. pp. 52–65, 83–88.

A.10   VOCABULARY STUDIES

Fr. Thureau-Dangin 1896 • W. T. Pilter 1914 • J. A. Montgomery 1923 • H. J. Polotsky 1932 • P. Joüon 1933 • P. Joüon 1934a • W. Henning 1935 • P. Joüon

1941a • G. Furlani 1948 • B. Couroyer 1952 • J. J. Rabinowitz 1956a • F. Rundgren 1957 • J. A. Fitzmyer 1957 • R. Yaron 1957, esp. p. 49 • J. J. Rabinowitz 1958a • J. J. Rabinowitz 1960 • E. Y. Kutscher 1961 • P. Grelot 1962 • T. C. Vriezen 1963 • F. C. Fensham 1963a • A. Dupont-Sommer 1964 • A. Shaffer 1965 • A. Shaffer 1965 • J. Swetnam 1965 • B. Uffenheimer 1965–55 • F. Rundgren 1965–66 • Ḥ. Farzat 1967 • R. Schmitt 1967 • R. Yaron 1967 • B. Z. Bergman 1968 • W. Eilers 1968 • W. Henning 1968 • J. C. Greenfield 1970 • E. M. Yamauchi 1970 • F. Altheim and R. Stiehl 1971, esp. pp. 2:233–42 • E. Puech 1971 • J. Blau 1972 • A. R. Millard 1972a • P. Grelot 1973 • Y. Muffs 1973 • M. Weinfeld 1973 • M. Weinfeld 1973–74 • M. Mayrhofer 1974 • N. M. Waldman 1974 • S. Wikander 1974 • J. C. Greenfield 1975 • Y. Avishur 1975–76 • M. M. Bravmann 1977a • M. M. Bravmann 1977b • H. F. Fuhs 1977 • J. C. Greenfield 1977a • J. Naveh 1978 • B. Grossfeld 1979, esp. p. 121 • F. Bron and A. Lemaire 1979–84, esp. pp. 23–25 • J. C. Greenfield 1979a • Z. Ben-Ḥayyim 1980–81 • P. T. Daniels 1981 • M. Eskhult 1981 • S. Qohut 1981–82 • 'A. Bahnassi 1982 • C. Cohen 1982 • L. Díez Merino 1982, esp. pp. 137–38 • L. Díez Merino 1982a, esp. pp. 210–11 • J. C. Greenfield 1982 • J. C. Greenfield 1982b, esp. pp. 8–11 • B. A. Levine 1982 • E. Puech 1982a • R. Zadok 1982a • J. L. Cunchillos 1983 • L. Díez Merino 1983 • J. C. Greenfield 1983 • J. Huehnergard 1983, esp. pp. 589–90 • M. Kaddari 1983 • N. Lohfink 1983 • J. Ribera i Florit 1983 • B. Zuckerman 1983 • Y. Avishur 1984 • L. Díez Merino 1984 • F. M. Fales 1984 • R. Murray 1984 • J. W. Wesselius 1984a • F. de Blois 1985 • J. W. Wesselius 1985a • L. Kataja 1986 • M. L. Brown 1987, esp. pp. 211–13 • F. M. Fales 1987b • A. Lemaire and H. Lozachmeur 1987 • A. R. Millard 1987 • J. Ribera i Florit 1987 • E. Will 1987 • K. Beyer 1988 • L. Díez Merino 1988 • S. Parpola 1988 • T. Petit 1988 • P.-E. Dion 1989a • E. Lipiński 1989 • M. O'Connor 1989, esp. pp. 28–29 • J. Ribera 1989.

A.11   ONOMASTICA

H. Derenbourg 1893 • G. B. Gray 1903 • W. Spiegelberg 1912 • E. König 1913 • M. Löhr 1913 • W. Spiegelberg 1913a • J. Friedrich 1930 • O. Eissfeldt 1930 • G. R. Driver 1939 • G. Garbini 1956b • 'A. Fāḍil 1958 • E. Vogt 1958a • I. as-Samarra'i 1960 • M. Liverani 1962 • K. Deller 1965 • F. Vattioni 1966 • N. G. Cohen 1966–67 • M. H. Silverman 1969 • M. H. Silverman 1969b • M. H. Silverman 1970 • J. Teixidor 1971, esp. pp. 461–62 • F. M. Fales 1973, esp. p. 135 n. 15 • J. Teixidor 1973, esp. p. 406 • A. van Selms 1974 • F. M. Fales 1974 • W. Kornfeld 1974 • M. D. Coogan 1975 • P.-R. Berger 1975, esp. pp. 226–34 • E. Lipiński 1975a, esp. pp. 58–76 • W. Kornfeld 1976 • A. R. Millard 1976 • J. Teixidor 1976, esp. p. 311, 313 • R. Zadok 1976 • R. Zadok 1976a • F. M. Fales 1977 • A. R. Millard 1977, esp. pp. 72–73 • A. R. Millard 1977a • R. Zadok 1977 • R. Zadok 1977a • F. M. Fales 1978 • S. A. Kaufman 1978 • W. Kornfeld 1978 • E. Lipiński 1978d • F. M. Fales 1979 • J. Teixidor 1979, esp. pp. 362–63 • E. Lipiński 1980 • R. Zadok 1980 • M. H. Silverman 1981 • J. A. Tvedtnes 1981 • K. P. Jackson 1983 • P. Swiggers 1983a • B. W. W. Dombrowski 1984 • E. Lipiński 1985b • M. H. Silverman 1985 • R. Zadok 1985a • R. Zadok 1985b • R. Zadok 1986 • J. D. Fowler 1988, esp. Ch. 4, Apps. 1–2 • M. Maraqten 1988 • A. R. Millard 1988 • R. M. Whiting 1988 • F. M. Fales 1989 • G. Vittmann 1989.

A.12   EPISTOLOGRAPHY

J. A. Fitzmyer 1974 • J. D. Whitehead 1974 • P.-E. Dion 1977 • P. S. Alexander 1978 • P.-E. Dion 1979 • B. Porten 1981 • P.-E. Dion 1982 • P.-E. Dion 1982a • P.-E. Dion 1982b • J. C. Greenfield 1982b • B. Porten 1983b • F. M. Fales 1987.

A.13   LAW

L. M. Epstein 1927 • U. Türck 1928 • P. Koschaker 1935 esp. pp. 20–22 • C. B. Welles 1949 • J. J. Rabinowitz 1953 • J. J. Rabinowitz 1955 • E. Volterra 1956 • J. J. Rabinowitz 1956 • E. Pritsch 1957 • E. Volterra 1957 • J. J. Rabinowitz 1957, esp. pp. 271–74 • R. Yaron 1957a • J. J. Rabinowitz 1957b • F. Rundgren 1958 • R. Yaron 1958a, esp. pp. 18–19 • R. Yaron 1958b • J. J. Rabinowitz 1959 • R. Yaron 1959 • R. Yaron 1960a • R. Yaron 1961 • R. Yaron 1961a • A. Verger 1964 • A. Verger 1964a • A. Verger 1965 • B. Porten 1968 • B. Porten and J. C. Greenfield 1969 • Y. Muffs 1969 • E. Lipiński 1975a, esp. pp. 77–82 • B. Porten and H. Szubin 1982 • H. Szubin and B. Porten 1982 • B. Porten and H. Szubin 1982a • H. Szubin and B. Porten 1983 • H. Szubin and B. Porten 1983 • B. Porten 1983c • B. Porten and H. Szubin 1987a • H. Szubin and B. Porten 1988 • A. Lemaire 1988b • J. C. Greenfield 1990a • D. R. Hillers 1990.

See also Part B, s.v. ElPap.

A.14   ARAMAIC LITERATURE

J.-B. Chabot 1910 • F. Rosenthal 1946 • K. R. Veenhof 1963a • M. Weinfeld 1965 • F. Vattioni 1967 • M. Weinfeld 1970 • H.-J. Zobel 1971 • M. Weinfeld 1971–72 • J. C. Greenfield 1971a • J. C. Greenfield 1971b • H. Tawil 1972 • H. Tawil 1973 • H. Tawil 1974 • M. Weinfeld 1975 • H. Tawil 1977 • J. C. Greenfield 1979 • H. Tawil 1980 • D. W. Gooding 1981 • B. Porten 1981 • M. Weippert 1981 • W. H. Shea 1981 • H. Tadmor 1982 • G. H. Wilson 1985 • S. P. Vleeming and J. W. Wesselius 1985a • A. Lemaire 1985b • K. L. Younger, Jr. 1986 • S. Segert 1986 • J. C. de Moor 1988 • A. Lemaire 1988c • H. F. Van Rooy 1989 • J. C. Greenfield 1989 • D. R. Hillers 1990 • A. R. Millard 1990.

A.15   RELIGION

A. Lemonnyer 1920 • O. Eissfeldt 1930 • A. Vincent 1937 • J. P. Hyatt 1939, esp. pp. 84–85 • M. D. Cassuto 1942 • G. Garbini 1960 • F. Vattioni 1965a • E. Seidl 1968, esp. pp. 86–88 • H. Donner 1968 • B. Porten 1969 • J. F. Ross 1970 • J. C. Greenfield 1973 • J. C. Greenfield 1976a • B. Uffenheimer 1977 • S. A. Kaufman 1978 • S. P. Vleeming and J. W. Wesselius 1982 • S. P. Vleeming and J. W. Wesselius 1983–84 • J. C. Greenfield 1987a.

A.16   INTERFERENCE — Other Languages in Aramaic

E. Böhl 1860, esp. p. 45 • F. Selle 1890 • F. Müller 1897 • H. Bauer 1926 • E. S. Rimalt 1932 • E. Benveniste 1934 • J. Leibovitch 1935–36 • L. H. Gray 1951 • F. Altheim and R. Stiehl 1953 • B. Couroyer 1954 • E. Benveniste 1954 • J. de Menasce 1954 • M. J. Mashkur 1968 • R. Degen 1968–69 • E. M. Yamauchi 1970 • M. J. Dresden 1971 • A. Hurvitz 1972 • E. Ebeling 1972 • H. Humbach 1972 • H. Tawil 1972 • H. Humbach 1974 • J. C. Greenfield 1974 • S. A. Kaufman 1974 • M. Sokoloff 1976a • D. Pardee 1977 • W. von Soden 1977 • A. Bausani 1980 • J. Oelsner 1980 • M. Nordio 1980 • G. Itō 1981 • A. Hurvitz 1982a • J. C. Greenfield 1982a • R. Lemosín 1984 • F. M. Fales 1985.

A.17   INFLUENCES — Aramaic on Other Languages

S. Fraenkel 1886 • F. Miller 1897 • E. Kautzsch 1903 • E. Littmann 1903 • U. Meltzer 1924 • U. Meltzer 1925 • U. Meltzer 1927 • E. S. Rimalt 1932 • R. Gordis 1952 • J. Lewy 1959 • W. von Soden 1959–60 • E. Y. Kutscher 1964 • M. Wagner 1966 • M. Wagner 1967 • A. Hurvitz 1968 • R. Degen 1970 • S. Parpola 1974–79 • F. Zimmermann 1975 • R. Schmitt 1975 • W. Lentz 1975 • R. Polzin 1976, esp. pp. 61–69 • F. M. Fales 1980 • G. Garbini 1980 • M. Nordio 1980 • F. Vattioni 1981 • J. Blau 1983 • J. F. Healey 1983 • F. M. Fales 1984 • R. S. Tomback 1984 • F. M. Fales 1985 • F. Rosenthal, J. Greenfield and S. Shaked 1986 • E. Jenni 1988 • H. Tadmor 1989 • M. O. Wise 1990.

B. TEXTS (Old and Official Aramaic)

B.1 Syria/Palestine

B.1.1   Bar-Hadad Stele (Brēdsh/Aleppo, ca. 850)   BarH

Basalt stele (1.15 x .43 m.) beneath a relief. Aleppo Museum.

נצבא | זי | שם ברה 1
דד בר עתרסמך
מלך ארם למראה למלקר
ת זי נזר לה ושמע לקל
ה 5

Ed. Pr.   M. Dunand 1939.

EASY ACCESS

Editions: *AC* 4 ● *AaG*Deg 8 ● *AaG*Seg 15 ● *EAS* 246 ● *KAI* 201 ● *TSSI* 2.1.

Translations: *ANET*^{3} 655 ● *DOTT* 239–41 ● *RTAT* 246–47 ● *NERTOT* 228–29.

Illustrations: *ANEP*^{2} pl. 499 ● *DOTT* pl. 15 ● *NSR* 2, fig. 66 ● *SW* fig. 76 ● *TSSI* 2, fig. 1 ● J. Naveh 1982, fig. 72 ● H. L. Ginsberg 1971, p. 515.

LITERATURE

E. Kraeling 1918, esp. p. 4 ● R. de Vaux 1934 ● R. de Vaux 1941, esp. p. 9, n. 1 ● W. F. Albright 1942 ● A. Jepsen 1942–43 ● M. Dunand 1942–43 ● G. Levi della Vida and W. F. Albright 1943 ● H. L. Ginsberg 1945 ● A. Herdner 1946–48 ● G. R. Driver 1948, esp. pp. 121, 127, 249 ● A. Dupont-Sommer 1949a, esp. p. 33 and n. 13 ● P. K. Hitti 1951, esp. pp. 169–70 ● F. M. Cross and D. N. Freedman 1952, esp. p. 24 ● A. Jepsen 1952–53 ● E. Meyer 1953, esp. p. 273, 332 ● K. Galling 1953, esp. pp. 183–86 ● W. F. Albright 1956, esp. p. 149 ● G. Garbini 1956a, esp. pp. 244–51 ● M. Unger 1957, esp. pp. 56, 59–60 ● G. Garbini 1958, esp. p. 202 ● M. Heltzer 1958 ● R. du Mesnil du Buisson 1963 ● G. Levi della Vida 1964, esp. pp. 312–13 ● D. Diringer and R. Regensburger 1968, pl. 2.186d ● R. Degen 1969, esp. p. 8 ● H. L. Ginsberg 1971 ● E. Lipiński 1971 ● F. M. Cross 1972 ● J. Teixidor 1974, esp. p. 329 ● S. Segert 1975, esp. p. 435 ● E. Lipiński 1975, esp. pp. 246–47 ● E. Lipiński 1975a, esp. pp. 15–19 ● E. Lipiński 1978a, esp. pp. 228–29 ● W. H. Shea 1978–79 ● J. Naveh 1982, fig. 72, p. 80 ● J. A. Dearman and J. M. Miller 1983 ● P. Bordreuil and J. Teixidor 1983 ● A. Lemaire 1984b ● G. G. G. Reinhold 1986 ● B. Zuckerman 1987, esp. pp. 11–16 + photo ● S. C. Layton 1988, esp. p. 176 ● W. T. Pitard 1988.

B.1.2   Ein Gev Jar (ca. 850)   EinGev

Inscribed store-jar (41.5 cm. ht.). Israel Museum.

לשקיא

Ed. Pr.   B. Mazar et al. 1964, esp. pp 27–29, pl. 13B.

EASY ACCESS
    Editions: *AaG*Deg 23 • *TSSI* 2.3.

    Illustrations: *IR* 122.

LITERATURE
    H. Cazelles 1962, esp. pp. 330–31 • B. Mazar 1962a, esp. p. 400 • G. Rinaldi
    1965 • J. Naveh 1964–65, esp. p. 183 • J. Naveh 1966, esp. p. 19 • M. Weippert
    1966, esp. pp. 278–79 • N. Avigad 1966 • J. Teixidor 1967, esp. p. 179 • N. Avi-
    gad 1968a, esp. p. 43.

B.1.3   Tell Dan Bowl (ca. 850)   TDan

       Inscribed bowl base (10.5 cm. diam.). Bet Ussishkin, Kibbutz Dan.

לטב[ח]יא

Ed. Pr.   N. Avigad 1968a.

EASY ACCESS
    Editions: *TSSI* 2.4.

    Illustrations: *IR* 123.

LITERATURE
    N. Avigad 1966 • J. Teixidor 1969, esp. p. 346 • A. Biran 1977, esp. pp. 260–61 •
    A. Biran and V. Tzaferis 1977–78 • A. Biran 1980, esp. pp. 171, 179–80 •
    A. Biran 1981.

B.1.4   Hazael Ivory Inlays (Arslan Tash, ca. 850–800) ArslanTash

       Two fragmentary ivory plaques. Louvre.

[...] זֹת.ח].....[ח בֹּר עמא | למראן | חזאל | בשנת [...] (1
למר]אן חזאל ... [(2

Ed. Pr.   1) F. Thureau-Dangin et al. 1931, esp. pp. 88, 91–92, 135–38, pl. 47,
                fig. 49.
                2) A. R. Millard 1962, esp. p. 41.

EASY ACCESS
    Editions: 1) *AC* 5 • *AaG*Deg 23 • *KAI* 232 • *TSSI* 2.2.

    Illustrations: 1) *SW* fig. 74

1, 2) *NESE* 3: 39, 48.

LITERATURE
1) A. Dupont-Sommer 1949a, esp. pp. 38–40, 49 and nn. 22, 50, 53, 80 • H. T. Norris 1951 • E. Meyer 1953 • S. A. Birnbaum 1954–57, 1971 • S. E. Loewenstamm 1955–82 • J. A. G. Larraya 1963–65 • F. Vattioni 1969, esp. p. 366 • J. Teixidor 1973, esp. pp. 433–34 • W. Röllig 1974, esp. pp. 38–39 • E. Puech 1981, pl. 12 • I. J. Winter 1981, esp. p. 103.

2) M. E. L. Mallowan 1966, esp. p. 598, fig. 582 • W. Röllig 1974, esp. p. 48.

B.1.5   Hamath Graffiti (9th–8th c.)   HamGr
Fifty graffiti scratched on red polished paving slabs. Damascus Museum.

Ed. Pr.   1, 4, 6, 8, 9, 11–14, 16, 18) H. Ingholt 1938.
                  3, 5, 7, 10, 15, 17, 19–50) B. Otzen 1990.

EASY ACCESS
    Editions: *KAI* 203–13 (Ingholt).

    Illustrations: J. Naveh 1982, fig. 74.

LITERATURE
R. du Mesnil du Buisson 1930, esp. p. 325 • G. R. Hughes, R. M. Engberg, and W. H. Dubberstein 1938, esp. p. 328 • A. Dupont-Sommer 1949a, esp. p. 30 • G. Garbini 1956a, esp. p. 252 • A. de Maigret 1979 • A. Lemaire 1987a, esp. pp. 214–16 • B. Otzen 1988.
13) R. Degen 1969, esp. p. 8.

B.1.6   Zakur Stele (Afis, 800–775)   Zak
Fragmentary basalt stele (2m. x 29 cm. wide). Louvre.

Ed. Pr.   H. Pognon 1907–8, esp. pp. 156–78, pls. 9, 10, 35, 36.

EASY ACCESS
    Editions: *AC* 8 • *AH* 1/1: 1–2 • *Aag*Deg 5–7 • *AaG*Seg 16 • *EAS* 206–10 •
                     ESE 3:1–11 • *KAI* 202 • *TSSI* 5.

    Translations: *ANET*[3] 655 • *ATAT* 443–44 • *DOTT* 242–50 • *RTAT* 247–50 •
                     NERTOT 229–32.

    Illustrations: *KAI* pls. 13, 14 • *NSR* 2, fig. 21 • J. Naveh, 1982, fig. 73 • *TSSI* 2
                     pl. 1(A); fig. 2 (B,C).

LITERATURE
> E. Sachau 1892 • M. Hartmann 1908 • P. Dhorme 1908, esp. p. 503 • R. Dussaud
> 1908 • S. R. Driver 1908 • S. Ronzevalle 1908 • J. Halévy 1908a • T. Nöldeke
> 1908a, esp. pp. 375–84 • J. Halévy 1908c, esp. pp. 255–58 • J. Halévy 1908d •
> A. J. Wensinck 1909, esp. pp. 12–15, 21–24 • I. Löw 1909 • J. A. Montgomery
> 1909 • J. Barth 1909 • S. Schiffer 1909 • P. Dhorme 1911 • E. Ebeling 1913 • S.
> Schiffer 1913 • C. C. Torrey 1915 • E. Kraeling 1918, esp. pp. 95–104 • R. Dus-
> saud 1922, esp. p. 176 • S. Mowinckel 1923 • E. Honigmann 1923–24 • W.
> Baumgartner 1924 • W. F. Albright 1926, esp. pp. 85–88 • E. Sachsse 1927 • R.
> Dussaud 1927, esp. pp. 235–38 • M. Noth 1929 • R. Dussaud 1931, esp. p. 316 n.
> 4 • W. F. Albright 1934, esp. p. 46 • F. Rosenthal 1939, esp. p. 9 n. 5 • K. Elliger
> 1947, esp. pp. 87–89 • G. R. Driver 1948, esp. pp. 121, 249 • R. A. Bowman
> 1948, esp. p. 72 • A. Dupont-Sommer 1949a, esp. pp. 45–48, 112 • W. F. Albright
> 1950a • P. K. Hitti 1951, esp. pp. 169–70 • F. M. Cross and D. N. Freedman 1952,
> esp. pp. 24–27 • Y. Aharoni 1953 • I. N. Vinnikov 1955 • G. Garbini 1956a, esp.
> pp. 251–56 • J. Simons 1959, esp. p. 142 • M. Liverani 1961, esp. pp. 185–86 •
> S. Gevirtz 1961, esp. p. 144 • H. Tadmor 1961a • A. Goetze 1962 • A. R. Millard
> 1962, esp. p. 43 • G. Buccellati 1964 • B. Uffenheimer 1965–66 • J. Friedrich
> 1966 • R. Degen 1967–68 • D. Diringer and R. Regensburger 1968, pl. 2.186b •
> P. Artzi 1968, esp. p. 168, n. 2 • A. Jepsen 1969, esp. pp. 1–2 • J. Teixidor 1969,
> esp. p. 345 • B. Volkwein 1969, esp. pp. 34–37 • J. F. Ross 1970 • M. Weinfeld
> 1970 • H.-J. Zobel 1971 • J. Teixidor 1971, esp. pp. 477–79 • E. Lipiński 1971a •
> J. C. Greenfield 1971a • M. Noth 1971b • M. Weinfeld 1971–72 • E. Lipiński
> 1972, esp. pp. 157–58, n. 2 • J. Teixidor 1973, esp. pp. 428–29 • H. Tawil 1974,
> esp. pp. 51–57 • E. Lipiński 1975, esp. pp. 247–50 • J. Teixidor 1975, esp. p. 286
> • R. Brauner 1975 • S. Segert 1975, esp. pp. 319, 437 • E. Lipiński 1975a, esp. pp.
> 15–23 • E. Lipiński 1977, esp. p. 98 • J. Teixidor 1977, esp. pp. 271–72 • A. R.
> Millard 1978, esp. p. 23 • E. Lipiński 1978a, esp. pp. 229–32 • A. Cody 1979 • J.
> C. Greenfield 1981a, esp. pp. 113–14 • A. Lemaire 1985f, esp. p. 556 • A. Avan-
> zini 1987 • S. C. Layton 1988, esp. p. 177 • J. C. de Moor 1988 • A. R. Millard
> 1989c • A. R. Millard 1990.

B.1.7　　Zenjirli (Samalian) Dialect — General Discussions

LITERATURE
> D. H. Müller 1893, esp. pp. 113–40 • T. Nöldeke 1893 • J. Halévy 1893–94, esp.
> pp. 243–58 • J. Halévy 1894 • J. Halévy 1895, esp. p. 185 • C. R. Conder 1896,
> esp. pp. 72–74 • C. Niebuhr 1898 • J. Halévy 1899, esp. pp. 345–55 • T. Nöldeke
> 1899, esp. pp. 31–33 • C. Sarauw 1907, esp. pp. 61–67 • S. Ronzevalle 1909 • S.
> Schiffer 1911, esp. pp. 88–100 • W. F. Albright 1927, esp. p. 171 • F. Rosenthal
> 1939, esp. p. 57 • H. L. Ginsberg 1942, esp. pp. 235–37 • W. F. Albright 1945,
> esp. p. 18 n. 8 • B. Landsberger 1948 • J. Friedrich 1951, esp. pp. 153–62 • F. M.
> Cross and D. N. Freedman 1952, esp. pp. 61–64 • G. Garbini 1956a, esp. pp.
> 256–64 • S. Moscati 1956b, esp. pp. 206–13 • S. Segert 1958a • O. Eissfeldt
> 1963 • O. Eissfeldt 1964 • R. D. Barnett 1964 • J. Friedrich 1965 • G. Garbini
> 1969 • P.-E. Dion 1974 • F. Rosenthal 1976 • G. Garbini 1976 • P.-E. Dion 1978
> • J. P. Healey 1984.

B.1.8   Kilamuwa Scepter (Zenjirli, 850–800)   Kil

Golden scepter or sheath (6.7 x 2.2 cm.). Staatliche Museen, Berlin.

1 סמר ז קן
כלמו
בר חי
לרכבאל
5 יתן לה ר
כבאל
ארך חי

Ed. Pr.   F. von Luschan 1943 p. 102, Abb. 124, pl. 47f,g.

EASY ACCESS
Editions: *AC* 2 • *AaG*Seg 12 • *EAS* 160 • *KAI* 25 • P.-E. Dion 1974, pp. 26–43.

Translations: *ANET* 501 • *ANET*[3] 655.

LITERATURE
F. von Luschan 1911, esp. pp. 374–77 • J. Halévy 1912a, esp. pp. 408–10 • J. Friedrich 1922 • A. Poebel 1932, esp. pp. 33–43 • B. Landsberger 1948, esp. pp. 42 nn. 102, 59–60 • A. Dupont-Sommer 1948a • K. Galling 1950 • J. Hoftijzer 1957–58, esp. p. 117 • G. R. Meyer 1965, esp. pp. 21, 78–79 • Y. Yadin 1967a, esp. pp. 29–34, א1 • D. Diringer and R. Regensburger 1968, pl. 2.186a • M. O'Connor 1977 • P. Swiggers 1982 • S. C. Layton 1988, esp. pp. 181–82 • A. Lemaire 1990a.

B.1.9   Hadad (Panamuwa I) Stele (Zenjirli, ca. 770)   Had

Fragmentary statue (2.85 m. ht. x 2.94 m. at bottom). Staatliche Museen, Berlin.

Ed. Pr.   F. von Luschan 1893 p. 51, pls. 6, 7.

EASY ACCESS
Editions: *AC* 9 • *AaG*Seg 13 • *EAS* 160–65 • *ESE* 1:56–58 • *HNE* 440–42 • *KAI* 214 • *NSI* 61 • P.-E. Dion 1974 • *TSSI* 2.13.

Translations: *ERS* 492–94.

Illustrations: *HNE* pl. 22 • *NSR* 2, fig.104 • *TSSI* pl. 3.

LITERATURE
E. Sachau 1892 • A. H. Sayce 1893 • C. Belger 1893 • D. H. Müller 1893, esp. pp. 50–70 • H. Derenbourg 1893 • J. Halévy 1893, esp. pp. 81–84 • T. Nöldeke 1893, esp. pp. 97–98 • J. Halévy 1893–94, esp. pp. 140–67; 319–24 • H. Winckler 1893 • H. Winckler 1893a • D. H. Müller 1894 • G. Steindorff 1894 •

M. J. de Goeje 1894 • M. Jastrow 1894 • J. G. Troickiy 1895 • J. V. Prašek 1895 • C. R. Conder 1896, esp. pp. 61–66 • H. L. Strack 1896 • J. Halévy 1899, esp. pp. 333–41 • C. Sarauw 1907, esp. pp. 60–61 • S. Schiffer 1911, esp. pp. 97–99 • J. A. Montgomery 1917 • E. Kraeling 1918 • D. D. Luckenbill 1925 • J. Friedrich 1930, esp. pp. 363–65 • A. Poebel 1932, esp. pp. 43–49 • J. A. Montgomery 1934, esp. pp. 421–23 • F. M. T. de Liagre Böhl 1937, esp. p. 45 • G. R. Driver 1945, esp. p. 11 • K. Elliger 1947, esp. pp. 87–89 • B. Landsberger 1948, esp. pp. 63–64 • R. A. Bowman 1948 • A. Dupont-Sommer 1949a • C. Brockelmann 1954, esp. p. 135 • L. A. Snijders 1954 • S. Moscati 1954, esp. p. 38 • G. Garbini 1956 • K. Galling 1956, esp. pp. 146–48 • S. Moscati 1956a • B. Kienast 1957 • G. Garbini 1957 • F. Vattioni 1965a, esp. p. 57 • J. C. Greenfield 1967–68, esp. pp. 359–60 • Y. Yadin 1967a, esp. p. 38 • H. Tawil 1973 • J. C. Greenfield 1973 • H. Tawil 1974, esp. pp. 41–50 • J. Teixidor 1974, esp. p. 328 • S. Segert 1975, esp. pp. 319, 433, 434, 436, 444 • E. Lipiński 1977, esp. pp. 101–3 • P.-E. Dion 1978 • E. Lipiński 1983 • J. P. Healey 1984, esp. pp. 9–60 • A. Faber 1987 • S. C. Layton 1988, esp. p. 181.

B.1.10   Panamuwa (Panamuwa II) Stele (Zenjirli, ca. 730)   Pan

Fragmentary statue (1.93 m. ht.). Staatliche Museen, Berlin.

Ed. Pr.   E. Sachau 1893.

EASY ACCESS

Editions: *AC* 11 • *AH* I/1: 6–8 • *AaG*Seg 14 • *EAS* 165–69 • *ESE* 3:218–38 • *HNE* 442–43 • *KAI* 215 • *NSI* 62 • P.-E. Dion 1974 • *TSSI* 2.14.

Translations: *ERS* 495–98 • *TUAT* 1:628–30 • *RTAT* 272–82 • *NERTOT* 256–66.

Illustrations: *HNE* pl. 23 • *TSSI* pl. 4.

LITERATURE

J. Halévy 1891 • P. Berger 1891, esp. pp. 206–12 • E. Sachau 1892 • A. H. Sayce 1893 • C. Belger 1893 • D. H. Müller 1893, esp. pp. 37–49 • H. Derenbourg 1893 • J. A. Craig 1893 • J. Halévy 1893, esp. pp. 84–87 • T. Nöldeke 1893, esp. pp. 97–98 • P. Rost 1893, esp. pp. 56–59, 27 • H. Winckler 1893a • J. Halévy 1893–94, esp. pp. 218–41 • D. H. Müller 1894 • G. Steindorff 1894, esp. pp. 456–57 • M. J. de Goeje 1894 • M. Jastrow 1894 • J. G. Troickiy 1895 • J. Halévy 1895, esp. p. 185 • J. V. Prašek 1895 • C. R. Conder 1896, esp. pp. 66–70 • H. L. Strack 1896 • C. Clermont-Ganneau 1897 • J. Halévy 1899, esp. pp. 341–45 • A. Šanda 1904 • C. Sarauw 1907, esp. p. 59 • S. Schiffer 1911, esp. pp. 97–99 • H. Bauer 1914 • E. Kraeling 1918, esp. pp. 122–26 • J. Friedrich 1930, esp. pp. 363–65 • J. A. Montgomery 1934, esp. pp. 423–24 • D. Diringer 1937, esp. p. 418 • B. Landsberger 1948, esp. pp. 68–70 • G. R. Driver 1948, esp. pp. 121, 127 • R. A. Bowman 1948, esp. p. 72 • A. Dupont-Sommer 1949a, esp. pp. 55–63 • L. Palacios 1953, esp. pp. 129–30 • C. Brockelmann 1954, esp. pp. 135–36 • S. Moscati 1954, esp. pp. 38–39 • H. Donner 1955 • G. Garbini 1956 •

S. Moscati 1956a • G. Garbini 1957, esp. p. 422 • H. T. Bossert 1958 • M. Dahood 1960a • R. D. Barnett 1964 • J. Friedrich 1965 • J. Swetnam 1965, esp. pp. 34–36 • Y. Yadin 1967a, esp. p. 38 • J. Teixidor 1974, esp. pp. 328–29 • S. A. Kaufman 1974, esp. p. 80 • J. Teixidor 1975, esp. pp. 285–86 • S. Segert 1975, esp. pp. 320, 434, 435 • E. Lipiński 1977, esp. pp. 99–101 • P.-E. Dion 1978 • J. Teixidor 1979, esp. p. 390 • J. P. Healey 1984, esp. pp. 61–88 • K. L. Younger, Jr. 1986 • S. C. Layton 1988, esp. p. 181.

B.1.11   Sefire Treaty (ca. 750)   Sf

Three fragmentary basalt stelae. Damascus (1–2), Beirut (3).

Ed. Pr.   1,2) S. Ronzevalle 1930–31.
                   3) A. Dupont-Sommer and J. Starcky 1956.

EASY ACCESS
   Editions: *AC* 10 • *AH* I/1: 3–6 • *AaG*Deg 9–23 • *AaG*Seg 18 • *EAS* 120–36
                   • *KAI* 222–224 • *TSSI* 2.7–9.

   Translations: *ANET* 503–5 • *ANET*[3] 659–61 • *TUAT* 1:178–86 • *NERTOT* 256–66.

   Illustrations: *KAI* pls. 15–18 • *TSSI* figs. 3–4, pl. 2 • J. A. Fitzmyer, 1967, pls. 2–17.

LITERATURE
General
R. Dussaud 1932 • H. Bauer 1932–33 • F. Rosenthal 1939, esp. pp. 10, 13 • G. R. Driver 1948, esp. pp. 121, 127 • J. M. A. Janssen 1955–56, esp. p. 68 • A. Pohl 1956, esp. p. 159 • G. Garbini 1956 • G. Garbini 1956b • H. Donner 1957, esp. p. 162 • A. Dupont-Sommer 1958 • A. Pohl 1958, esp. pp. 290–91 • D. J. Wiseman 1958 • A. Dupont-Sommer 1960b • C. Picard 1961 • H. Tadmor 1961a • I. J. Gelb 1962 • D. J. McCarthy 1963, esp. pp. 51–67, 189–94 • F. C. Fensham 1963, esp. pp. 156, 159, 164–72 • W. L. Moran 1963 • K. R. Veenhof 1963a • F. C. Fensham 1964 • S. Segert 1964 • D. R. Hillers 1964a • H. Klengel 1965, esp. p. 92 • J. C. Greenfield 1965 • J. M. Grintz 1966, esp. pp. 119 n. 28, 123 • M. E. Sherman 1966, esp. pp. 18–22 • R. Degen 1967 • J. A. Fitzmyer 1967 • J. Teixidor 1967, esp. pp. 178–79 • D. B. Weisberg 1967, esp. pp. 29–42 • J. A. Soggin 1968 • J. C. Greenfield 1968 • J. Coppens 1968 • J. Teixidor 1968, esp. pp. 355, 377 • S. P. Brock 1968 • H. Tadmor 1970 • Z. Ben-Ḥayyim 1970–71 • D. R. Hillers 1971 • J. Teixidor 1971, esp. p. 477 • L. A. Bange 1971 • D. J. McCarthy 1972 • M. Weinfeld 1972, esp. pp. 59, 103, 105, 110, 124–26, 136, 141–42 • A. R. Millard and H. Tadmor 1973, esp. pp. 59–60 • M. Weinfeld 1973 • E. Lipiński 1975, esp. pp. 272–82 • M. Parnas 1975 • H. Tadmor 1975, esp. pp. 42–43 • J. Teixidor 1975, esp. p. 264 • M. Weinfeld 1975, esp. pp. 52, 60, 62, 64, 70, 72, 73 • A. Malamat 1976 • J. A. Fitzmyer 1977 • N. Na'aman 1977–78 • D. Pardee 1978 • E. Lipiński 1978a, esp. pp. 256–66 • D. J. McCarthy 1979 • Y. Ikeda 1979 • A. Moriya 1980 • J. W. Wesselius 1980 • J. D. Hawkins 1980–83 • J. C. Greenfield

1981a, esp. pp. 110–13 • J. D. Hawkins 1982, esp. p. 402 • Y. Muffs 1982, esp. pp. 91–92 • H. Tadmor 1982 • H. Tadmor 1982a, esp. pp. 455–58 • M. L. Barré 1983 • R. Zadok 1984 • S. A. Kaufman 1985 • W. von Soden 1985 • J. C. Greenfield 1986 • E. Lipiński 1986a • J. Huehnergard 1987, esp. p. 531 • K. Watanabe 1987 • B. Couroyer 1988 • S. C. Layton 1988, esp. pp. 178–80 • H. F. Van Rooy 1989 • F. M. Fales 1990.

Text 1
R. Dussaud 1928 • G. Dossin 1930 • R. Dussaud 1930, esp. pp. 155–56 • J. Cantineau 1931 • R. Dussaud 1931 • J. Hempel and H. Bauer 1932 • E. Weidner 1932–33 • G. R. Driver 1932–33 • E. Herzfeld 1933 • J. Friedrich and B. Landsberger 1933 • S. Langdon 1933 • A. Alt 1934 • J. A. Montgomery 1934, esp. pp. 424–25 • E. Littmann 1935 • F. Rosenthal 1936, esp. pp. 5–6 n. 2 • J. Friedrich 1936 • K. F. Euler 1937 • H. Torczyner, L. Harding, A. Lewis and J. L. Starkey 1938, esp. pp. 60–61 • A. Parrot 1939, esp. pp. 33–34 • J. N. Epstein 1942 • G. Dossin 1944 • K. Elliger 1947, esp. pp. 89–90, 93–94, 107 • B. Landsberger 1948, esp. n. 147 • A. Dupont-Sommer 1949a, esp. pp. 55–60, 70–71 • Z. Ben-Ḥayyim 1951 • F. M. Cross and D. N. Freedman 1952, esp. pp. 27–29 • O. Eissfeldt 1955 • G. Garbini 1956a, esp. pp. 264–70 • H. Donner 1957–58 • A. Dupont-Sommer 1958 • G. Garbini 1958a • A. Dupont-Sommer 1959 • M. Tsevat 1959 • A. Dupont-Sommer and J. Starcky 1960, pls. 1–29 • M. Tsevat 1960, esp. pp. 83, 85, 86, 88 • P. Sacchi 1960–61, esp. pp. 127–31 • G. Garbini 1961 • J. A. Fitzmyer 1961 • M. Liverani 1961, esp. pp. 185–86 • M. Noth 1961 • M. V. Seton Williams 1961 • P. Sacchi 1961 • S. Gevirtz 1961, esp. p. 144 • V. Korošec 1961 • W. von Soden 1961, esp. pp. 578–79 • A. Caquot 1962 • B. Mazar 1962, esp. pp. 116–20 • F. C. Fensham 1962 • H. Cazelles 1962, esp. p. 337 • H. Donner 1962 • J. L'Hour 1962 • R. Lack 1962 • F. C. Fensham 1962a • C. Brekelmans 1963 • T. C. Vriezen 1963 • F. C. Fensham 1963a • W. L. Moran 1963a • F. C. Fensham 1963b, esp. pp. 137–38 • D. R. Hillers 1964 • J. C. Greenfield 1964–65 • A. González Nuñez 1965 • E. Gerstenberger 1965 • E. von Schüler 1965, esp. p. 67 • J. A. Thompson 1965 • M. Weinfeld 1965 • M.-L. Chaumont 1965 • F. Vattioni 1966 • J. C. Greenfield 1966 • M. Delcor 1966 • O. Loretz 1966 • B. L. Haines 1967 • F. C. Fensham 1967 • F. O. Garcia-Treto 1967 • F. Vattioni 1967, esp. pp. 194–95, 199–200, 202 • K. Galling 1967, esp. pp. 134–35 • J. C. Greenfield 1967–68 • G. Garbini 1967a, esp. pp. 90–92 • J. C. Greenfield 1967a • R. Degen 1969, esp. pp. 9–17 • A. R. Millard 1970 • F. Stolz 1970, esp. pp. 133–37, 149–51 • H. Donner 1970a • F. E. Deist 1971 • J. Renger 1971, esp. p. 496 • P. Garelli 1971 • N. C. Habel 1972, esp. pp. 321–23 • A. R. Millard 1973 • M. Fox 1973 • M. Weinfeld 1973–74 • G. Garbini 1974 • M. Cogan 1974, esp. pp. 40–64 • S. Parpola 1974–79 • J. C. Greenfield 1974a • S. Segert 1975, esp. pp. 431, 432, 435, 437, 440 • E. Lipiński 1975a, esp. pp. 24–76 • B. Uffenheimer 1977 • E. Lipiński 1977, esp. p. 98 • H. Tawil 1977 • R. A. Oden, Jr. 1977 • J. A. Rimbach 1978 • J. C. Greenfield 1978, esp. pp. 94–95 • T. Wittstruck 1978 • J. C. Greenfield 1978c • K. A. Kitchen 1979 • M. C. Astour 1979, esp. p. 6, n. 36 • S. Dalley 1979 • H. Tawil 1980 • B. Menzel 1981, esp. p. 117 • A. Lemaire 1981a • A. Hurvitz 1982, esp. p. 265 • D. J. McCarthy 1982 • E. Puech 1982, esp. pp. 576–83 • H. Cazelles 1982, esp. pp. 133–37 • M. Weinfeld 1982, esp. p. 49 n. 107 • S. A. Kaufman 1982, esp. pp. 170–72 • E. Puech 1982–84 • A. Lemaire and J.-M. Durand 1984 • A. Lemaire 1984a • A. Moriya 1985 • M. L. Barré 1985

• A. Lemaire 1985d, (A:24) esp. pp. 33–35 • B. Mazar 1986 • A. K. Grayson 1987 • S. Parpola 1987 • J. Huehnergard 1987a.

Text 2
K. Elliger 1947 • B. Landsberger 1948 • Z. Ben-Ḥayyim 1951 • M. Tsevat 1959 • A. Dupont-Sommer and J. Starcky 1960 • J. A. Fitzmyer 1961 • M. Liverani 1961, esp. pp. 185–86 • M. Noth 1961 • V. Korošec 1961 • B. Mazar 1962 • H. Donner 1962 • J. L'Hour 1962 • W. L. Moran 1963a • E. von Schüler 1965, esp. p. 70 • H. B. Huffmon 1966, (C 8) • J. A. Fitzmyer 1967 • R. Degen 1967, esp. pp. 57–58 • J. C. Greenfield 1967–68 • R. Degen 1969, esp. pp. 17–19 • G. Garbini 1969a, esp. p. 12 • A. R. Millard 1970 • H. Donner 1970a • J. Renger 1971 • B. Soyez 1972 • M. Cogan 1974, esp. pp. 40–64 • J. C. Greenfield 1974a • E. Lipiński 1975a, esp. pp. 90–91 • J. C. Greenfield 1978 • J. C. Greenfield 1978c • K. A. Kitchen 1979 • D. J. McCarthy 1982 • H. Cazelles 1982 • A. Lemaire and J.-M. Durand 1984 • A. Moriya 1985 • A. K. Grayson 1987 • S. Parpola 1987.

Text 3
K. Elliger 1947 • B. Landsberger 1948 • Z. Ben-Ḥayyim 1951 • A. Dupont-Sommer 1957a • E. Vogt 1958 • J. A. Fitzmyer 1958 • J. J. Rabinowitz 1958 • P. Mouterde 1958 • A. Dupont-Sommer 1959 • A. Pohl 1959 • M. Tsevat 1959 • G. Garbini 1959a, esp. pp. 41–54 • P. Nober 1959a • F. Rosenthal 1960 • M. Noth 1961 • V. Korošec 1961 • B. Mazar 1962 • H. Donner 1962 • J. L'Hour 1962 • F. Vattioni 1963 • W. L. Moran 1963a • J. C. Greenfield 1964–65 • E. von Schüler 1965, esp. p. 79 • F. Vattioni 1965 • F. O. Garcia-Treto 1967 • J. C. Greenfield 1967–68 • J. A. Fitzmyer 1969 • J. Limburg 1969 • R. Degen 1969, esp. pp. 19–23 • D. Sperling 1969–70 • A. R. Millard 1970 • G. Schuttermayr 1970, esp. pp. 515–16 • H. Donner 1970a • H. Cazelles 1971 • J. Renger 1971 • H. Tawil 1973, esp. p. 478 • M. Cogan 1974, esp. pp. 40–64 • J. C. Greenfield 1974a • M. Dahood 1975 • S. Segert 1975, esp. pp. 319, 320, 432, 433, 438, 441 • E. Lipiński 1975a, esp. pp. 92–93 • J. C. Greenfield 1978 • J. C. Greenfield 1978c • K. A. Kitchen 1979 • D. J. McCarthy 1982 • E. Puech 1982, esp. pp. 583–86 • H. Cazelles 1982 • A. Lemaire and J.-M. Durand 1984 • J. W. Wesselius 1984 • A. Moriya 1985 • A. K. Grayson 1987 • S. Parpola 1987.

B.1.12   Hamath Weight (ca. 750)   HamWt
Bronze weight (26 g.) in shape of sphinx. Bibliothèque Nationale, Paris.

שקלי חמת

Ed. Pr.   P. Bordreuil and E. Gubel 1983, pp. 340–41.

LITERATURE
F. Bron and A. Lemaire 1983 • P. Bordreuil and E. Gubel 1990, esp. p. 489.

B.1.13   Emar Stone (Meskéné ca. 750)   EmarSt

Fragmentary limestone block, possibly part of a stele (4.6 x 6.8 cm.). Aleppo Museum.

1 צלמא זנה
פרעבדי

Ed. Pr.   J. Margueron and J. Teixidor 1983.

B.1.14   Bar-Rakkab Inscriptions (Zenjirli, ca. 730)   BarRak

Eight inscriptions:
1. Orthostat ("Bauinschrift") with relief (1.31 m. x 62 cm.). Museum of Antiquities, Istanbul.
2. Orthostat with relief (1.06m ht.). Staatliche Museen, Berlin.
3–5. Fragmentary orthostats. Staatliche Museen, Berlin.
6. Three silver bars. Staatliche Museen, Berlin.
7. Seal. Staatliche Museen, Berlin.
8. Fragmentary orthostat (44.5 x 45.5 cm.). Staatliche Museen, Berlin.

Ed. Pr.   1,3) F. von Luschan 1893.
               2, 4–5) E. Sachau 1895, pp. 27–30, pl. 14.
               6–7) F. von Luschan 1943: 6) pp. 119–20, pl. 58 t,u,v; 7) p. 73, pl. 38b.
               8) H. Donner 1955.

EASY ACCESS
     Editions: 1) *AC* 12 • *AH* I/1:8 • *AaGDeg* 8–9 • *AaGSeg* 17 • *EAS* 169–71 • *KAI* 216 • *NSI* 63 • *TSSI* 2.15.
                  2) *AaGDeg* 8–9 • *EAS* 169–71 • *HNE* 444, no. 4 • *KAI* 218 • *TSSI* 2.17.
                  3) *HNE* 444, no. 5 • *KAI* 219.
                  4) *HNE* 444, no. 6 • *KAI* 220.
                  5) *HNE* 444, no. 7 • *KAI* 221.
                  8) *KAI* 217 • *TSSI* 2.16.

     Translations: 1) *ANET* 501a • *ANET*[3] 655 • *ATAT* 445 • *TUAT* 1:631–32.

     Illustrations: 1) *ANEP*[2] pl. 281 • *HNE* pl. 24 • *KAI* pl. 32 • *LA* 67, fig. 10 • J. Naveh 1982, fig. 71 • *NSR* 2, fig. 55 • *SW* pl. 31(i).
                  2) *HNE* pl. 24/2 • *ANEP* pl. 460 • *SW* pl. 31.
                  3) *HNE* pl. 24/3.
                  4) *HNE* pl. 24/4.
                  5) *HNE* pl. 24/5.

LITERATURE
     G. Steindorff 1894, esp. pp. 456–57 • H. Winckler 1896 • C. Clermont-Ganneau 1897 • A. J. Wensinck 1909, esp. pp. 9–10 • A. Dupont-Sommer 1949a, esp. p. 7 • L. Palacios 1953 • G. Garbini 1956a, esp. pp. 273–4 • J. Friedrich 1957–58 •

H. T. Bossert 1958 • J.-G. Février 1959, esp. p. 234 • R. D. Barnett 1964 • S. C. Layton 1988, esp. pp. 182–83.

Text 1
C. Clermont-Ganneau 1885–1924, esp. 2 pp. 101–7 • D. H. Müller 1893, esp. pp. 117–18 • F. von Luschan 1893, esp. pp. 73, 119–201, pl. 38 • J. Halévy 1893–94, esp. pp. 242–43 • M. Jastrow 1894 • J. Halévy 1895b • D. H. Müller 1896 • E. Sachau 1896, esp. pp. 1051–56 • G. Hoffmann 1896a • J. Halévy 1896a • J. Halévy 1897 • F. E. Peiser 1898 • R. Koldewey 1898, esp. pp. 163, 167–69 • J. Halévy 1899, esp. p. 355 • J. Barth 1908a • F. von Luschan 1911, esp. pp. 377–80 • C. C. Torrey 1912, esp. pp. 89–90 • A. Poebel 1932, esp. pp. 49–52 • G. R. Driver 1945, esp. p. 11 • B. Landsberger 1948, esp. p. 71 • G. R. Driver 1948, esp. pp. 121, 127, 249 • F. M. Cross and D. N. Freedman 1952, esp. pp. 29–31 • M. Liverani 1961, esp. pp. 186–87 • J. Swetnam 1965, esp. pp. 35–36 • Y. Yadin 1967a, esp. pp. 34, 37, 2א • D. Diringer and R. Regensburger 1968, pl. 2.186c • R. Degen 1969, esp. p. 8 • S. Segert 1975, esp. p. 319 • J. Naveh 1982, fig. 71, p. 79 • K. L. Younger, Jr. 1986 • S. Paul 1986, esp. p. 202.

Text 2
C. Clermont-Ganneau 1880–97, esp. 2 pp. 213–15 • F. von Luschan 1893, esp. pp. 44–54 • J. Halévy 1893 • E. Sachau 1895 • J. Halévy 1895a • D. H. Müller 1896 • R. Koldewey 1898, esp. pp. 162–63 • F. von Luschan 1911, esp. pp. 345–49 + 2 pls. • A. Dupont-Sommer 1949a, esp. p. 67 • G. R. Meyer 1965, esp. pp. 21, 80–81 • Y. Yadin 1967a, esp. pp. 43–44, 2ב • R. Degen 1969, esp. p. 9.

Text 3
J. Halévy 1893–94, esp. p. 243 • E. Sachau 1895, esp. p. 27, pl. 14 • R. Degen 1969, esp. p. 9 • J. Teixidor 1979, esp. p. 390.

Text 7
Y. Yadin 1967a, esp. pp. 34–35.

Text 8
G. Garbini 1957a, esp. pp. 427–28 • M. E. Sherman 1966, esp. pp. 16–17 • Y. Yadin 1967a, esp. pp. 39–41, 1ב • R. Degen 1969, esp. pp. 8–9.

B.1.15 Tell Sifr Stele (near Aleppo, ca. 700)   TSifr
  Fragmentary basalt relief (28 x 72 cm.). Aleppo Museum.

רשף [...] 1
[...וכבב] [...]

Ed. Pr.   F. Michelini Tocci 1962.

LITERATURE
  J. Naveh 1965–66, esp. p. 157 • J. Naveh 1966, esp. pp. 19–20.

B.1.16   Nerab Stelae (ca. 700)   Nerab

Two stelae with reliefs and text (93 x 35 cm. [1], 95 x 45 cm. [2]).
Louvre.

Ed. Pr.   G. Hoffmann 1896.

EASY ACCESS
  Editions: 1) *AC* 17 • *AH* I/1:9 • *ESE* 1:192–3, 318–19 • *HNE* 445 • *KAI*
                  225 • *NSI* 64 • *TSSI* 2.18.
                  2) *AC* 18 • *AH* I/1:9 • *AaG*Seg 19 • *HNE* 445 • *KAI* 226 • *NSI* 65
                  • *TSSI* 2.19.

  Translations: 1,2) *ERS* 500–1 • *ANET* 504–5 • *TUAT* 2:573–74 • S. Gevirtz
                  1961: 147–48.

  Illustrations: 1,2) *HNE* pl. 25 • *LA* 115–16 • *SW* pl. 59 • *NSR* 2, figs. 117–8 •
                  KAI pls. 24–5.
                  1) *ANEP* 280 • J. Naveh 1982, fig 76.
                  2) *ANEP* 635.

LITERATURE
  Text 1
  C. Clermont-Ganneau 1880–97, esp. 2 pp. 182–223 • C. Clermont-Ganneau 1896
  • J. Halévy 1896, esp. pp. 280–82 • J. Halévy 1896b, esp. pp. 369–70 • J. Halévy
  1897a, esp. p. 189 • P. Kokovtsov 1899 • T. Nöldeke 1899, esp. pp. 31–33 • P.
  Kokovtsov 1900 • P. Dhorme 1928 • A. Parrot 1939 • G. R. Driver 1945, esp. p.
  11 • G. R. Driver 1948, esp. pp. 121, 127, pl. 59/1 • A. Dupont-Sommer 1949a,
  esp. pp. 115–16 • H. T. Bossert 1951, pl. 491 • S. Gevirtz 1961, esp. p. 148 • F.
  Altheim and R. Stiehl 1964–69, esp. pp. 3:105–6 • E. Y. Kutscher 1965, esp. p. 42
  • M. E. Sherman 1966 • H. Tawil 1974 • J. Naveh 1982, fig. 76, p. 83 • S. C. Layton 1988, esp. pp. 184–85 • J. Oelsner 1989.

  Text 2
  C. Clermont-Ganneau 1880–97, esp. 2 pp. 182–223 • J. Halévy 1896, esp. pp.
  282–84 • J. Halévy 1896b, esp. pp. 370–71 • J. Halévy 1897a, esp. p. 190 • P.
  Kokovtsov 1899 • P. Kokovtsov 1899a • C. C. Torrey 1912, esp. p. 90 • G. R.
  Driver 1948, esp. pp. 121, 127, pl. 59/2 • A. Dupont-Sommer 1949a, esp. pp. 87,
  116 • H. T. Bossert 1951, pl. 492 • S. Gevirtz 1961, esp. p. 147 • M. Bogaert
  1964, esp. p. 227 • J. Swetnam 1965, esp. p. 33 • M. E. Sherman 1966, esp. pp.
  427–28 • S. A. Kaufman 1970 • H. Tawil 1974, esp. pp. 57–65 • J. Teixidor
  1975, esp. p. 286 • S. Segert 1975, esp. pp. 319, 434, 439 • S. Parpola 1985 • S. C.
  Layton 1988 • J. Oelsner 1989, esp. p. 190.

B.1.17   Hazael Bridles (unknown, ca. 810–805)   HazBrid

Identical text on two bronze headstalls. National Museum, Athens.

זי נתן הדד למראן חזאל מן עמק בשנת עדה מראן נהר

Ed. Pr.   1) A. Charbonnet 1986.
                 2) H. Kyrieleis and W. Röllig 1988.

LITERATURE
        1) F. Bron and A. Lemaire 1989 • I. Eph'al and J. Naveh 1989.
        2) I. Eph'al and J. Naveh 1989.

B.1.18   Tell Zeror Ostracon (N. Sharon Valley, ca. 700)   TZerB

בעל עלסמך

Ed. Pr.   M. Kochavi 1965, p. 549.

LITERATURE
        K. Ohata 1967 • K. Gotō 1973.

B.1.19   Deir 'Alla Plaster Text (ca. 700)   DA
        Two groups of plaster fragments with ink inscription. Amman.

Ed. Pr.   J. Hoftijzer and G. van der Kooij 1976.

EASY ACCESS

        Translations: *TUAT* 2:138–48.

LITERATURE
        H. J. Franken 1967 • J. Naveh 1967 • F. M. Cross 1969b, esp. p. 14, n. 2 • J. Hof-
        tijzer 1973 • H. J. Franken 1976 • J. Hoftijzer 1976 • J. Hoftijzer 1976a • A.
        Caquot and A. Lemaire 1977 • E. Hammershaimb 1977 • H. Ringgren 1977 • H.
        J. Franken and M. M. Ibrahim 1977–78 • A. Caquot 1978 • A. Lemaire 1978 • A.
        R. Millard 1978, esp. pp. 24–25 • G. Rinaldi 1978 • H.-P. Müller 1978 • J. A.
        Fitzmyer 1978 • J. B. Segal 1978 • J. Naveh 1978 • O. Loretz 1978 • A. Rofé
        1979 • D. Pardee 1979 • G. Garbini 1979 • H. J. Franken 1979 • A. Lemaire
        1979–84 • J. Naveh 1979b • J. C. Greenfield 1980 • L. G. Herr 1980 • P. K.
        McCarter, Jr. 1980 • S. A. Kaufman 1980 • S. Segert 1980a • B. A. Levine 1981 •
        J. Koenig 1981 • J. Naveh 1981 • M. Delcor 1981 • M. Weippert 1981 • M.
        Weinfeld 1981–2 • A. R. Millard 1982 • H. Weippert and M. Weippert 1982 •
        H.-P. Müller 1982 • M. Delcor 1982 • H. Ringgren 1983 • J. Koenig 1983 • J.
        Hackett 1984 • J. Naveh 1984, esp. p. 65 • J. Hackett 1984a • A. Lemaire 1984d •
        A. Lemaire 1985f, esp. pp. 556–57 • A. Lemaire 1985 • A. Rofé 1985 • B. A.
        Levine 1985 • E. Puech 1985 • F. M. Cross 1985 • H. Rouillard 1985 • J. Balensi
        1985, esp. p. 368 • J. C. Greenfield 1985 • M. Weinfeld 1985 • V. Sasson 1985 •
        W. E. Aufrecht 1985 • W. R. Garr 1985 • B. Z. Luria 1985–86 • A. R. Millard
        1985a • E. Puech 1985a • A. Lemaire 1985b • A. R. Millard 1985b • J. Naveh

1985b • A. Lemaire 1985c • E. Puech 1986 • G. van der Kooij 1986 • J. Hackett 1986 • V. Sasson 1986 • A. Lemaire 1986a • V. Sasson 1986a • E. Puech 1986b • B. Halpern 1987 • E. Puech 1987 • J. W. Wesselius 1987 • S. A. Kaufman 1988 • S. C. Layton 1988, esp. p. 183 • A. Wolters 1988 • A. Lemaire 1988c • W. E. Aufrecht 1989 • A. Lemaire 1990 • G. I. Davies 1991 • M. Dijkstra 1991 • H. J. Franken 1991 • J. C. Greenfield 1991 • J. Hackett 1991 • J. Hoftijzer 1991 • J. Hoftijzer and G. van der Kooij 1991 • J. Huehnergard 1991 • M. M. Ibrahim and G. van der Kooij 1991 • F. Israel 1991 • A. Lemaire 1991 • B. A. Levine 1991 • P. K. McCarter, Jr. 1991 • H.-P. Müller 1991 • D. Pardee 1991 • E. Puech 1991 • G. van der Kooij 1991 • M. Weippert 1991 • A. Wolters 1991 • B. A. Levine forthcoming.

B.1.20　　Deir 'Alla Epigraphs (ca. 700)　　　　　　　　DAEpig

Six short texts on a variety of surfaces.
1) Jar (DA 1818)
2) Flint nodule (DA 2000).
3) Bowl rim alphabet (DA 2230).
4) Jar (DA 2003).
5) Jar fragments (DA 2530).
6) Ostracon (DA 2600, unpublished).
7) Jar fragment with four letters (DA 2555, unpublished).
8) Fragmentary ostracon (unpublished).

(1　זי שרעא
(2　אבן שרעא
(3　אבגדזח
(4　ר / ת̇
(5　לשאׄול

Ed. Pr.　　1–4) J. Hoftijzer and G. van der Kooij 1976.
　　　　　　5–8) H. J. Franken and M. M. Ibrahim 1977–78 (descriptions only for 6,7,8).

LITERATURE
　　J. Hoftijzer 1977–78 • A. Lemaire 1984, esp. pp. 254–55.

B.1.21　　Tell Jemmeh Ostracon (7th c.)　　　　　　　　Jemmeh

Fragmentary account (5 x 5.4 cm.). Israel Department of Antiquities.

1 עעעעעע [a series of 'ayins or open circles]
על יד .[....]
ח 2 פ [........]
ב[............]

Ed. Pr.　　J. Naveh 1985, pp. 19–20.

B.1.22   Olympian Bowl (7th c.)   Olymp

Bronze dish. Varvakian Museum [Coll. 574], Athens.

לנגד בר מיפע

Ed. Pr.   J. Euting 1871.

EASY ACCESS
Editions: *CIS* 112.

Illustrations: *CIS* pl. 8.

B.1.23   Beirut Decree (ca. 600)   Decree

Inscribed stone (28.5 x 28.5 cm.). French Institute of Archeology, Beirut.

Ed. Pr.   A. Caquot 1971.

LITERATURE
J. Teixidor 1972a, esp. p. 437 • S. A. Kaufman 1974, esp. pp. 43, 49, 55 • P.-E. Dion 1974a • E. Lipiński 1975a, esp. pp. 77–82 • F. M. Fales 1978a.

B.1.24   Louvre (Starcky) Tablet (570)   LouvTab

Clay tablet, witnessed loan contract (5 x 7 cm.). Louvre [AO 21.063].

recto
1 [........]
.[.] ביתאלעשני
27 שקלן
34 בשנת
5 נ[נ]בוכדרצר מלך
[ב]בל שהד געלא
verso
1 [בר] סוה שהד
[ב]יתאלדלני בר
.[.]יזכה שהד
ביתאלדלני בר
5 [.]דיחוט שהד
[..]ילא ספרא
[..........]

Ed. Pr.   J. Starcky 1960.

EASY ACCESS
Editions: *AaG*Seg 48 • *KAI* 227 • *TSSI* 2.22.

LITERATURE
> J. Naveh 1964–65, esp. pp. 185–86 • J. Naveh 1966, esp. pp. 23–24 • S. J. Lieberman 1968, esp. p. 26 • E. Lipiński 1977, esp. p. 104 • J. Naveh 1982, pl. 8A.

B.1.25   Elath Ostraca (7th–5th c.)   ElathOstr
> Six ostraca.

Ed. Pr.   1) N. Glueck 1938, p. 17.
                2–6) N. Glueck 1940, 1941.

LITERATURE
> C. C. Torrey 1941 • W. F. Albright 1941 • C. C. Torrey 1941a • F. Rosenthal 1942 • J. Naveh 1966a • J. Naveh 1966b • P. Colella 1973, esp. pp. 547–49 • E. A. Knauf 1990, esp. p. 205.
> 2) R. A. Bowman 1948, esp. p. 82, n. 100 • N. Glueck 1971, esp. p. 232.
> 3) N. Glueck 1971, esp. pp. 232–33 • A. Lemaire and B. Delavault 1975, esp. pp. 32–34.
> 4) N. Glueck 1971, esp. pp. 233–34.

B.1.26   Tell es-Saidiyeh Ostraca (6th c.?)   SaidOstr
> Two sherds with black ink epigraphs, evidently barley receipts.

1 [..]..[...] 1
שׂעׂרׂן כרן 300[+1
פקיד לאחרן זׄי עׄלֹכׄ ..]
4 ינוחי שמה ..]
5 אחרן. . . . כל]
ליד . . .]

1 שׂ[עריא זי]‎ 2
ענ[זיא מן .]
[לויה . . .]
6+20 לשבד]‎ . . .
5 [ר פלה שערן כרן]
[א שׁון שעׄרׂן]

Ed. Pr.   J. B. Pritchard 1985, pp. 87–88, fig. 175.1,2 + photos.

B.1.27   Nerab Tablets (Reign of Nabonidus)   NerTab
> Aramaic dockets on five of 27 cuneiform economic documents. Louvre.

יכ[...]‎ (1
שטר נושכלני כס]ף]‎ (2
נ[ח]סי בר אבא‎ (3

4) נושכלנ[י]י / שער[ן]
5) לסנאל

Ed. Pr.   P. Dhorme 1928, pp. 56–64, nos. 3, 7, 12, 15, 18.

EASY ACCESS
    Editions: Vat. 137–41.

LITERATURE
    F. M. Fales 1973 ● I. Eph'al 1978 ● L. Cagni 1990.

B.1.28   Moussaief Bowl (unknown, 6th c.?)   MousBowl
Bronze bowl (11.7 x 4.9 cm.). S. Moussaief Collection, London.

לאחרם בר שאל

Ed. Pr.   P. Bordreuil and E. Gubel 1986.

B.1.29   Samaria Sherds (6th–4th c.)   SamSh
Seventeen ostraca and jar inscriptions.

Ed. Pr.   1–11) G. A. Reisner et al. 1924, pl. 58.
                   12–14, 17) S. A. Birnbaum 1957, pp. 25–32, pl. 3.
                   15–16) E. L. Sukenik 1933a.

LITERATURE
    B. Mazar (Maisler) 1948.

B.1.30   Qadum Bowl (6 km. w. of Shechem, 6th–5th c.)   Qadum
Decorated jar with painted text. Israel Department of Antiquities.

מתרא

Ed. Pr.   E. Stern and Y. Magen 1982.

LITERATURE
    E. Stern and Y. Magen 1984, esp. pp. 10–14.

B.1.31   Ashdod Ostracon (mid-5th c.)   AshdodOstr
Sherd with ink epigraph (4.3 x 4.3 cm.).

1 כרם זבדיה
פ ג

Ed. Pr.   J. Naveh 1971b.

EASY ACCESS
     Editions: *IR* 165.

LITERATURE
     J. Naveh 1971, esp. p. 31 • J. Naveh 1972 • J. Teixidor 1973, esp. p. 429.

B.1.32   Khan Sheikhoun Jar (N. Syria, 5th c.?)   KhShJar
        Jar with inscription on shoulder (74 cm. wide).

לבנין

Ed. Pr.   R. Mesnil du Buisson 1930.

B.1.33   Yoqneam Ostracon (early 4th c.)   Yoqneam
        List of five names (5 x 6 cm.). Israel Department of Antiquities.

1 עקביה
אסיתון
[....]ע
מזדגי
5 [.]עֿבדֿ[.]

Ed. Pr.   J. Naveh 1985a, pp. 119–20, pl. 20.

B.1.34   Ein Gedi Ostraca (1st half 4th c.)   EinGedi
        Two unpublished ostraca.

LITERATURE
     B. Mazar and I. Dunayevsky 1964 • B. Mazar and I. Dunayevsky 1965 • B. Mazar, T. Dothan and I. Dunayevsky 1966.

B.1.35   Ketef Yeriḥo Papyrus (Cave w. of Jericho, 4th c.)   KetefYer
        Two fragments of a single papyrus with an account list. Israel Department of Antiquities. Also an additional small fragment (K 10215, text: הב).

Recto
1 חנניה בר [...] זֿי ש 2
תחנה בר גרפא ש 2
[...]ש דלוי
יהוחנן בר שפנה ש 2
5 יהוחנן בר אביאור ש 2

נריה בר פדיה ש 1
יהוחנן בר גרפא ש 2
שלמיה נגרא ש 1
יהועזר בר שוה ר 2
10 יהוסף בר שוה ר 2
תחנה בר שלומה ש 1
[ת]חנ[ה] בר עקוב ר 2

[כ]ל ש 21

Verso
1

[...] יהוחנן ב[ר א]ביאור ר 2   [...] בר יהוחזי ר 2
עבדא בר [ע]קוב ר 2   [...] גרפא ש 1
תחנה חטלא ר 2   [...] בר אחוהי ש 2
שֹמעֹון בר יהורם ר 2   5 [יהוחנן] בר שפנה ר 2
[יהו]עזר בר שוה מ 4   [...]ה ר 2

כל [...]מ 4 שאר ש 8 מֹ[]   [...]נ[גֹוֹ]רֹא ר 2

Ed. Pr.   H. Eshel and H. Misgav 1986–87.

LITERATURE
H. Eshel 1988 • H. Eshel and H. Misgav 1988.

B.1.36   Tell Arad Ostraca (4th c.)   AradOstr

85 administrative texts, 45 legible. Israel Museum, Jerusalem.

Ed. Pr.   J. Naveh 1975a.

EASY ACCESS
Editions: 1, 3, 5, 6, 38) *IR* 159–63.
                 38) *TSSI* 2.31.

Illustrations: *IR* 159–63.

LITERATURE
General
Y. Aharoni and R. Amiran 1962 • Y. Aharoni 1963b • K. R. Veenhof 1966 • Y. Aharoni 1964, esp. p. 283 • Y. Aharoni 1965, esp. p. 250 • J. Teixidor 1967, esp. p. 179 • Y. Aharoni 1967 • Y. Aharoni 1967a, esp. pp. 243–44 • Y. Aharoni 1968a, esp. pp. 9–11 • Y. Aharoni 1969 • J. Naveh 1971, esp. p. 31 • J. Teixidor 1971, esp. p. 479 • C. H. J. De Geus 1979–80, esp. pp. 62–63 • A. N. Temerev 1980.

38) Y. Aharoni and R. Amiran 1963, esp. pp. 227–29, pl. viii.2 • Y. Aharoni and R. Amiran 1964, esp. pp. 141–42, pl. 38B • J. Naveh 1964–65, esp. p. 192 • J. Naveh 1966, esp. pp. 31–32.

B.1.37   Tell Beer-Sheba Ostraca (mid-4th c.)   BeershebaOstr

66 administrative texts. Israel Museum, Jerusalem.

Ed. Pr.   1–26) J. Naveh 1973.
                27–67) J. Naveh 1979 [no. 54 is a jar fragment, see below].

EASY ACCESS
   Editions: 1, 3, 6) *IR* 156–158.

LITERATURE
   J. Naveh 1971, esp. p. 31 • Y. Aharoni 1974, esp. p. 39 • J. Naveh 1975 • J. Teixidor 1975, esp. p. 285.

   33) J. Naveh 1982, pl. 10B.

B.1.38   Tell Beer-Sheba Jar (mid 4th c.)   BeershebaOstr.54

Fragment of jar. Israel Department of Antiquities (7119/1).

לביתא]לדלני[

Ed. Pr.   J. Naveh 1979.

B.1.39   Samaria Papyri (Wādi ed-Dāliyeh, 375–335)   SamPap

Twenty-seven fragmentary conveyance deeds.

Ed. Pr.   1) F. M. Cross 1985.
               2–9) D. Gropp 1986.

LITERATURE
   F. M. Cross 1963 • K. R. Veenhof 1963 • F. M. Cross 1963a • P. W. Lapp 1963a
   • K. R. Veenhof 1964 • M. Weippert 1964, esp. pp. 172–74 • I. H. Eybers 1966 •
   F. M. Cross 1966a • F. M. Cross 1969a • F. M. Cross 1974 • F. M. Cross 1978 •
   P. W. Lapp 1978 • J. Naveh 1982, fig. 80, p. 87 • D. Gropp 1990.

   1) B. Zuckerman 1987, esp. pp. 37–41 + photo • D. N. Freedman and F. I. Andersen 1989.

B.1.40 Jar Handle Stamps and Inscriptions JarH

type	provenance	date	quantity	texts
1	Damascus	Old Aram.	1	למרא
	Engedi	ca. 600	1	
2	Tell en-Naṣbeh	6th–5th	30	מצה, מוצה
	Gibeon		3	
	Ramat Rachel		1	
	Jericho		1	
	Beth Hanina		1	
	Belmont Castle		1	
3	Jericho, Jerusalem	Persian–Hellenistic	over 250	יהד, יהוד, יה
	Ramat Rachel			
	Moṣah, Gezer			
	Engedi			
	Tell en–Naṣbeh			
4	Ophel	Persian–Hellenistic	22	יהוד ט, יהד ט
	Tyropeon		3	
	Jew. Quarter		??	
	Bethany		2	
	Ramat Rachel		21	
	Gezer		2	
	Tell en-Naṣbeh		2	
	unknown		2	
5	Ramat Rachel	Persian	4	יהוד פחוא, יהד פחוא
6	Beth Shemesh	Persian	1	לבכי לשלם
7	Jericho	5th. c.	1	ליהעזר
	Ramat Rachel		2	

Remarks:Type 3: Some erringly read the divine name יה and יהו for a number of יהד
impressions. Over 100 impressions read only יי, while 5 read only ה.

Type 4: Three subgroups have been determined (E. Stern, 1982, p. 203), apparently from
different periods. Some erringly read העיר instead of יהד ט.

Type 5: F. M. Cross reads פחרא instead of פחוא.

LITERATURE

General) C. Clermont-Ganneau 1883a • N. Avigad 1957 • Y. Yadin 1957 • Y.
Yadin 1961 • Y. Aharoni 1963 • A. F. Rainey 1965 • H. D. Lance 1971 • J. Teixidor 1975, esp. p. 286 • G. Garbini 1979a • J. W. Betlyon 1986.

1) B. Mazar, T. Dothan and E. Dunayevski 1963, pp. 50–52 (fig. 12) • B. Mazar
1967, p. 225 • M. Heltzer 1983.

2) E. Sellin and C. Watzinger 1913, p. 518 (pl. 42.k) • M. Lidzbarski 1902–15,
3:45 • *RES* no. 1812 • C. C. McCown 1947, pp. 165–67 (pls. 56.15–28;
57.15–16) • S. Moscati 1951, p. 72, n. 1 • N. Avigad, 1958a • N. Avigad 1960, p.
25 • J. Naveh 1971c, pp. 61–62 • E. Stern 1971, pp. 6, 8 • E. Stern 1982, p. 208 •
A. R. Millard 1989a, pp. 60–61 (fig. 13).

3) E. Sellin 1908, p. 39 (fig. 17–18) • M. Lidzbarski 1902–15, 3:45 • *RES* nos.
1814, 1815 • L.-H. Vincent 1910 • L.-H. Vincent 1910a, p. 412 • E. Sellin and C.
Watzinger 1913, p. 159 (pl. 42.ll–3, m and m1) • R. S. A. Macalister and J. G.

Duncan 1926, pp. 189–90 (fig. 203) • D. Diringer 1934, pp. 128–29, 132–37 • W. F. Albright 1934a • E. L. Sukenik 1934, pp. 182–84 (pl. III.1) • C. C. McCown 1947, pp. 164–65 (pl. 57.1–3, 13–14, 17–19) • L.–H. Vincent 1949, pp. 279–94 • S. Moscati 1951, p. 72, n. 1 • Y. Aharoni 1956, pp. 148–49 • W. F. Albright 1957a • G. Garbini 1962 • P. W. Lapp 1963 • B. Mazar and I. Dunayevsky 1964, p. 125 (pl. 27.A–C) • B. Mazar 1967, p. 227 • F. M. Cross 1969, p. 23 • E. Stern 1971, pp. 6–9, 15–16 • J. Naveh 1971c, pp. 58–61 • F. Vattioni 1971a, (no. 101–102) • N. Avigad 1976, p. 23 • E. Stern 1982, pp. 202–7 • M. Kochman 1982, pp. 3–9.

4) R. S. A. Macalister 1907, pp. 264–65 (fig. 6) • R. S. A. Macalister 1909, p. 22 (fig. 5) • R. S. A. Macalister 1912, p. 225 (fig. 375–376) • E. L. Sukenik 1933 • R. S. A. Macalister and J. G. Duncan 1926, pp. 190–91 • D. Diringer 1934, pp. 129–30 • Y. Aharoni 1956, p. 149 (fig. 17; pl. 26.6) • N. Avigad 1960 • Y. Aharoni 1962a, p. 30 (fig. 22.1; pl. 31.2) • Y. Aharoni 1964a, pp. 20 and 43 (pl. 18.7–9) • S. J. Saller 1957, pp. 193–95 (fig. 37; pl. 111.b–c) • F. M. Cross 1968, pp. 231–32 • F. M. Cross 1969, p. 23 (pl. V.1–2) • F. M. Cross 1969c, pp. 19–20 (fig. 1) • P. Colella 1973, pp. 549–53 • N. Avigad 1974 • N. Avigad 1976, p. 23 • E. Stern 1982, p. 203.

5) Y. Aharoni 1960, p. 400 • Y. Aharoni 1962, p. 403 • Y. Aharoni 1962a, p. 9 (no. 2 and 4; fig. 9.2–3,6; pl. 9.1,3,6) • F. M. Cross 1969, p. 26 • J. Naveh 1971, p. 30 • S. A. Kaufman 1974, p. 82 • N. Avigad 1976, pp. 22–23 • M. Kochman 1982, pp. 23–30 • E. 1989.

6) C. C. Torrey 1935, pp. 309–10.

7) E. Sellin and C. Watzinger 1913, p. 158 (pl. 42.i) • M. Lidzbarski 1902–15, 3:45 • Y. Aharoni 1956, pp. 145–46 (figs. 13–14; pl. 25.5) • Y. Aharoni 1962a, pl. 31.8 • Y. Aharoni 1964a, pl. 19.10 • J. Naveh 1971c, p. 60.

B.1.41   Ḥorvat Dorban Jar Fragment (4th c.)   HorvDor

נתי

Ed. Pr.   Y. Aharoni 1963.

LITERATURE
  J. Naveh 1971, esp. p. 31.

B.1.42   Tell Abu Zeitun Ostracon (4th c.)   TAbuZeitun
  Sherd in two pieces with incised text (9 x 8 cm.).

חשוב

Ed. Pr.   J. Kaplan 1958.

LITERATURE
  J. Teixidor 1973, esp. p. 429.

B.1.43 **Tell Sheikh Ḥasan Ostracon (Syria, 4th c.?)** **ShHasOst**

Thick orange sherd with six faded lines (78 x 61 mm.). Raqqa Museum (TSH 87.2).

Ed. Pr. W. Röllig 1990 + drawing, photo.

B.1.44 **Kerak Altar Fragment (350–25)** **Kerak**

Limestone (37 x 25 x 20cm.). Jerusalem.

1 ‬וגר סרא מלכתא [ע]בד
2 ‬עבד כמש הלל בר עמא
3 ‬מדבחא דנה ונשכתה
4 ‬לזך ב[י]ת[א] שנת 15

Ed. Pr. J. T. Milik 1958–59.

EASY ACCESS
  Editions: *AaG*Seg 51.

  Translations: *NERTOT* 244–45 • *TUAT* 2:581.

LITERATURE
  R. Canova 1954, esp. p. 10 • Anon. 1960 • J. T. Milik 1960a • A. Spijkerman 1961–62, esp. pp. 326–28 • E. Lipiński 1975, esp. pp. 261–62 • E. Lipiński 1978a, esp. pp. 244–45.

B.1.45 **Nebī Yūnis Ostracon (2d half 4th c.)** **NebYun**

Israel Department of Antiquities.

1 ‬בעלצד תק]לן [...]
2 ‬דשנא

Ed. Pr. F. M. Cross 1964.

EASY ACCESS
  Editions: *TSSI* 2.32.

LITERATURE
  J. Naveh 1964–65, esp. pp. 192–93 • J. Naveh 1966, esp. p. 32 • M. Weippert 1966, esp. p. 296 • J. Teixidor 1967, esp. pp. 179–80 • N. Avigad 1968a, esp. p. 43.

B.1.46   Tell el-Fara' Ostraca (1: ca. 400, 2–6: ca. 300)   TFara

1) 3 line record of barley seed (8 x 6.5 cm.). Rockefeller Museum, Jerusalem (I 9742).
2) Illegible text (9 x 7 cm.). Rockefeller Museum, Jerusalem (I 1509).
3–6) Short administrative texts. Israel Department of Antiquities (IDAM 74-564, 74-559, 74-561).

Ed. Pr.   1) A. Cowley 1929, pp. 111–12.
2) A. Cowley 1932.
3–6) J. Naveh 1985a, pp. 116–17.

EASY ACCESS
    Editions: 1) *IR* 164.

LITERATURE
    Anon. 1929 • J. Naveh 1971, esp. p. 31 • J. Naveh 1972 • J. Naveh 1985a, esp. pp. 114–16.

B.1.47   Yatta Ostracon (357?)   Yatta

(8 x 6 cm.). Israel Department of Antiquities.

1 ב 6 לתמוז שנ[ת] 2
2 יתעו בר מרֹצ] [
3 ש ס 26 על יד
4 יתירו וצביחו

Ed. Pr.   J. Naveh 1985a, pp. 117–18, pl. 19.

B.1.48   Gaza Ostracon (ca. 300)   Gaza

Sherd with ink text (7 x 4 cm.).

1 [...]תא תבן פחלצן 1ô
2 [...]קֹרֹ בר עבדמראן

Ed. Pr.   J. Naveh 1972–73.

LITERATURE
    J. Teixidor 1974, esp. p. 328 • J. Naveh 1985a, esp. pp. 118–19.

B.1.49   Tel 'Ira Ostracon (ca. 300)   Ira

1 נתנו ש ס 11
2D

Ed. Pr.   A. Biran and R. Cohen 1979, p. 125 pl. 16c.

LITERATURE
J. Naveh 1985a, esp. p. 118, pl. 20.

B.1.50   Khirbet el-Kom Ostraca (4th–3d c.)   KhElKom

Seven ostraca, five with Aramaic inscriptions, one Aramaic-Greek bilingual, one Greek only.

Ed. Pr.   L. T. Geraty 1972.

LITERATURE
J. Teixidor 1976, esp. p. 333 • A. Lemaire 1977 • A. Skaist 1978 • J. Naveh 1979
• L. T. Geraty 1983.
1) L. T. Geraty 1975 • L. T. Geraty 1981.

B.1.51   Jerusalem Ostracon (mid-3d c.)   JerusOstr

List of commodities. Israel Department of Antiquities.

הֹמצין מתלחי[ן] 1
סקן אסתרבלֹט[...]
חרתס 10+1

Ed. Pr.   F. M. Cross 1981.

B.1.52   Tell Dan Bilingual (3d[?] c.)   TDanBil

Greek-Aramaic votive inscription on limestone slab (15.5 x 26.5 cm.).

[...]לאן זילס נדר [...]

Ed. Pr.   A. Biran 1976, pp. 204–5, p. 35D.

LITERATURE
J. Teixidor 1979, esp. pp. 388–89.

B.1.53   Philotas Bilingual (unknown, 3d c.?)   PhilBil

Basalt bas-relief with Greek-Aramaic text (69 x 56 x 10 cm.). Moussaieff Collecton, London.

פלתא שמה 1
זי כמרא 2

(On the basis of the Greek, שמה is probably to be understood as 'he
erected it' rather than 'his name'.)

Ed. Pr.   P. Bordreuil and P.-L. Gatier 1990.

B.2 Mesopotamia

NB: The terminology used in the literature to refer to Aramaic epigraphs on clay tablets from Mesopotamia is somewhat confusing. The term "docket" has been regularly but inconsistently used. We use it here strictly to refer to Aramaic labels or summaries on tablets whose main text is cuneiform. Other documents, written only in Aramaic, range in size from "labels," through small triangular corn-loan (i.e. barley) records (termed "dockets" by Fales in *AECT* and others) to normally sized, rectangular tablets.

B.2.1   Tell Halaf "Altar" (ca. 900)   HalAlt

Fragmentary limestone block. Formerly in Berlin, now destroyed.

Ed. Pr.   J. Friedrich 1940.

EASY ACCESS

Editions: *AC* 3 ● *AaG*Deg 23 ● *EAS* 21 ● *KAI* 231 ● *TSSI* 2.10.

Illustrations: *KAI* pl. 12 ● *SW* fig. 73 ● *TSSI* fig. 5.

LITERATURE

R. T. O'Callaghan 1948 ● G. Garbini 1956a, esp. pp. 270–72 ● R. A. Bowman 1941 ● A. Malamat 1949–50a ● F. M. Cross and D. N. Freedman 1952, esp. pp. 23–24 ● W. F. Albright 1956a, esp. pp. 82–83 ● R. Degen 1969, esp. p. 23 ● J. Teixidor 1973, esp. p. 428 ● G. Dankwarth and Ch. Müller 1988.

B.2.2   Tell Fakhariyeh Bilingual Statue (ca. 850)   Fakh

Akkadian-Aramaic bilingual text on statue of HDYS'Y, "king" of Gozan. Damascus.

Ed. Pr.   A. Abou Assaf 1981.

EASY ACCESS

Editions: *EAS* 14–20.

Translations: *TUAT* 1:634–37.

LITERATURE

H. Yalon (cf. כנן!) 1935 ● "A. Mikaya" 1981 ● A. Spycket 1981 ● A. Shaffer and J. C. Greenfield 1981–82 ● J. Naveh 1981–82 ● J. C. Greenfield 1981a, esp. pp. 112–13 ● A. Abou Assaf 1982 ● A. Abou Assaf, P. Bordreuil, and A. Millard 1982 ● A. R. Millard and P. Bordreuil 1982 ● Anon. 1982 ● P.-E. Dion 1982c ● F. M. Fales 1982 ● F. M. Fales 1982a, esp. pp. 80–83 ● D. F. Graf 1982 ● S. A. Kaufman 1982 ● W. von Soden 1982 ● R. Zadok 1982 ● P.-E. Dion 1983 ● C. Dohmen 1983 ● F. M. Fales 1983 ● J. C. Greenfield and A. Shaffer 1983 ● F. Israel 1983 ● A. R. Millard 1983 ● J. M. Sasson 1983 ● J. W. Wesselius 1983 ● T. Muraoka

1983–84 • E. Lipiński 1983a, esp. p. 132 n. 12 • F. Israel 1983a • J. C. Greenfield and A. Shaffer 1983a • A. Angerstorfer 1984 • A. Angerstorfer 1984a • P.-E. Dion 1984 • J. C. Greenfield 1984, esp. pp. 220–21 • S. A. Kaufman 1984a • A. R. Millard 1984 • D. Pardee and R. D. Biggs 1984 • J. C. Greenfield 1984–86, esp. pp. 149–52 • B. F. Batto 1985 • P.-E. Dion 1985 • P.-E. Dion and D. Fraikin 1985, esp. column 373 • W. R. Garr 1985 • D. M. Gropp and T. J. Lewis 1985 • J. C. Greenfield and A. Shaffer 1985 • D. R. Hillers 1985, esp. p. 107 • A. Lemaire 1985e, esp. pp. 278–79 • V. Sasson 1985a • S. Segert 1985 • A. Spycket 1985 • J. Huehnergard 1986 • P. Garelli 1986 • F. I Andersen and A. D. Forbes 1986, esp. pp. 33–34, 43–44, 52, 55, 59–60, 133 • F. Leemhuis 1986 • F. Vattioni 1986 • S. A. Kaufman 1986 • E. Attardo 1987 • F. Deblauwe 1987, esp. p. 353 • J. Blau 1987, esp. pp. 3–6 • J. Huehnergard 1987a • J. Naveh 1987 • P.-E. Dion 1987 • F. I. Andersen and D. N. Freedman 1988 • G. A. Rendsburg 1988 • S. C. Layton 1988, esp. p. 176 • W. E. Aufrecht and G. J. Hamilton 1988 • G. A. Rendsburg 1988a • P. Bordreuil and E. Gubel 1988 • G. Herrmann 1989, esp. pp. 106–9 • I. J. Winter 1989, esp. pp. 324–36 • V. Brugnatelli forthcoming.

B.2.3   Tell Halaf Alphabet (end 8th c.)   HalAlph

Alphabet on limestone disk fragment (10.5 x 8.1 x 1.5 cm.). British Museum.

Ed. Pr.   R. Degen 1978a.

LITERATURE

B. Hrouda 1962, esp. pp. 9, 21, pl.8, no. 44.

B.2.4   Nineveh Lion Weights (ca. 700)   NinLiW

Fourteen inscribed weights (of 16 total) in lion shape. British Museum.

Ed. Pr.   H. Layard 1853 (unabridged ed.), nos. 1–5, 8–16.

EASY ACCESS

Editions: *AC* 13 • *AaG*Seg 22 • *CIS* 1–14 • *NSI* 66.

Illustrations: *ANEP* 119 • *CIS* pl. 1.

LITERATURE

E. Norris 1856 • A. Aurès 1884 • E. Ledrain 1884 • J. Halévy 1890, esp. pp. 224–27 • C. H. W. Johns 1901, esp. 2 pp. 256 ff. • S. Schiffer 1911, esp. pp. 36, 174–77 • I. Henninger 1927, esp. p. 195 • M. E. Sherman 1966, esp. pp. 427–28 • J. Teixidor 1969, esp. pp. 346–47 • J. Naveh 1971c • R. Degen 1978.

B.2.5   Tablets from Nineveh and Environs   AECT.1–42

(R = H. C. Rawlinson, 1865; J = C. H. W. Johns 1925–26; d. = docket)

	Editio princeps	*EA*	*ABC*	*CIS*	Vat.	Description	Date
1	R 8	1	1	16	1	Conveyance d.	687
2	CIS	28	19	32	28	Conveyance d.	684
3	P. Berger 1886	21	2	38	21	Corn loan	682
4	*ABC*	13	3		13	Conveyance d.	681
5	R 2 pl. 14	14	4	17	14	Conveyance d.	680
6	R 11 pl. 14	22	25	40	22	Corn loan	ca. 680
7	CIS	24		41	24	Corn loan	ca. 680
8	R 16 pl. 14	3	47	25	3	petition, d.	Esarh.
9	R 13 pl. 15	23		39	23	Corn loan	674
10	R 5 pl. 15	18	23	27	18	Conveyance d.	670?
11	CIS	31		35	31	Legal record(?) d.	670?
12	A. R. Millard 1983					?	670?
13	P. Berger 1886	26		43	26	Loan pledge	670?
14	*ABC*	15	5		15	Conveyance d.	671/666
15	CIS	25	6	42	25	Corn loan	665
16	CIS	30	18	31	30	Conveyance d.	668–660
17	R 6 pl. 15	12	7	19	12	Conveyance d.	659
18	*ABC*	32	8		32	Conveyance d.	653
19	CIS	16	9	29	16	Conveyance d.	652
20	CIS	5	20	33	5	Conveyance d.	ca. 650
21	CIS	19	10	30	19	Loan envelope d.	ca. 646
22	*ABC*	29	24		29	Conveyance d.	ca. 646
23	G. Smith 1875, p. 424	11	22	28	11	Conveyance d.	ca. 646
24	R 3 pl. 15	9	15	18	9	Conveyance d.	after 648
25	*ABC*	33	21		33	Conveyance d.	after 648
26	CIS	6	26	36	6	Conveyance d.	ca. 640
27	R 1 pl. 15	8	14	22	8	Conveyance d.	after 648
28	R 12 pl. 15	7	16	20	7	Loan envelope d.	after 648
29	*ABC*	27	27		27	Conveyance d.	ca. 630
30	R 7 pl. 15	4	11	15	4	Conveyance d.	after 648
31	R 4 pl. 22	10	12	23	10	Conveyance d.	after 648
32	R 9 pl. 22	17	13	24	17	Conveyance d.	after 648
33	R 14 pl. 22	2	17	21	2	Conveyance d.	after 648

	Editio princeps	EA	ABC	CIS	Vat.	Description	Date
34	*EA*	34			34	Conveyance d.	after 648
35	R 3 pl. 22	20	28	37	20	Conveyance d.	
36	J p. 273					Fragmentary	
37	A. R. Millard 1972					Conveyance d.	ca. 665
38	A. R. Millard 1972					Conveyance d.	
39	J pl. 14					Loan d.	619
40	*AECT*					Conveyance d.	
41	*AECT*					Court (?) document d.	
42	*AECT*					Conveyance, no legible text!	ca. 665
FI	*AECT*, p. 268					Conveyance d.	
FII	*AECT*, p. 269					Contract envelope(?) d.	

For the texts of the above the reader is referred to *AECT* and S. A. Kaufman 1989.

LITERATURE

General) H. C. Rawlinson 1870, esp. 3:46 ● E. Schrader 1878 ● T. Nöldeke 1879 ●
T. G. Pinches 1910 ● M. Rostovtzeff 1932, esp. pp. 18–19, 37, 94–97 ● S. J.
Lieberman 1968 ● E. Lipiński 1985 ● E. Lipiński 1988, esp. pp. 510–12 ● S. A.
Kaufman 1989.
1) S. Guyard 1879, esp. pp. 441–43 ● E. Ledrain 1885.
2) S. Schiffer 1911, esp. pp. 179–80 ● R. Zadok 1981–82, esp. p. 136 n. 24.
3) S. A. Kaufman 1989, esp. p. 98.
5) S. Schiffer 1911, esp. p. 178 ● I. Eph'al 1973, esp. p. 202 ● S. A. Kaufman
1989, esp. p. 98.
9) S. Schiffer 1911, esp. p. 181 ● S. A. Kaufman 1989, esp. p. 98.
13) S. A. Kaufman 1989, esp. p. 98.
14) S. Schiffer 1911, esp. p. 177.
15) S. A. Kaufman 1989, esp. p. 98.
19) A. R. Millard 1971.
21) S. Schiffer 1911, esp. p. 178.
23) S. Schiffer 1911, esp. p. 178.
30) S. Schiffer 1911, esp. p. 177 ● S. A. Kaufman 1989, esp. p. 99.
37) J. N. Postgate 1970, esp. pp. 139–42, pls. 22, 31 ● J. Teixidor 1973, esp. p.
428.
38) J. N. Postgate 1970, esp. pp. 144–45, pl. 23 ● S. A. Kaufman 1989, esp. p. 99.

B.2.6   Nimrud Labels (ND 2346 and 2347) (?)   AECT.43–44

Two triangular clay labels.

1) להיכלא
2) לבי[ן]ת ...[

Ed. Pr.   A. R. Millard 1972, 131–32, p. 53a–c.

EASY ACCESS
  Editions: Vat. 161–62.

LITERATURE
  J. Teixidor 1973, esp. pp. 427–28.

B.2.7   Nimrud Bullae (ND 2348 and 2349) (?)   AECT.45
  Two ovoid clay bullae.

בין עוזא (1
ולבבא (2

Ed. Pr.   A. R. Millard 1972, pp. 132–33, pl. 53d–f.

EASY ACCESS
  Editions: Vat. 163–64.

LITERATURE
  J. Teixidor 1973, esp. pp. 427–28 • S. A. Kaufman 1989, esp. p. 100.

B.2.8   Assur Tablets (Assur, ca. 659)   AECT.46–51.
  Six triangular loan tablets. Staatliche Museen, Berlin.

Ed. Pr.   M. Lidzbarski 1921, pp. 15–20, pl. 2.

EASY ACCESS
  Editions: 1–6) Vat. 143–48.
                   2) *KAI* 234.
                   3) *KAI* 235.
                   4) *KAI* 236.

LITERATURE
  E. Lipiński 1975a, esp. pp. 90–113 • S. A. Kaufman 1977 • J. Teixidor 1977, esp.
  p. 272 • S. A. Kaufman 1989, esp. p. 100.

B.2.9   Freydank Assur Tablet (Mid 7th c.)   AECT.52
  Rectangular tablet, list of loans.

Obv.
1 4?+10? [שקלן ...שקל]ן על משיה
1 שקל על ננִי
1 שקל עַל בֹננִי בר ננִי
1 שקל על [........]

5 2 שקלן ע]ל [.......]
Side
[.] שקלן חזרן
Rev.
[.] שקל]ן] כנני

Ed. Pr.   H. Freydank 1975.

EASY ACCESS
  Editions: Vat. 191.

B.2.10   Tell Halaf Tablets (614–612)   AECT.53–57
Five triangular corn-loan tablets. Formerly in Berlin, now destroyed.

Ed. Pr.   J. Friedrich 1940.

EASY ACCESS
  Editions: *NESE* 1:50–56 • Vat. 149–53.

LITERATURE
  C. H. W. Johns 1901, esp. p. 2 • R. Degen 1972c • E. Lipiński 1975a, esp. pp.
  115–42 • S. A. Kaufman 1989, esp. p. 100.

B.2.11   A Judicial Settlement (??, 635)   AECT.58
Rectangular clay tablet (6.5 x 4.2 cm.).

Ed. Pr.   P. Bordreuil 1973.

EASY ACCESS
  Editions: Vat. 190.

LITERATURE
  E. Lipiński 1974, esp. pp. 377–79 • J. Teixidor 1974, esp. p. 330 • F. M. Fales
  1976 • S. A. Kaufman 1977 • J. Teixidor 1979, esp. pp. 390–92 • J. W. Wesselius
  1985 • S. A. Kaufman 1989.

B.2.12   AECT 59 (??, ca. 658)   AECT.59
Fragment of triangular corn-loan. Private collection, Hamburg.

קשת [................]

Ed. Pr.   J. N. Postgate 1973, pp. 34–35.

EASY ACCESS
   Editions: Vat. 189.

B.2.13   Assur Ostracon (ca. 650)   AssOstr
   Ostracon in six fragments (ca. 42 x 60 cm.). Staatliche Museen, Berlin.

Ed. Pr.   M. Lidzbarski 1917–18a.

EASY ACCESS
   Editions: *AC* 14 • *AaG*Seg 20 • *ESE* 2:1–33 • *KAI* 233 • *TSSI* 2.20.

   Illustrations: *KAI* pl. 26 • *SW* pl. 60 • *TSSI* pl. 5.

LITERATURE
   M. Lidzbarski 1917 • D. H. Baneth 1919 • M. Lidzbarski 1921, esp. pp. 5–15, I •
   B. Gemser 1924 • R. A. Bowman 1936 • F. Rosenthal 1939, esp. p. 34 • J. L.
   Palache 1939 • A. Dupont-Sommer 1943 • A. Dupont-Sommer 1944–45 • G. R.
   Driver 1948, esp. p. 121, pl. 60/1 • A. Dupont-Sommer 1949a, esp. p. 85 • E.
   Weidner 1952–53, esp. p. 14 • E. Y. Kutscher 1965, esp. p. 42 • M. Dietrich 1970,
   esp. pp. 32, 177 • S. Segert 1975, esp. pp. 320, 321 • A. R. Millard 1976, esp. pp.
   4–7, 9.

B.2.14   Loan Settlement (??, 617)   AECT.60
   Assyrian *egirtu ša šulmu* with Aramaic endorsement. Manchester
   Museum.

                                                        1 ספר שלם זי
                                                           חזאל

Ed. Pr.   A. R. Millard 1972.

EASY ACCESS
   Editions: Vat. 167.

LITERATURE
   W. von Soden and T. Fish 1952, esp. p. 19 (Akk.) • J. Teixidor 1973, esp. p. 428.

B.2.15   Copenhagen Conveyance (??, 622)   AECT.61
   Rectangular tablet. National Museum (No. 8612), Copenhagen. Finger-
   nail impression with illegible Aramaic!

Ed. Pr.   J. N. Postgate 1976, p. 116 no. 18.

B.2.16   Nimrud Jar Inscriptions (??)   NimJar

Fragmentary text in ink on two pottery fragments. British Museum.

Ed. Pr.   H. Rawlinson 1865.

EASY ACCESS
  Editions: *CIS* 44–45.

B.2.17   Bilingual Tablet (7th c.)   BilTab

Tablet with Babylonian text on obverse, fragmentary Aramaic on the
reverse and edges. British Museum.

Ed. Pr.   *CIS* II, pp. 40–41 (No. 34), pl. 2.

B.2.18   Brussels Tablets (7th c.)   BrusTab

Twenty-four unpublished loan documents; 23 entirely in Aramaic, 1 bilingual. Les Musées Royaux d'Art et d'Histoire, Brussels.

LITERATURE
  E. Lipiński 1974, esp. p. 2 • E. Lipiński 1975b • D. Homès-Fredericq 1978 • E.
Lipiński 1979 • E. Lipiński 1979b • F. M. Fales 1984 • E. Lipiński 1985 • F. M.
Fales 1986, pp. 269–73.

B.2.19   Babylonian Dockets in the British Museum   **BMDoc**

	Museum #	Editio princeps	*CIS/ESE*	*EA*	*ABC*	Vat.
1	BM 30267	H. C. Rawlinson 1884	62	43	29	44
2	BM 92723	*CIS*	63	90	30	94
3	BM 56353	*CIS*	61	41	31	42
4	BM 33091	P. Berger 1886	64	91	32	95
5	82-9-18 403	cf. S. A. Kaufman 1974, p. 69				
6	BM 74572	*ABC*		96	39	100
7	BM 55794	*CIS*	67	54	40	55
8	BM 132642	M. W. Stolper 1976				292
9	BM 43754	*ABC*		106	44	110
10	BM 49277	T. G. Pinches 1910		45	46	46
11	BM 49288	T. G. Pinches 1910		44		45
12	BM 49536	T. G. Pinches 1910		37		37
13	BM 50151	*ABC*	*ESE* 2:202(F)	82	43	86
14	BM 78922	T. G. Pinches 1910		36		36
15	BM 92734	*CIS*	68	40	33	41
16	BM 79708	T. G. Pinches 1910	*ESE* 2:201(C)	81	34	85
17	K 5424c	H. C. Rawlinson 1865, p. 222	26	103	41	107
18	BM 92722	*CIS*	65	101		105
19	BM 64065	*ABC*		92	35	96
20	BM 92733	*CIS*	71	97	36	101
21	BM 74333	*CIS*	70	98	38	102
22	BM 39404	*ABC*		102	45	106
23	BM 78707	*CT* 4, pl. 20	*ESE* 2:202	99		103

LITERATURE
     5) S. A. Kaufman 1974, p. 34.
     6) S. A. Kaufman 1974, p. 60.
     Texts of the above will be treated in a forthcoming volume by E. Cussini.

B.2.20 Late Babylonian Contracts from Babylon **BabDoc**

21 relatively lengthy Aramaic endorsements, mostly on date harvest taxation contracts, excavated in Babylon, 1913. Staatliche Museen, Berlin.

Ed. Pr. L. Jakob-Rost and H. Freydank 1972.

EASY ACCESS
 Editions: Vat. nos. 168–188.

J-R. & F.	Museum #	Date	Text
1	VAT 13377	415	שטר מֹקֹשׁר זי שׁערי זי סאת אלבני על נבובלסו אקב
2	VAT 13393	417	שטר כסף מנ'[ן] קדם בלאטר בר נבואֹתֹן [מן] יום 1 לטבת שנת 3+3+1
3	VAT 13402	410	כ .. מ נבוכצרש עֹל
4	VAT 13407	414	שטר .מ . נבו חן 12 ... ... לאמ......חנ ס שׁ 10+5 שת 6 לשׁנתא 10
5	VAT 13409	455	[כ]רן 20+10+5 שׁנת 10+.
6	VAT 13410	???	... א זי בֹּאבֹל ...] קד[ס תבשׁב. תמרן כרן 20+10+1
7	VAT 13411 + 13422	451	שׁטר דנתבל רמנֹאילי גנֹנֹיא . בר [...] תמרן כרן 10+4 [...] שׁנת 10+4 ..א..
8	VAT 13416	417	שׁ[טר ת]מרן כרן 10+3 זי קדם ...] זֹי ...
9	VAT 13419	???	[שׁ]טר כסֹ[פ]א זי אפלי קֹ.ם מתנגזך זי ...... זֹי לשׁנתא שׁערן כרן תמרן כרן
10	VAT 13420	???	שׁ.....
11	VAT 13421	406	[ ] זי שׁנת 10+3+3[+2]
12	VAT 13424	Darius II	[ ] 3+3+10+20+20+20 [ ] ומקֹצת [ ] זֹי. ....

J-R. & F.	Museum #	Date	Text
13	VAT 15755	418	שטר כסף מנ[ה ...] [...] 10 זי יום
14	VAT 15866	???	. שטר אגורן זי ... בלאצרש בר
15	VAT 15896	???	.. [ש]נֹת 10... [קד]ם רא
16	VAT 15993	404	. נבו]
17	VAT 16062	???	[ ] [ש]טר[ ] [ ] [נתמנ א]
18	VAT 16002	???	...... י..נ בֹר א
19	VAT 16114	Darius II	שטר נ[...] זי שנ[ת ...]
20	VAT 17983		תמרן כרן 20+20+10+3 ... זי שנֹת 3 ... א ... . ש...
21	VAT 13190	414	. פפא זי שנת 7??

LITERATURE
    14) S. A. Kaufman 1974, p. 33.

B.2.21   Bricks from Babylon (ca. 600)   BabBrick

    Clay bricks with stamped and inscribed texts.

Ed. Pr.   1) E. Ledrain 1884c.
               2) E. Ledrain 1884d
               3–7) *CIS* 54–58.
               8,9) R. Koldewey 1914, pp. 42–43, 79–81.

EASY ACCESS
    Editions: 1) *CIS* 59.
                 2) *CIS* 60.

LITERATURE
    8,9) G. R. Driver 1945, esp. p. 12.

B.2.22 Murashû Dockets (Nippur, 2nd half 5th c.) **MurDoc**

Endorsements lightly scratched in often difficult cursive script on contracts and receipts of the Murashû banking family. Mostly in the University Museum, Philadelphia, some in Istanbul. (See also BMDoc.8.) Numbering follows Clay 1908 for 1–50. This enumeration is repeated in Clay 1912, pls. 116–23, which adds items 51–54.

Ed. Pr. A: H. V. Hilprecht and A. T. Clay 1898.
B: A. T. Clay 1904.
C: A. T. Clay 1912.
D: M. W. Stolper 1985.

A. T. Clay 1908 republished the Aramaic of those texts already presented in **A** and **B** as well as the Aramaic alone of those whose cuneiform texts were to be published in full in **C** (except for numbers 51–54) and **D**. See the discussion in Stolper 1985, p. 13.

	Ed. pr.	*EA*	*ESE*	Vat.	Text
1	A 2	68	3:12A	71	שטר אחושן בר בלש... לאלל..
2	D 58	46	3:12B	47	אחתר זי תמרן כרן 1 100
3	D 16	85	3:13C	89	שטר [.]. על אחיל[ן 2+1[...]
4	A 64	58	3:13D	60	שטר שיטא
5	A 66a	84	3:13E	88	שטר סאת ארקא זי אריבי בר אנדבלתי ˆפריעˆ מן אללשואדן
6	A 108	74	3:13F	77	שטר נידבל בר לבני זי שערן כרן 10+3+3+1 X בˆ2+3 למרחסו[ן] בשנת 2+20+20
7	A 68	49		50	שטר אור[ן
8	A 71	83	3:14G	87	שטר סאת ארקא זי נבואתן עלים X פרען
9	D 99	94	3:14H	98	[סימא ש]טר ר.שכן.. זי כֹסֹת
10	A 87	55		57	שטר חנון
11	D 37	69	3:15K	72	שטר אחושן זי פריע [ס]את ארקא
12	D 112	48		49	שטר אורא[ד]ן
13	D 86	47		48	יהונתן [ש]ערן כרן 10
14	B 29	62	2:204A	64	שֹטֹרֹ אושתאדן אשתיֹמֹא
15	B 46	107	2:205D	111	סא]ת ארˈקא ..

	Ed. pr.	*EA*	*ESE*	Vat.	Text
16	B 52	105	2:205E 3:15P	109	ח ..זי קמש א] . בר תירן
17	B 56	93	2:205G	97	בשנת 1 שטר בתא
18	C 49	59		61	שטר תתן
19	B 59	56	2:205H	58	שטר לבש
20	B 60	76	2:206J 3:15N	79	שטר בלאדן אשתימ]ם משח כרן 3+3
21	D 4	86	3:15O	90	ש]טר ס את ארקא
22	C 149	104		108	שערן כרן 20+3+20+2 קדם שנ.. שנת 2 בדריהוש מלכא
23	B 68	72	2:206K	75	שטר רחימאל .. תמרן כרן ..
24	B 74	87	2:206L	91	שטר] ראש[.
25	C 73	52		53	...אֹנֹושת...
26	B 78	79	2:206M	82	שטר בנה זי כסף X הלכא זי פריע זי שנת 3 דריהוש
27	B 87	75	2:204B	78	שטר אנושת..לט בר .. שזב תמרן כרן 10+3+2
28	C 92	80		84	שטר בנה זֹ. כסף ש 20?+3+1 זי שנת פריע
29	B 99	77	2:206N	80	שטר ארקת | נגריא זי יהב הידורי בר חבצ.ר לריבת בר בלאריב בסאה
30	B 104	64	2:207O	66	שטר בלאטר בר גוזי
31	C 129	51		52	שטר אֹנֹושתאבלט
32	B 105	50	2:207P	51	... אורפחר
33	B 106	71	2:207Q	74	שטר זבדננא זי קנא
34	C 118	53		54	שטר בלאטר
35	B 115	73	2:208R	76	שטר בלאבצר בר בלא]ן יא.... ה]לכא זי שנת 3+3

	Ed. pr.	*EA*	*ESE*	Vat.	Text
36	B 116	38	2:208S	38	בלאטרשוש
37	B 120	42	2:208U	43	נבורפ.
38	B 121	57	2:208V	59	שטר מרדכא
39	B 125	95	2:208W	99	בלת ביבא שנת 3+3+1
40	B 126	70	2:209X	73	שטר בלאצרש סגן בנשיא כסף ש 10 זי ארק בנשיא ..
41	B 131	63	2:209Y	65	שטר אחושן בר בלאטר
42	B 132	66	2:209Z	68	שטר חנני ב]ר[טבי
43	B 55	35	2:205F	35	אדגשירזבד
44	C 154	60	3:16U	62	שטר בלאבצר וארדנרב]ל[
45	C 157	61		63	שטר .לרת. ושוש
46	C 170	39		40	בלשואדן
47	D 35	100		104	זי פריע זי] .... שנת 3+10+20
48	C 46	78		81	שטר בנה הלכא ..... ש]נת 2 ...
49	D 3	109		113	...]ת כצר בר בלנצר לאללחתן
50	C 145	65		67	שטר דחלתה בר חזהאל
51	C 69	79bis		83	שטר חנטן כר 1 קדם אדי
52	C 215	38bis		39	בלאטרשוש
53		54bis		56	שטר אדי.
54		66bis		69	שטר כר/דן רב ת.י

LITERATURE

General) S. Daiches 1910 ● A. T. Clay 1912a ● J. Augapfel 1917 ● C. S. Knopf 1933 ● G. Cardascia 1951, pp. 25, 175 ● R. Zadok 1986a, esp. pp. 287–88 ● J. Oelsner 1987.

5) A. T. Clay 1906–7.

14) A. T. Clay 1907.

20) A. R. Millard 1971.

26,35) G. Cardascia 1951, esp. pp. 110–12 ● S. A. Kaufman 1974, p. 58.

51) M. W. Stolper 1976.

B.2.23   Miscellaneous Babylonian Tablets and Dockets   MiscBab

#	collection	editio princeps	editions
1	Louvre BN 2689	*CIS* 69	*EA* 89 • Vat. 93
2	Louvre AO 10301	TC 13:208	Vat. 156
3	Louvre AO 6847	TC 12:58	Vat. 155
4	Louvre AO 7672	V. Scheil 1914	Vat. 131
5	J. Offord Collection	T. G. Pinches 1900, pp. 266–68	*ESE* 1:194 • *RES* 1830 • Vat. 130
6	????	F. M. T. de Liagre Böhl 1946	Vat. 159
7	Mus. Nat. Hist., Torquay, U.K.	G. R. Driver 1937	Vat. 142; cf. F. Rosenthal 1939, p. 298
8	Berlin ?????	F. E. Peiser 1890, p. 92 (no. 67), pl. 43	M. San Nicolò and A. Ungnad 1935, pp. 219–20
9	11 N 26	S. A. Kaufman 1975, p. 152	Vat. 269
10	11 N 28	S. A. Kaufman 1975, p. 152	Vat. 270
11	??	G. F. Grotefund 1839, p. 177	J. Oelsner 1976a, pp. 316–19

#	provenance	date	text
1	"Forti d'Urban"	416	*
2	Nippur	???	*
3	Uruk	561	*
4	Uruk	552	*
5		Darius II	*
6	Sippar	492	*
7	??	5th. c.	שטר נבוכצר בר כדס זי תמרן כרן 3[1+] לֹנֹלֹאתן בירח מרחשון שנת 1+3+3
8		???	שלב בר אדנא
9	Nippur	558/7	ל תתן
10	Nippur	Murashû tablet!	לשלואלל קֹל קֹיֹף[...]
11	??	407	שטר ...

* Text to be published by E. Cussini.

LITERATURE
    7) B. Meissner 1941.

B.2.24   Hilprecht Dockets (Nippur[3&4], 5th c.)   HilprDock

Four endorsements on Babylonian legal tablets. Jena, Hilprecht Collection.

זי רשׁי (1
שׁושׁבלט בר שׁושׁא[חדן] (2
שׁטר בלאחתן (3
שׁטר בי>ס<דה (4

Ed. Pr.   O. Krückmann 1933, nos. 19,90,99,146.

EASY ACCESS
    Editions: Vat. 133–36.

B.2.25   Larsa Ostracon (5th c.)   LarOstr

Grey sherd (13 x 10 cm.). Louvre (A0 16922, L. 297).

Ed. Pr.   A. Dupont-Sommer 1945–46.

EASY ACCESS
    Editions: *AC* 39.

B.2.26   Nippur Ostracon (5th c.)   NipOstr

Sherd with text on convex side (7.5 x 6.5 cm.). Univ. of Pennsylvania Museum.

Ed. Pr.   J. A. Montgomery 1908.

EASY ACCESS
    Editions: *AC* 38 • *ESE* 3: 63–64 • *RES* 957.

    Illustrations: *SW* pl. 62,2.

LITERATURE
    A. T. Clay 1907 • J. Halévy 1911, esp. pp. 340–42 • G. A. Barton 1926 • G. R. Driver 1948, pl. 62/2 • A. R. Millard 1976, esp. p. 5.

B.2.27   Tello Bricks (4th c.)   TelBr

Several bricks with the same bilingual impression. Louvre and Berlin Museum.

הדדנדנאח (Greek: ADADNADINAXHS).

Ed. Pr.   E. Ledrain 1885.

EASY ACCESS
   Editions: *CIS* 72 • *HNE* 446.

   Illustrations: *CIS* pl. 5 • *HNE* pl. 26/4.

B.2.28   Uruk Bricks (end 4th c.)   UrukBr
A single inscription written seriatim on 15 glazed bricks in the Seleucid temple at Uruk

אנאבלט [זי שמה א[חרן קפ]ל[ל]ון [א[נאבלט ז[י ש[מה א[ח[רן קפל[ו]ן

Ed. Pr.   A. von Haller 1935.

LITERATURE
   T. Nöldeke et al. 1936 • R. A. Bowman 1939 • W. Röllig 1960.

B.2.29   Uruk Cuneiform Incantation (3d c.)   UrukInc
Aramaic text in syllabic cuneiform on baked clay tablet (9 x 7 cm.). Louvre (AO 6489).

Ed. Pr.   F. Thureau-Dangin 1922, p. 58, pl. 105.

EASY ACCESS
   Editions: *AC* 56.

   Translations: *ANET*^{3} 658 • *TUAT* 2:432–34.

LITERATURE
   E. Ebeling 1925 • G. R. Driver 1926 • P. Jensen 1926 • P. O. Bostrup 1927 • E. Littmann 1929 • C. H. Gordon 1937–39 • B. Landsberger 1937–39 • F. Rosenthal 1939, esp. p. 35 • C. H. Gordon 1940 • Cyrus H. Gordon 1941 • A. Dupont-Sommer 1942–44 • J. N. Epstein 1960, esp. pp. 11–12 • G. Garbini 1971 • J. W. Wesselius 1982.

B.3 Egypt

B.3.a Early

B.3.a.1 Bel-shar-uṣur Statuette (??, ca. 660)   BelStat
Granite statue (40 cm. ht.). Cairo Museum (J. 31919).

בלסראצר

Ed. Pr.   *ESE* 3.117–18 (+ drawing).

EASY ACCESS
  Editions: *RES* 965.

B.3.a.2 RES 1791 (Saqqara, late 7th c.)   TADC3.1
Fragmentary account of wine. Cairo Museum (J. 36449).

Ed. Pr.   A. H. Sayce and A. Cowley 1929, no. 15.

EASY ACCESS
  Editions: *ESE* 3.128–29 ● *RES* 1791.

B.3.a.3 Göttingen Papyrus (late 7th c.)   TADC3.2
Fragmentary account. Göttingen University Library.

Ed. Pr.   R. Degen 1974.

B.3.a.4 Bauer-Meissner Land Lease (515)   TADB1.1
Padi b. Daganmelek leases his field to Aḥa b. Ḥapio. Bayerische
Staatsbibliothek (Pap. aram. mon. 1).

Ed. Pr.   H. Bauer and B. Meissner 1936 (+ 2 plates).

EASY ACCESS
  Editions: *AC* 19.

  Translations: *DAE* 1.

LITERATURE
  C. C. Torrey 1938 ● F. Rosenthal 1939, esp. pp. 36–37 ● H. L. Ginsberg 1939–40
  ● A. Dupont-Sommer 1944 ● E. Y. Kutscher 1954, esp. p. 247, n. 131 ● J. J. Rabinowitz 1956, esp. pp. 121, 142–52 ● G. Garbini 1957, esp. p. 423 ● R. Yaron
  1958a, esp. pp. 18–19 ● R. Yaron 1961, esp. pp. 1–2, 10, 13–15, 17, 25–29, 33,
  115, 127, 129–30, 135, 141–42, 159, 172 ● M. E. Sherman 1966 ● B. Porten and

J. C. Greenfield 1969, esp. p. 155 ● P. Grelot 1971a ● B. Couroyer 1973a, esp. p. 467 ● B. Porten 1985a, esp. p. 41 ● B. Porten 1990, esp. p. 18.

B.3.a.5 Adon Letter (end 7th c.) TADA1.1

Ed. Pr. A. Dupont-Sommer 1948b (+ photo).

EASY ACCESS
Editions: *AaG*Seg 41 ● *AC* 16 ● *KAI* 266 ● *TSSI* 21.

Translations: *DOTT* 251–55 ● *TUAT* 633–34.

LITERATURE
E. F. Weidner 1939, esp. p. 932 ● H. L. Ginsberg 1940 ● E. Zaki Saad 1945 ● H. L. Ginsberg 1948a ● A. Bea 1949 ● A. Pohl 1949 ● J. Bright 1949 ● A. Malamat 1949–50 ● A. Dupont-Sommer 1949a, esp. p. 89 ● R. Dussaud 1949a ● A. Malamat 1950, esp. pp. 222–23 ● D. Winton Thomas 1950, esp. pp. 8–13 ● A. Vaccari 1953 ● R. Meyer 1954 ● A. Malamat 1956, esp. p. 252 ● E. Vogt 1957, esp. pp. 85–89 ● J. D. Quinn 1961 ● K. Galling 1963 ● J. A. Fitzmyer 1965 ● M. E. Sherman 1966 ● F. Vattioni 1966a ● J. T. Milik 1967, esp. pp. 561–62 ● T. C. Mitchell 1967, esp. p. 416, 425 ● S. H. Horn 1968 ● J. Naveh 1971c, esp. p. 16, Fig. 3/1 ● J. Naveh 1971c, esp. p. 16, Fig. 3/1 ● S. Segert 1975, esp. pp. 436, 437, 445 ● W. H. Shea 1976 ● E. Lipiński 1977, esp. pp. 103–4 ● J. Teixidor 1977, esp. p. 271 ● W. Huss 1977 ● P. S. Alexander 1978, esp. p. 158, n. 2 ● C. R. Krahmalkov 1981 ● B. Porten 1981a ● J. Naveh 1982, Fig. 75, p. 82 ● P.-E. Dion 1982b, esp. pp. 530, 532, 540, 547–54 ● S. Paul 1986, esp. p. 203 ● E. J. Smit 1990.

B.3.a.6 Wâdi es-Saba´ Riggaleh Graffiti (6th–5th c.) WaSabRigGr
Six rock graffiti on the western bank of the Nile.

Ed. Pr. 1–2) W. M. F. Petrie 1888, pl. 16, nos. 519, 523.
3–6) A. H. Sayce 1895.

EASY ACCESS
Editions: 1) *CIS* 135.
2) *CIS* 136 ● *RES* 960.
3) *RES* 961.
4–6) *RES* 962.

Illustrations: 1–2) *CIS* pl. 11.

LITERATURE
S. de Ricci 1906, esp. p. 32.

B.3.b Hermopolis West

B.3.b.1 Hermopolis Letters (early 5th c.)   TADA2

A collection of eight family letters on papyrus, one very fragmentary (**Herm.8**). Univ. of Cairo.

Ed. Pr.   E. Bresciani and M. Kamil 1966.

EASY ACCESS
    Editions: 1–7) *TSSI* 27.

                   1) *TADA* 2.3.
                   2) *TADA* 2.2.
                   3) *TADA* 2.4.
                   4) *TADA* 2.1.
                   5) *TADA* 2.5.
                   6) *TADA* 2.6.
                   7) *TADA* 2.7.

    Illustrations: *TADA* 2.

    Translations: *DAE* 25–31 • *JEAS* VI.1–7.

LITERATURE
    General
    M. Kamil 1945–46 • S. Gabra 1945–46 • A. Bea 1946 • M. Kamil 1947 • S. Gabra 1947 • A. Bea 1948 • A. Pohl 1948 • M. Kamil 1949 • N. V. Pigulevskaja 1949 • M. Kamil 1952 • M. Dahood 1960 • E. Bresciani 1967 • P. Grelot 1967c • J. T. Milik 1967 • B. Porten and J. C. Greenfield 1968 • E. Hammershaimb 1968 • B. Porten 1968, esp. pp. 264–72 • B. Porten 1969 • J. Teixidor 1969, esp. pp. 330–31 • J. P. Hayes and J. Hoftijzer 1970 • R. du Mesnil du Buisson 1970 • E. Hammershaimb 1971 • E. Y. Kutscher 1971 • H. Donner 1971 • J. Naveh 1971a • J. Naveh 1971c, esp. pp. 16, 18 • J. C. Greenfield and B. Porten 1974 • M. Weippert 1975 • E. Lipiński 1977, esp. pp. 115–16 • P. S. Alexander 1978, esp. pp. 158–67 • P.-E. Dion 1979, esp. pp. 559–73 • J. C. Greenfield 1981a, esp. pp. 118–19 • P.-E. Dion 1982, esp. pp. 60–71 • P.-E. Dion 1982b, esp. pp. 556, 558, 560, 568 • P. Swiggers 1982a • J. Hoftijzer 1983.

    1) E. Lipiński 1975, esp. pp. 271–72 • E. Lipiński 1978a, esp. pp. 255–56 • P. Swiggers 1981 • P. Swiggers 1981a • P.-E. Dion 1982b, esp. pp. 558–60.

    2) P. Grelot 1967c, esp. p. 11 • J. Neuffer 1968 • D. R. Hillers 1979 • P. Swiggers 1981a • P.-E. Dion 1982b, esp. pp. 560–61, 565 • J. Hoftijzer 1989.

    3) J. C. Greenfield 1971b, esp. p. 266 • P. Swiggers 1982a • J. Naveh 1982, pl. 8B • P.-E. Dion 1982b, esp. pp. 560, 565.

4) E. Lipiński 1975, esp. pp. 271–72 ● E. Lipiński 1978a, esp. pp. 255–56 ● P. Swiggers 1981 ● P. Swiggers 1981a ● P.-E. Dion 1982b, esp. pp. 558–60.

5) P.-E. Dion 1982b, esp. p. 560.

6) B. Porten and J. C. Greenfield 1974 ● D. R. Hillers 1979 ● P.-E. Dion 1982b, esp. p. 557 ● J. W. Wesselius 1986 ● J. Hoftijzer 1989.

B.3.c Elephantine

B.3.c.1 Elephantine Texts: General Information

G. Steindorff 1894–72 • M.-J. Lagrange 1904, esp. p. 140 • A. H. Sayce 1904a •
H. Schäfer 1904 • M.-J. Lagrange 1905a, esp. p. 147–48 • W. Bacher 1906–7 •
C. J. M. de Vogüé 1906 • Anon. 1907 • S. A. Cook 1907 • G. A. Cooke 1907 • S.
Daiches 1907 • L. Desnoyers 1907 • J. Döller 1907 • G. Hoffmann 1907 • J.
Hontheim 1907 • C. H. W. Johns 1907 • I. Lévi 1907 • D. S. Margoliouth 1907 •
R. H. Mode 1907 • N. Peters 1907 • N. Peters 1907a • O. Rubensohn 1907 • E.
Schürer 1907 • E. Schürer 1907a • F. Schulthess 1907 • R. Smend 1907 • S.
Ronzevalle 1907 • L. Blau 1907–08 • N. Herz 1907–8 • N. Herz 1907–8(a) • E.
B. Knobel 1907–09 • I. Lévi 1907–8 • H. Bornstein 1908 • C. Bruston 1908 • F.
Buhl 1908 • S. A. Cook 1908 • L. Desnoyers 1908 • J. Döller 1908 • B. D. Eerd-
mans 1908 • J. Hontheim 1908 • D. Köberle 1908 • M.-J. Lagrange 1908 • J. M.
P. Smith 1908 • F. Stähelin 1908 • C. J. M. de Vogüé 1908 • O. C. Whitehouse
1908 • Ch. H. H. Wright 1908 • J. K. Fotheringham 1908–9 • O. C. Whitehouse
1908–9 • L. Belléli 1909 • L. Belléli 1909a • J.-B. Chabot 1909 • S. Daiches
1909 • F. Feldmann 1909 • J. K. Fotheringham 1909 • J. A. Kelso 1909 • E.
Sachau 1909 • A. H. Sayce 1909 • J. G. Smyly 1909 • C. Steuernagel 1909 • A.
van Hoonacker 1909 • A. van Hoonacker 1909a • T. Witzel 1909 • T. Witzel
1909a • W. Honroth, O. Rubensohn, and F. Zucker 1909–10 • A. Alt 1910 • E.
Revillout 1910 • D. Sidersky 1910 • F. Westberg 1910, esp. pp. 103–11 • J. K.
Fotheringham 1910–11 • M. Sprengling 1910–11 • W. F. Albright 1911 • R.
Dussaud 1911 • H. Grimme 1911 • H. Gunkel 1911 • J. Halévy 1911a • S. Jampel
1911 • M. Lidzbarski 1911 • E. Meyer 1911 • F. N. Nau 1911 • A. H. Sayce 1911
• A. H. Sayce 1911a • H. L. Strack 1911 • A. Ungnad 1911 • A. H. Sayce
1911–12 • L. Blau 1911–12 • M. L. Margolis 1911–12 • F. K. Ginzel 1911–14,
esp. pp. 2:45–53, 3:375–76 • H. Anneler 1912 • L. Blau 1912 • P. Boylan 1912 •
C. F. Burney 1912 • C. F. Burney 1912a • S. A. Cook 1912 • H. J. Elhorst 1912 •
H. Grimme 1912 • J. Halévy 1912 • J. Halévy 1912a, esp. p. 410 • A. Jirku 1912
• A. Jirku 1912a • J. Kohler 1912 • J. A. Knudtzon 1912 • P. Leander 1912 • I.
Lévi 1912 • A. S. Lewis 1912 • E. Mahler 1912 • D. S. Margoliouth 1912 • D. S.
Margoliouth 1912a • E. Meyer 1912 • E. Mittwoch 1912 • F. N. Nau 1912 • E.
Pritsch 1912 • F. Schwally 1912 • M. Seidel 1912 • C. van Gelderen 1912 • A.
Eberharter 1912–13 • L. Blau 1913 • J. K. Fotheringham 1913 • G. Jahn 1913 •
M. Löhr 1913 • J. W. Rothstein 1913 • W. Spiegelberg 1913 • U. Wilcken 1913,
esp. pp. 200–217 • G. B. Gray 1914 • G. Jahn 1914 • W. T. Pilter 1914 • A.
Lemonnyer 1914[–19] • S. A. Cook 1915 • E. König 1915 • I. Löw 1915 • E.
Meyer 1915 • J. Offord 1915 • A. van Hoonacker 1915 • R. Muuss 1916 • H.
Torczyner 1916, esp. pp. 288–89 • J. M. P. Smith 1916–17 • M. Sprengling 1917
• M. Sprengling 1918 • A. Strazzulli, P. Bovier-Lapierre and S. Ronzevalle
1918–19 • L. Blau 1919 • A. Lemonnyer 1920 • A. S. Hirschberg 1921 • J. A.
Montgomery 1923 • I. Scheftelowitz 1923 • J. Morgenstern 1924, esp. pp. 20–21
• R. Kittel 1925 • R. Kittel 1926 • D. Sidersky 1926 • W. Struve 1926 • L. M.
Epstein 1927 • F. X. Kortleitner 1927 • M. San Nicolò 1927 • W. Stein 1927–30
• J. Hempel 1927–31 • U. Türck 1928 • C. G. Wagenaar 1928 • J. Gutmann
1928–34 • G. Ricciotti 1929–39 • O. Eissfeldt 1930 • A. T. Olmstead 1931, esp.

pp. 585–610 *et passim* ● F. Dijkema 1931 ● H. Kees 1931 ● E. M. MacDonald 1931 ● L. Borchardt 1932 ● P. Joüon 1933 ● E. Benveniste 1934 ● L. Hennequin 1934 ● P. Joüon 1934 ● K. G. Kuhn 1935, esp. pp. 26–28 ● R. Müller 1935 ● J. Leibovitch 1935–36 ● C. C. Torrey 1939 ● C. C. Torrey 1940 ● P. Joüon 1941a ● R. A. Parker 1941a ● M. D. Cassuto 1942 ● J.-B. Chabot 1944 ● E. Neufeld 1944 ● P. Korngruen 1948 ● R. Dussaud 1949 ● C. B. Welles 1949 ● F. S. Pericoli Ridolfini 1949–54 ● R. Dussaud 1950 ● E. Y. Kutscher 1950 ● E. G. Kraeling 1952 ● A. Sachs 1952 ● L. Rost 1952–53 ● W. F. Albright 1953, esp. pp. 168–75 ● A. Dupont-Sommer 1953, esp. p. 292, n. 27 ● J. J. Rabinowitz 1953 ● E. Vogt 1953 ● D. Colombo 1953–58 ● E. Benveniste 1954 ● H. Cazelles 1954 ● B. Couroyer 1954 ● B. Couroyer 1954a ● Z. W. Falk 1954 ● S. H. Horn and L. H. Wood 1954 ● E. Y. Kutscher 1954 ● J. de Menasce 1954 ● J. T. Milik 1954 ● C. C. Torrey 1954 ● E. Vogt 1954 ● W. Eilers 1954–56 ● H. Cazelles 1955 ● C. H. Gordon 1955 ● E. Hammershaimb 1955 ● R. A. Parker 1955 ● J. J. Rabinowitz 1955a ● S. Segert 1956 ● S. Segert 1956a ● E. Volterra 1956 ● R. Borger 1957 ● J. A. Fitzmyer 1957 ● E. Hammershaimb 1957 ● E. G. Kraeling 1957 ● E. Pritsch 1957 ● J. J. Rabinowitz 1957b ● F. Rundgren 1957 ● A. Vincent 1957 ● R. Yaron 1957a ● W. Eilers 1957–58 ● Z. Ben-Ḥayyim and S. E. Loewenstamm 1958 ● E. Bresciani 1958b ● C. G. Tuland 1958 ● R. Yaron 1958 ● R. Yaron 1958b ● H. L. Ginsberg 1959, esp. pp. 148–49 ● S. Greengus 1959 ● J. J. Rabinowitz 1959 ● R. Yaron 1959 ● R. Stiehl 1959–62 ● H. Bardtke 1960 ● J. J. Rabinowitz 1960 ● H. Ricke 1960 ● R. Yaron 1960a ● B. Porten 1961 ● J. J. Rabinowitz 1961 ● R. Yaron 1961 ● R. Yaron 1961a ● E. Hammershaimb 1962 ● J. Körner 1962 ● B. Porten 1963 ● E. Volterra 1963 ● P. Grelot 1964 ● A. Verger 1964 ● A. Verger 1964a ● E. Volterra 1964a ● R. Yaron 1964 ● A. Verger 1965 ● B. A. Ayad 1967 ● E. Seidl 1967, esp. pp. 531–32 ● R. Yaron 1967 ● B. Couroyer 1968 ● E. C. B. MacLaurin 1968 ● B. Porten 1968 ● E. Seidl 1968, esp. pp. 86–88 ● D. Sperling 1968 ● Y. Muffs 1969 ● B. Porten and J. C. Greenfield 1969 ● B. Porten 1969 ● R. A. Bowman 1970a ● A. Charbel 1970 ● B. Couroyer 1970b ● P. Grelot 1970a ● E. Stern 1970 ● J. Teixidor 1970 ● K. R. Veenhof 1970 ● R. Yaron 1970 ● H. Bardtke 1971 ● P. Grelot 1971 ● P. Grelot 1971a ● W. T. In der Smitten 1971 ● G. Nahon 1971 ● B. Porten 1971 ● J. B. Segal 1971 ● S. Segert 1971 ● R. Yaron 1971 ● Z. Shunnar 1971, 1973 ● B. A. Ayad 1972 ● P. Grelot 1972 ● B. Couroyer 1973 ● B. Couroyer 1973a ● S. A. Kaufman 1973 ● M. H. Silverman 1973 ● S. A. Kaufman 1974, esp. p. 66 ● G. Nahon 1974 ● B. A. Ayad 1975 ● E. Bresciani 1975 ● B. A. Levine 1975 ● S. Segert 1975a ● H. Shirun 1975–86 ● L. Habachi 1975–86 ● A. Ammassari 1976 ● J. C. Greenfield 1976 ● S. Segert 1976 ● J. Teixidor 1976a ● W. Witakowski 1976 ● J. C. Greenfield 1977 ● P. Zivie 1978 ● W. Witakowski 1978–79 ● B. Porten 1979 ● A. N. Temerev 1979 ● P. Grossmann 1980 ● H. Jaritz 1980 ● W. Müller 1980 ● B. Porten 1980 ● A. N. Temerev 1980 ● I. Gottlieb 1981 ● J. C. Greenfield 1981a, esp. pp. 119–26 ● E. Lipiński 1981 ● E. Lipiński 1981a ● M. H. Silverman 1981a ● S. P. Vleeming 1981 ● B. Porten 1983d ● A. Skaist 1983 ● A. N. Temerev 1983 ● J. C. Greenfield 1984–86, esp. p. 153 ● J. C. Greenfield 1984a ● A. M. Mann 1985 ● P. Grelot 1986 ● B. Porten 1986 ● F. M. Fales 1987a ● D. R. Hillers 1990 ● B. Porten 1990.

Elephantine: Literary Texts

B.3.c.2   Bisitūn Inscription (510?)   TADC2.1

Two papyrus sheets and 36 papyrus fragments of the Aramaic version of Darius I's Bisitun Inscription. Staatliche Museen, Berlin (P. 13447a-d, P. 13442).

Ed. Pr.   *APO*, pp. 185–210 (+ pls. 52, 54–57).

EASY ACCESS
   Editions: *AaG*Seg 33 • *AC* 32 • *AP* pp. 248–71.

   Illustrations: J. C. Greenfield and B. Porten 1982.

LITERATURE
   F. H. Weissbach 1911 • J. Halévy 1912b • J. Halévy 1912c • L. H. Gray 1913, esp. pp. 281–84 • G. R. Driver 1932, esp. pp. 89–90 • A. Poebel 1938 • A. T. Olmstead 1938 • F. W. König 1938 • E. Meyer 1953, esp. pp. 98–101 • J. Lewy 1954 • G. G. Cameron 1960 • O. Klíma 1967 • S. A. Kaufman 1974, esp. p. 58 • W. Hinz 1974 • S. Segert 1975, esp. p. 437 • E. N. von Voigtlander 1978 • N. Sims-Williams 1981 • J. C. Greenfield and B. Porten 1982 • R. Borger 1982 • R. N. Frye 1982 • J. C. Greenfield 1984–86, esp. pp. 152–53 • J. W. Wesselius 1984c • E. Lipiński 1986 • W. Vogelsang 1986 • W. Hinz 1988 • M. O. Wise 1990, esp. p. 252.

B.3.c.3   Aḥiqar (end 5th c.)   TADC1.1

Eleven fragmentary papyrus sheets containing 14 columns of text. Staatliche Museen, Berlin. NB: The order of the columns has been rearranged in the *TADC* publication on the basis of the undertext of the palimpsest, TADC3.9.

Ed. Pr.   *APO*, pp. 147–82 (+ pls. 40–50).

EASY ACCESS
   Editions: *AaG*Seg 34 • *AC* 31 • *AH* I/1, II.C.1 • *AP* pp. 204–48 • *APE* 50–63 • *ESE* 3.253–55.

   Translations: *ATAT* 454–62 • *ANET*[3] 427–30 • *DAE* 106–108 • *DOTT* 270–75.

LITERATURE
   F. C. Conybeare, J. R. Harris, and A. S. Lewis 1898 • R. Smend 1908 • F. N. Nau 1909 • F. Perles 1911–12, esp. pp. 14:500–503, 15:54–57 • M. L. Margolis 1911–12, esp. pp. 440–41 • H. Grimme 1911a • J. Barth 1912, esp. p. 11 • J. N. Epstein 1912, esp. pp. 132–37 • J. Halévy 1912, esp. pp. 37–78 • D. S. Margoliouth 1912, esp. p. 70 • J. A. Montgomery 1912 • F. N. Nau 1912a • A. Schollmeyer 1912a • H. Torczyner 1912, esp. pp. 402–3 • A. J. Wensinck 1912 •

J. A. Montgomery 1912–13 • J. N. Epstein 1913, esp. pp. 225–33 • J. N. Epstein 1913a, esp. pp. 310–11 • J. Halévy 1913 • J. R. Harris, A. S. Lewis, and F. C. Conybeare 1913 • T. Nöldeke 1913 • T. Nöldeke 1913a • D. H. Baneth 1914 • F. Stummer 1914 • F. Stummer 1914a • F. N. Nau 1914–15 • S. A. Cook 1915, esp. pp. 367–68 • I. Löw 1915 • F. Stummer 1915 • J. N. Epstein 1916 • B. Meissner 1917 • F. Bork 1918 • F. N. Nau 1918–19 • F. N. Nau 1920 • G. Dossin 1932 • G. R. Driver 1932, esp. pp. 87–89 • W. von Soden 1936, esp. pp. 9–13 • A. Yellin 1937 • A. H. Krappe 1941 • C. I. K. Story 1945 • G. Haddad 1953 • E. G. Kraeling 1953, esp. pp. 97–99 • W. F. Albright 1957, esp. p. 331 • R. Tournay 1957 • A. E. Goodman 1958 • P. Grelot 1961 • P. Grelot 1962 • E. G. Kraeling 1962 • H. J. Lenzen 1962 • F. Altheim and R. Stiehl 1963, esp. pp. 182–95 • M. Dietrich 1963–65 • P. Termes 1963–65 • D. R. Dumm 1967 • F. Altheim and R. Stiehl 1968, esp. pp. 3–9 • M. Held 1968, (on 48, 49, 71, 72) • L. Rost 1969 • A.-M. Denis 1969–70 • A.-M. Denis 1970 • W. McKane 1970 • J. C. Greenfield 1971, (156) • M. E. Stone 1971 • J. Gutmann 1971–72 • S. A. Kaufman 1974, esp. p. 96 • H. G. Andersen 1975 • S. Segert 1975, esp. pp. 319, 432, 434, 436, 437, 440, 445 • G. P. Bahnam 1976, esp. pp. 69–93 • A. R. Millard 1976, esp. pp. 9, 13 • K. T. Zauzich 1976 • S. Abramson 1976–77, esp. pp. 191–92 • J. H. Charlesworth 1981, esp. pp. 75–77, 273 • J. C. Greenfield 1981 • F. Pennacchietti 1981 • H. P. Rüger 1981 • R. Zadok 1981 • E. Martínez Borobio 1982 • J. M. Lindenberger 1982 • J. M. Lindenberger 1983 • Y. Avishur 1984, esp. pp. 470–72 • D. Metzler 1984 • W. G. E. Watson 1984 • J. M. Lindenberger 1985 • A. Lemaire 1985a • S. A. Kaufman 1986a • E. Puech 1988 • J. C. Greenfield 1990 • F. Israel 1990 • I. Kottsieper 1990.

Elephantine: Letters

B.3.c.4   The Yedaniah Archive   **TADA4**

Ten documents from the communal archive of Yedaniah b. Gemariah.

The "Passover" Letter (419)   **TADA4.1**

Ḥananiah enjoins the observance of the Festival of Unleavened Bread on the Jews of Elephantine. Staatliche Museen, Berlin (P. 13464).

Ed. Pr.   *APO*, pap. 6, pp. 38–40, pl. 6.

EASY ACCESS
    Editions: *AaG*Seg 28 • *AP* 21 • *APE* 6.

    Translations: *ANET³* 491 • *ATAT* 453 • *DAE* 96 • *DOTT* 258–60 • *JEAS* III.1 • *TUAT* 253.

LITERATURE
    C. Steuernagel 1911 • F. Perles 1911–12, esp. p. 14:498 • M. L. Margolis 1911–12, esp. pp. 436–38 • J. Halévy 1911a, esp. pp. 488–94 • A. H. Sayce 1912 • A. Schollmeyer 1912 • C. Steuernagel 1912 • I. Lévi 1912, esp. pp. 164–71 • J. Barth 1912, esp. p. 10 • S. Daiches 1912 • W. R. Arnold 1912 • H. J. Elhorst 1912a • J. Halévy 1912e • S. A. Cook 1915, esp. pp. 356–58 • G. R. Driver 1932, esp. p. 79 • L. Borchardt 1932, esp. p. 301 • L. Hennequin 1934, esp. pp. 997–98 • H. G. May 1936, esp. pp. 74, 80–81 • A. Vincent 1937, esp. pp. 265–66 • C. C. Torrey 1940, esp. pp. 120–22 • R. Dussaud 1945, esp. pp. 174–76 • A. Dupont-Sommer 1946–47(b) • P. Grelot 1954 • P. Grelot 1955 • S. Talmon 1958, esp. pp. 71–73 • P. Grelot 1967a • P. Grelot 1967b • P. Grelot 1967c • B. Porten 1968, esp. pp. 279–82, 311–14 • J. Naveh 1971c, esp. pp. 25, 33 • E. Lipiński 1975, esp. pp. 270–71 • P. S. Alexander 1978, esp. pp. 158, 167 • B. Porten 1978–79 • E. Lipiński 1978a, esp. pp. 254–55 • B. Porten 1979, esp. pp. 90–92, pl. pp. 88–89 • P.-E. Dion 1979, esp. p. 556 • M. H. Silverman 1981a, esp. pp. 289–90 • P.-E. Dion 1982b, esp. pp. 529–33, 539–40 • B. Porten 1986, esp. pp. 7 + photo, drawing • B. Porten 1990, esp. pp. 19–20.

Request for Assistance (late 5th c.)   **TADA4.2**

The writer reports a conflict with the Egyptians to Yedaniah and appeals for assistance. Cairo Museum (J. 43471).

Ed. Pr.   *APO*, pap. 10, pp. 51–54, pl. 11.

EASY ACCESS
    Editions: *AP* 37 • *APE* 10.

Translations: *DAE* 97 • *JEAS* III.2.

LITERATURE
> E. Meyer 1911, esp. p. 1042 • H. Torczyner 1912, esp. p. 400 • J. N. Epstein 1912, esp. p. 129 • J. N. Epstein 1913, esp. pp. 143–44 • S. A. Cook 1915, esp. p. 360 • G. R. Driver 1932, esp. pp. 79–80 • J. Naveh 1971c, esp. p. 33 • S. Segert 1975, esp. p. 434 • P. S. Alexander 1978, esp. pp. 162, 164, 166 • P.-E. Dion 1979, esp. p. 566 • B. Porten 1980, esp. p. 43 • P.-E. Dion 1982, esp. p. 60 • B. Porten 1982, esp. pp. 15–17 + 1 pl. • P.-E. Dion 1982b, esp. pp. 529–33, 539–40, 549, 554–60, 569 • B. Porten 1990, esp. p. 17.

A Recommendation (late 5th c.)   TADA4.3

> Mauziah asks that Yedaniah and the community welcome Ṣeḥa and Ḥor. Cairo Museum (J. 43472).

Ed. Pr.   *APO*, pap. 11, pp. 55–57, pl. 12.

EASY ACCESS
> Editions: *AP* 38 • *APE* 11.

> Translations: *DAE* 98 • *JEAS* III.3.

LITERATURE
> H. Torczyner 1912, esp. pp. 400–1 • J. Barth 1912, esp. p. 11 • J. N. Epstein 1913, esp. p. 144 • S. A. Cook 1915, esp. pp. 360–61 • G. R. Driver 1932, esp. pp. 81–82 • J. C. Greenfield 1967, esp. p. 91 • B. Porten 1968, esp. p. 41 • R. Yaron 1968, esp. pp. 204–5 • J. Naveh 1971c, esp. p. 33 • P. S. Alexander 1978, esp. pp. 158, 162–67 • P.-E. Dion 1979, esp. p. 569 • B. Porten 1980, esp. p. 47, pl. p. 103 • P.-E. Dion 1982b, esp. pp. 529–33, 539–40, 550, 557, 565–70 • B. Porten 1982, esp. pp. 11–15 • M. O. Wise 1990, esp. p. 252.

Report of Imprisonment (late 5th c.)   TADA4.4

> Islaḥ reports the imprisonment of Jewish leaders. Staatliche Museen, Berlin (P. 13456), Cairo Museum (J. 43476).

Ed. Pr.   *APO*, pap. 43, p. 138 + pap. 15, pp. 63–65, pl. 37; pl. 15.

EASY ACCESS
> Editions: *AP* 56 + 34 • *APE* 44 + 16.

> Translations: *DAE* 100 • *JEAS* III.4.

LITERATURE
> H. Torczyner 1912, esp. p. 401 • J. N. Epstein 1912, esp. p. 130 • J. N. Epstein 1913, esp. pp. 144–45, 225 • S. A. Cook 1915, esp. pp. 364–65 • B. Porten 1968, esp. pp. 288–89 • J. Naveh 1971c, esp. pp. 24, 33, 35 • P.-E. Dion 1979, esp. p.

566 • B. Porten 1980, esp. p. 48 • P.-E. Dion 1982, esp. p. 60 • B. Porten 1982, esp. pp. 17–20 • P.-E. Dion 1982b, esp. pp. 529–32, 541, 554–65.

Draft Petition (410?)   TADA4.5

> The Jewish community petitions for the reconstruction of the temple. Bibliothèque Nationale et Universitaire, Strasbourg (Aram. 2).

Ed. Pr.   J. Euting 1903, pp. 297–311 + photo.

EASY ACCESS
>   Editions: *AP* 27 • *APA* 78 • *APE* 2a • *APO* pp. 26–27 • *ESE* 2. 210–17 • *RES* 361, 498.

>   Illustrations: *APO* pl. 75.

>   Translations: *DAE* 101 • *JEAS* III.5.

LITERATURE
> C. Clermont-Ganneau 1903 • W. Spiegelberg 1904 • P. Kokovtsov 1904–5 • J. Halévy 1904a • J. Halévy 1906 • F. Schwally 1904 • S. de Ricci 1906, esp. p. 29 • E. Meyer 1911, esp. p. 1041 • S. A. Cook 1915, esp. p. 362 • J. Hoftijzer 1959, esp. pp. 316–17 • P. Naster 1968 • B. Porten 1968, esp. pp. 284–85 • M. N. Bogolyubov 1969 • J. Naveh 1971c, esp. p. 35 • B. Porten 1978, esp. pp. 171–3 • P.-E. Dion 1979, esp. p. 569 • P.-E. Dion 1982b, esp. pp. 547, 550–52, 563, 567.

Fragmentary Letter Concerning Imprisonment (5th c.)   TADA4.6

> Staatliche Museen, Berlin (P. 13445).

Ed. Pr.   *APO* 72 72, pp. 216–20, 226, pl. 59, 61/12.

EASY ACCESS
>   Editions: *AP* 68/12 + 66 • *APE* 72.

LITERATURE
> H. Torczyner 1912, esp. p. 403 • J. N. Epstein 1913, esp. p. 234 • B. Porten 1980, esp. p. 50.

The Bagohi Temple Petition (first draft) (408)   TADA4.7

> The Jewish community petitions the governor Bagohi for permission to rebuild the temple of YHW. Staatliche Museen, Berlin (P. 13495).

Ed. Pr.   E. Sachau 1907 + 1 pl.

EASY ACCESS
     Editions: *AaG*Seg 23 ● *AH* I/1, II.A.1 ● *AP* 30 ● *AC* 28 ● *APE* 1 ● *APO* 1.

     Illustrations: *APO* pl. 1.2 ● *DOTT* pl. 16.

     Translations: *ANET*^{3} 491–92 ● *ATAT* 450–52 ● *DAE* 102 ● *DOTT* 260–65 ● *JEAS* III.6 ● *TUAT* 254–256.

LITERATURE
     D. H. Müller 1907 ● J. Barth 1907, esp. pp. 324–28 ● M. Lidzbarski 1907 ● R. Smend 1907, esp. pp. 708–11 ● I. Lévi 1907–8, esp. pp. 54:153–58 ● J. Barth 1908 ● J. Halévy 1908 ● S. A. Cook 1908, esp. pp. 87–89 ● T. Nöldeke 1908, esp. pp. 197–201 ● S. Fraenkel 1908 ● M.-J. Lagrange 1908a ● K. Marti 1909 ● F. Perles 1911–12, esp. pp. 14:497–98 ● M. L. Margolis 1911–12, esp. pp. 425–30 ● J. Halévy 1911a, esp. p. 480 ● H. Torczyner 1912, esp. pp. 397–99 ● J. N. Epstein 1912, esp. pp. 128 f. ● G. Rauschen 1913, esp. pp. 41–51 ● J. N. Epstein 1913, esp. p. 138 ● S. A. Cook 1915, esp. pp. 361–62 ● J. Gutmann 1928–34, esp. pp. 447–48 ● G. Ricciotti 1929–39, 1 pl. ● H. Birkeland 1934 ● L. Hennequin 1934, esp. 2 pls. ● M. Vogelstein 1942 ● Z. Ben-Ḥayyim and S. E. Loewenstamm 1958, esp. pp. 3:431–34 ● J. Hoftijzer 1959, esp. pp. 317–18 ● D. Diringer and R. Regensburger 1968, pl. 2.187a ● J. P. Asmussen 1968 ● P. Naster 1968, esp. p. 69 ● B. Porten 1968, esp. pp. 110–14, 290–91 ● A. Charbel 1970 ● P. Grelot 1970c, esp. pp. 33–35 ● J. Naveh 1971c, esp. p. 32 ● J. C. Greenfield 1975, esp. p. 312 ● S. Segert 1975, esp. pp. 319, 433, 438, 445 ● B. Porten 1978, esp. pp. 165–71 ● P. S. Alexander 1978, esp. pp. 158–60, 162, 164, 166–67 ● W. Witakowski 1978–79 ● B. Porten 1980 ● J. Naveh 1982, Fig. 78, p. 85 ● P.-E. Dion 1982, esp. p. 60 ● P.-E. Dion 1982b, esp. pp. 529–33, 539–40, 547–54 ● B. Porten 1990, esp. p. 20.

The Bagohi Temple Petition (second draft) (408)   **TADA4.8**
     Second draft of TADA4.7. Cairo Museum (J. 43465).

Ed. Pr.   E. Sachau 1907.

EASY ACCESS
     Editions: *AaG*Seg 23 ● *AH* I/1, II.A.1 ● *AP* 31 ● *APE* 2 ● *APO* 2.

     Translations: *DAE* 102 ● *JEAS* III.7.

     Illustrations: *APO* pl. 3.

LITERATURE
     M. Lidzbarski 1907 ● I. Lévi 1907–8, esp. pp. 54:158–60 ● S. Fraenkel 1908, esp. pp. 158–60 ● M.-J. Lagrange 1908a, esp. pp. 158–60 ● J. Halévy 1911a, esp. pp. 480–81 ● J. N. Epstein 1912, esp. p. 128 ● J. N. Epstein 1913, esp. pp. 138–39 ● S. A. Cook 1915, esp. pp. 361–62 ● H. Holma 1918 ● J. Naveh 1971c, esp. p. 32 ●

S. Segert 1975, esp. p. 438 • B. Porten 1978, esp. pp. 165–71 • B. Porten 1980, esp. p. 44 • P.-E. Dion 1982b, esp. pp. 529–33, 539–40, 547–54 • B. Porten 1986, esp. pp. 2–3 + drawing.

Memorandum of Bagohi's Response (408?)   **TADA4.9**

Bagohi gives permission for the temple to be rebuilt. Staatliche Museen, Berlin (P. 13497).

Ed. Pr.   E. Sachau 1907.

EASY ACCESS
Editions: *AaG*Seg 24 • *AC* 29 • *AH* I/1, II.A.1a • *AP* 32 • *APE* 3 • *APO* 3.

Translations: *ANET*^{3} 492 • *ATAT* 452 • *DAE* 103 • *DOTT* 265–66 • *JEAS* III.8.

Illustrations: *APO* pl. 4.

LITERATURE
J. Barth 1907, esp. pp. 328–33 • M. Lidzbarski 1907 • I. Lévi 1907–8, esp. pp. 54:160–61 • S. Fraenkel 1908, esp. pp. 160–61 • M.-J. Lagrange 1908a, esp. pp. 160–61 • J. Halévy 1911a, esp. pp. 481–82 • J. N. Epstein 1913, esp. p. 139 • S. A. Cook 1915, esp. pp. 362–63 • J. H. Bondi 1918 • L. Hennequin 1934, esp. p. 978 • P. Grelot 1967d • B. Porten 1968, esp. p. 291 • J. Naveh 1971c, esp. p. 32 • B. Porten 1978, esp. pp. 173–5 • B. Porten 1979, esp. pp. 96–100, pl. p. 98 • P.-E. Dion 1982b, esp. p. 552 • B. Porten 1986, esp. pp. 4–5 + photo, drawing.

Offer of Payment (408?)   **TADA4.10**

The Jewish leaders offer payment for permission to rebuild the temple. Cairo Museum (J. 43467).

Ed. Pr.   *APO*, pap. 5, pp. 31–33, pl. 4.

EASY ACCESS
Editions: *AP* 33 • *APE* 4.

Translations: *ANET*^{3} 492 • *ATAT* 452–53 • *DAE* 104 • *DOTT* 266–69 • *JEAS* III.9 • *TUAT* 256–57.

LITERATURE
H. Torczyner 1912, esp. p. 399 • I. Lévi 1912, esp. pp. 171–75 • J. N. Epstein 1913, esp. pp. 139–40 • S. A. Cook 1915, esp. pp. 363–64 • P. Grelot 1967d • B. Porten 1968, esp. pp. 292–93 • P. Grelot 1970c, esp. pp. 35–36 • J. Naveh 1971c, esp. p. 32 • B. Porten 1978, esp. pp. 175–7 • B. Porten 1979, esp. pp. 100–101, pl. p. 100 • P.-E. Dion 1982b, esp. pp. 549, 552, 569 • B. Porten 1986, esp. p. 6 + photo.

B.3.c.5   Padua Letters (5th c.)   Pad

Ed. Pr.   E. Bresciani 1960.

Padua Papyrus Letter I   TADA3.3

Letter from Oshea to Shelomam. Padua Museum, Aramaic Papyrus 1.

EASY ACCESS
Editions: *TSSI* 2.28.

Translations: *DAE* 14.

LITERATURE
E. Bresciani 1960a • F. Díaz Esteban 1962 • J. A. Fitzmyer 1962, esp. pp. 16–22
• J. Naveh 1964–65, esp. pp. 186–89 • J. Naveh 1966, esp. pp. 25–29 • K. R.
Veenhof 1968, esp. pp. 135–36 • J. Naveh 1971c, esp. p. 36 • P. S. Alexander
1978, esp. pp. 162–67 • P.-E. Dion 1979, esp. pp. 563–73 • B. Porten 1980, esp.
p. 43–44 • P.-E. Dion 1982, esp. pp. 62–63, 69 • P.-E. Dion 1982b, esp. pp. 538,
554, 556 • B. Porten 1990, esp. pp. 16–17.

Padua Papyrus Letter II   TADA3.4

Letter from Shallum to his mother Yehoyishma. Padua Museum, Aramaic Papyrus 2.

LITERATURE
J. A. Fitzmyer 1962, esp. pp. 22–23 • J. Naveh 1964–65, esp. pp. 189–90 • J.
Naveh 1966, esp. pp. 29–30 • J. Naveh 1971c, esp. p. 36 • P.-E. Dion 1979, esp.
pp. 565–73 • B. Porten 1980, esp. p. 44, pl. p. 103 • P.-E. Dion 1982, esp. p. 62.

Padua Papyrus Letter III   Pad.3

Fragmentary. Padua Museum, Aramaic Papyrus 3.

LITERATURE
J. A. Fitzmyer 1962, esp. p. 24 • J. Naveh 1964–65, esp. pp. 190–91 • J. Naveh
1966, esp. p. 30 • B. Porten 1985.

B.3.c.6   Elephantine: Miscellaneous Letters

Petition for Rectification of Injustice (after 434)   TADA5.2
>   Nattun (?) petitions an official. Cairo Museum (J. 43468).

Ed. Pr.   *APO*, pap. 7, pp 41–43, pl. 7.

EASY ACCESS
>   Editions: *AP* 16 ● *APE* 7.

>   Translations: *DAE* 18.

LITERATURE
>   J. Halévy 1911a, esp. pp. 494–97 ● J. N. Epstein 1913, esp. p. 140 ● S. A. Cook
>   1915, esp. p. 360 ● J. Naveh 1971c, esp. p. 33 ● P.-E. Dion 1979, esp. pp. 577–79
>   ● B. Porten 1980, esp. pp. 46–47 ● B. Porten and H. Z. Szubin 1985, esp. p. 285.

Fragmentary Letter from an Officer (end 5th c.)   TADA5.5
>   A letter reporting disorder among the troops. Académie des Inscriptions
>   2–4.

Ed. Pr.   *RES* 247 + 248.

EASY ACCESS
>   Editions: *AP* 80 ● *APE* 90 ● *ESE* 2. 219–20 ● *RAO* 6: 248–70 ● *RES* 1797 +
>   1798.

LITERATURE
>   C. J. M. de Vogüé 1902a ● S. de Ricci 1906, esp. p. 30 ● G. R. Driver 1932, esp. p.
>   83 ● B. Porten and H. Z. Szubin 1985, esp. pp. 287–88 ● B. Porten 1986a.

Letter concerning 10 Asses (5th c.)   TADA3.1
>   Shezibnabu reports on 10 asses. Cairo Museum (J. 43493).

Ed. Pr.   *APO*, pap. 39, pp. 133–34, pl. 36.

EASY ACCESS
>   Editions: *AP* 54 ● *APE* 40.

LITERATURE
>   J. N. Epstein 1913, esp. p. 225 ● J. N. Epstein 1913a, esp. p. 311 ● J. Naveh 1971c,
>   esp. p. 35 ● P.-E. Dion 1982b, esp. pp. 529, 541, 560, 565.

Fragmentary Letter (5th c.)　　　　　　　　　　　　　　　　TADA3.2

> Cairo Museum (J. 43494).

Ed. Pr.　　　　　*APO*, pap. 40, p. 135, pl. 36.

EASY ACCESS
> Editions:　　　*AP* 55 ● *APE* 41.

Mauziah to Maḥseiah (late 5th c.)　　　　　　　　　　　TADA3.5

> Mauziah sends to his "brother," Maḥseiah, asking for news. Cairo Museum (J. 43474).

Ed. Pr.　　　　　*APO*, pap. 13, pp. 60–61, pl. 14.

EASY ACCESS
> Editions:　　　*AP* 41 ● *APE* 14.

LITERATURE
> J. N. Epstein 1912, esp. p. 130 ● J. Naveh 1971c, esp. p. 33 ● P. S. Alexander 1978, esp. pp. 163–66 ● P.-E. Dion 1979, esp. p. 566 ● B. Porten 1980, esp. p. 45 ● P.-E. Dion 1982, esp. pp. 65, 70 ● P.-E. Dion 1982b, esp. pp. 530, 533, 539–40, 554–60.

Hoshaiah to Pilti (425–400)　　　　　　　　　　　　　　TADA3.6

> A letter expressing sympathy. Cairo Museum (J. 43475).

Ed. Pr.　　　　　*APO*, pap. 14, pp. 59–60, pl. 13.

EASY ACCESS
> Editions:　　　*AP* 40 ● *APE* 13.

> Translations:　*DAE* 16.

LITERATURE
> J. N. Epstein 1913, esp. p. 144 ● G. R. Driver 1932, esp. p. 82 ● J. Naveh 1971c, esp. p. 33 ● S. Segert 1975, esp. p. 437 ● P. S. Alexander 1978, esp. pp. 158, 161, 166–67 ● P.-E. Dion 1979, esp. p. 566 ● B. Porten 1980, esp. p. 45 ● P.-E. Dion 1982b, esp. pp. 529–33, 539–40, 554–60.

Hoshea to Shalwah (425–400)　　　　　　　　　　　　　TADA3.7

> A fragmentary letter with a reference to gold. Cairo Museum (J. 43473).

Ed. Pr.   *APO*, pap. 12, pp. 58–59, pl. 13.

EASY ACCESS
    Editions: *AP* 39 ● *APE* 12.

    Translations: *ATAT* 454 ● *DAE* 15.

LITERATURE
    J. N. Epstein 1912, esp. p. 130 ● G. R. Driver 1932, esp. p. 82 ● J. Naveh 1971c,
    esp. p. 33 ● P. S. Alexander 1978, esp. pp. 162, 165 ● P.-E. Dion 1979, esp. p. 566
    ● B. Porten 1980, esp. p. 47 ● P.-E. Dion 1982, esp. p. 60 ● P.-E. Dion 1982b, esp.
    pp. 529–35, 539–40, 554–60.

Hoshea to Haggus (425–400)   **TADA3.8**
        Instructions on various commercial transactions. Cairo Museum (J.
        43477).

Ed. Pr.   *APO*, pap. 16, pp. 66–68, pl. 16.

EASY ACCESS
    Editions: *AP* 42 ● *APE* 17.

    Translations: *DAE* 17.

LITERATURE
    H. Torczyner 1912, esp. pp. 401–2 ● J. N. Epstein 1912, esp. p. 130 ● J. N. Epstein
    1913, esp. p. 145 ● J. Naveh 1971c, esp. p. 33 ● S. Segert 1975, esp. p. 432 ● P. S.
    Alexander 1978, esp. pp. 162, 164, 166–67 ● B. Porten 1980, esp. p. 45 ● P.-E.
    Dion 1982b, esp. pp. 537–40, 554, 558, 560–65 ● B. Porten 1990, esp. p. 17.

Letter Fragments (end 5th c.)   **AP.57**

Ed. Pr.   *APO*, pap. 45, p. 140, pl. 38.

EASY ACCESS
    Editions: *AP* 57 ● *APE* 46.

LITERATURE
    G. R. Driver 1932, esp. p. 83 ● B. Porten 1980, esp. p. 50.

Shewa to Islaḥ (399)   **TADA3.9**
        A fragmentary letter mentioning the change of ruler in Egypt. Brooklyn
        Museum (47.218.151).

Ed. Pr.   *BMAP* 13, pp. 283–90, pl. XIII.

EASY ACCESS

     Translations: *DAE* 105.

LITERATURE
     H. Cazelles 1955, esp. pp. 86–87 • J. Naveh 1971c, esp. p. 36 • P. S. Alexander
     1978, esp. pp. 158, 162, 166–67 • P.-E. Dion 1979, esp. p. 566 • B. Porten 1980,
     esp. p. 44 • P.-E. Dion 1982, esp. p. 60 • P.-E. Dion 1982b, esp. pp. 530, 533, 539,
     541, 554–61 • B. Porten 1990, esp. p. 17.

Spentadata to Ḥori and Petemachis (375–50)   **TADA3.10**
     A letter mentioning a boat and some commercial transactions. Ägyp-
     tisches Museum, Berlin (23000).

Ed. Pr.   Z. Shunnar 1970 (+ 2 plates).

EASY ACCESS
     Editions: *NESE* 1. 9–22.

     Illustrations: *NESE* 1, pl. 1.

     Translations: *DAE* 109.

LITERATURE
     J. Naveh and S. Shaked 1971 • R. Degen 1972b • R. Macuch 1973 • D. Golomb
     1975 • P. S. Alexander 1978, esp. pp. 158, 162, 167 • B. Porten 1980, esp. pp.
     48–49 • P.-E. Dion 1982, esp. p. 60 • P.-E. Dion 1982b, esp. pp. 529–31, 540,
     560–65 • B. Porten and A. Yardeni 1988.

Letter Fragments (end 5th c.)   **AP.58**

Ed. Pr.   *APO*, pap. 42, pp. 137–38, pl. 37.

EASY ACCESS
     Editions: *AP* 58 • *APE* 43.

Elephantine: Legal Texts

B.3.c.7   The Mibtaḥiah Archive   TADB2

Eleven documents from the family archive of Mibtaḥiah, daughter of Maḥseiah.

LITERATURE
B. Porten 1968, pp. 235–62.

Grant of a Built Wall (471)   TADB2.1

Konaiah b. Ṣadaq waives right to a wall he built on Maḥseiah's property. Bodleian (MS Heb. b. 19 [P]).

Ed. Pr.   *APA* A, pp. 35–36, 62 + 2 plates.

EASY ACCESS
Editions: *AP* 5 ● *ESE* 3.129.

Translations: *DAE* 32 ● *JEAS* I.1.

LITERATURE
M.-J. Lagrange 1907, esp. pp. 259–60 + 1 pl. ● S. Gutesmann 1907, esp. p. 195 ● J. K. Fotheringham 1908–9, esp. p. 14 ● M. H. Pognon 1911, esp. pp. 345 f. ● S. A. Cook 1915, esp. p. 352 ● D. Sidersky 1926, esp. pp. 68 f. ● G. R. Driver 1932, esp. p. 77 ● L. Borchardt 1932, esp. p. 300 ● S. H. Horn and L. H. Wood 1954, esp. pp. 6–8 ● R. A. Parker 1955, esp. p. 271 ● R. Yaron 1961, esp. pp. 109, 117–33 ● A. F. Rainey 1965 ● A. Verger 1965, esp. pp. 83, 91, 103, 110, 137, 153 ● R. Yaron 1968 ● J. Naveh 1971c, esp. pp. 25, 31 ● S. A. Kaufman 1974, esp. p. 57 ● B. Porten 1979, esp. p. 79, pl. p. 100 ● B. Porten 1981, esp. p. 169 ● B. Porten and H. Z. Szubin 1982, esp. p. 124 ● H. Z. Szubin and B. Porten 1982, esp. pp. 3–4 ● B. Porten and H. Z. Szubin 1982a, esp. p. 652 ● B. Porten 1983, esp. pp. 527–28, 531–32, 535–37 ● B. Porten 1983c, esp. p. 564 ● B. Porten 1984, esp. pp. 380–81, 385, 394–96 ● B. Porten 1985a, esp. pp. 41–42, 48–49 ● B. Porten and H. Z. Szubin 1987, esp. pp. 232, 237 ● B. Porten and H. Z. Szubin 1987a, esp. pp. 49–50 ● B. Porten 1987a, esp. p. 90 ● B. Porten and H. Z. Szubin 1987b, esp. pp. 185–87 ● B. Porten 1990, esp. p. 20.

Withdrawal from Land (464)   TADB2.2

Dargamana the Khwarezmian renounces a claim to Maḥseiah's land. Cairo Museum (J. 37107).

Ed. Pr.   *APA* B, pp. 36–37, 63 + 2 plates.

EASY ACCESS
      Editions: *AP* 6 • *AH* I/1, II.B.1 • *ESE* 3.129.

      Translations: *DAE* 33 • *JEAS* I.2.

LITERATURE
      M.-J. Lagrange 1907, esp. p. 259 • J. K. Fotheringham 1908–9, esp. p. 14 • M. H.
      Pognon 1911, esp. pp. 344 f. • S. A. Cook 1915, esp. pp. 351–52 • D. Sidersky
      1926, esp. p. 68 • L. Borchardt 1932, esp. p. 300, 2 pls. • S. H. Horn and L. H.
      Wood 1954, esp. pp. 8–9, pl. 1 • R. A. Parker 1955, esp. pp. 272, 274 • J. J. Rabi-
      nowitz 1957, esp. pp. 271–74 • J. Friedrich 1957c • R. Yaron 1961, esp. pp. 44ff.,
      101–23 • A. F. Rainey 1965, esp. pp. 344 f. • A. Verger 1965, esp. pp. 40, 85,
      137, 153, 181, 188, 191f. • B. Porten 1968, esp. p. 152 • Y. Muffs 1969, esp. pp.
      32, 83, 188, 192 • P. Grelot 1971a, esp. pp. 110–12 • J. Naveh 1971c, esp. p. 32 •
      J. Naveh 1971c, esp. pp. 25, 31 • B. Porten 1979, esp. pp. 79, 81 • B. Porten 1981,
      esp. p. 169 • B. Porten and H. Z. Szubin 1982, esp. p. 124 • H. Z. Szubin and B.
      Porten 1982, esp. pp. 3–4 • B. Porten and H. Z. Szubin 1982a, esp. p. 652 • H. Z.
      Szubin and B. Porten 1983, esp. pp. 281–83 • B. Porten 1983c, esp. pp. 565–66 •
      A. Skaist 1983 • B. Porten 1984, esp. pp. 380–82, 385, 394, 396 • B. Porten
      1985a, esp. pp. 41–42, 49 • B. Porten and H. Z. Szubin 1987, esp. p. 237 • B. Por-
      ten and H. Szubin 1987a, esp. pp. 45, 48–50, 56, 65–66 • B. Porten 1987a, esp.
      pp. 89–91 • B. Porten and H. Z. Szubin 1987b, esp. p. 187 • B. Porten 1990, esp.
      p. 21.

Deed of Donation (459)   **TADB2.3**
      Maḥseiah bequeaths house and land to Mibtaḥiah. Cairo Museum (J.
      37114).

Ed. Pr.   *APA* D, pp. 39–40, 65 + 4 plates.

EASY ACCESS
      Editions: *AH* I/1, II.B.2 • *AP* 8.

      Translations: *DAE* 34 • *JEAS* I.3.

LITERATURE
      M.-J. Lagrange 1907, esp. pp. 260–61 • J. K. Fotheringham 1908–9, esp. p. 15 •
      M. H. Pognon 1911, esp. pp. 356–58 • J. K. Fotheringham 1913, esp. p. 571 • S.
      A. Cook 1915, esp. p. 353 • D. Sidersky 1926, esp. p. 69 • L. Borchardt 1932, esp.
      p. 300 • S. H. Horn and L. H. Wood 1954, esp. pp. 9–10 • J. J. Rabinowitz 1955 •
      R. A. Parker 1955, esp. p. 272, pl. 2 • J. Hoftijzer 1959, esp. pp. 312–14 • J. J.
      Rabinowitz 1961, esp. pp. 65, 74 • R. Yaron 1961, esp. pp. 36f., 40ff., 80ff., 95ff.,
      100–34 • A. F. Rainey 1965, esp. pp. 356–58 • A. Verger 1965, esp. pp. 40, 85,
      94, 100, 153, 183ff. • Y. Muffs 1969, esp. pp. 23, 34, 41, 182ff. • J. Naveh
      1971c, esp. pp. 25, 31 • J. C. Greenfield 1977b, esp. p. 91 • B. Porten 1979, esp.

pp. 76–81, 96, pl. p. 77 • B. Porten 1981, esp. pp. 169–74 • B. Porten and H. Z. Szubin 1982, esp. pp. 123–24 • H. Z. Szubin and B. Porten 1982 • H. Z. Szubin and B. Porten 1982, esp. pp. 3–5 • B. Porten 1983, esp. pp. 528–29, 531, 533–35, 537, 541 • H. Z. Szubin and B. Porten 1983a, esp. pp. 35–36, 38–43, 45 • B. Porten 1983c, esp. pp. 565–66 • B. Porten 1984, esp. pp. 380–81, 385, 394–96, 398, 400 • B. Porten 1985a, esp. pp. 41–42, 49 • B. Porten and H. Z. Szubin 1987, esp. pp. 233–37 • B. Porten and H. Z. Szubin 1987a, esp. pp. 55–56 • B. Porten 1987a, esp. pp. 89, 91 • B. Porten 1990, esp. p. 23.

Grant of Usufruct to Son-in-law (460)   **TADB2.4**

Maḥseiah grants usufruct of house and land to Yezaniah b. Uriah, Mibtaḥiah's husband. Cairo Museum (J. 37106).

Ed. Pr.   *APA* C, pp. 38, 64 + 2 plates.

EASY ACCESS
   Editions: *AP* 9.

   Translations: *DAE* 35 • *JEAS* I.4.

LITERATURE
   M.-J. Lagrange 1907, esp. p. 261 • S. Gutesmann 1907, esp. p. 196 • T. Nöldeke 1907, esp. p. 146 • J. K. Fotheringham 1908–9, esp. pp. 14–15 • S. A. Cook 1915, esp. p. 353 • G. R. Driver 1932, esp. p. 77 • S. H. Horn and L. H. Wood 1954, esp. p. 10 • J. Hoftijzer 1959, esp. pp. 312–14 • R. Yaron 1961, esp. pp. 36f., 80ff., 100–34 • A. Verger 1965, esp. pp. 40, 93, 100, 111, 118, 137, 153 • Y. Muffs 1969, esp. pp. 133ff. • J. Naveh 1971c, esp. pp. 25, 31 • J. C. Greenfield 1977b, esp. p. 91 • B. Porten 1979, esp. p. 94, pl. p. 78 • B. Porten 1981, esp. p. 169 • B. Porten and H. Z. Szubin 1982, esp. pp. 123–24 • B. Porten 1983, esp. pp. 527–28, 530, 533–36, 541 • H. Z. Szubin and B. Porten 1983a, esp. pp. 35–36, 39–41, 43 • B. Porten 1983c, esp. p. 565 • B. Porten 1984, esp. pp. 380, 394–95, 398, 400 • B. Porten 1985a, esp. pp. 41–42, 49 • B. Porten and H. Z. Szubin 1987, esp. pp. 234–35 • B. Porten 1987a, esp. pp. 89, 91.

Marriage Contract (?) (mid 5th c.)   **TADB2.5**

Fragment of a betrothal contract. Cairo Museum (J. 43492).

Ed. Pr.   *APO*, pap. 38, p. 132, pl. 35.

EASY ACCESS
   Editions: *AP* 48 • *APE* 39.

LITERATURE
> R. Yaron 1961, esp. pp. 2–3 • B. Porten 1971, esp. pp. 256–57 • H. Z. Szubin and B. Porten 1982, esp. pp. 3–4.

Marriage Contract (449?)   **TADB2.6**
> Marriage document for Eshor b. Ṣeḥa and Mibtaḥiah. Cairo Museum (J. 37110).

Ed. Pr.   *APA* G, pp. 43–44, 68 + 4 plates.

EASY ACCESS
> Editions: *AP* 15.

> Translations: *TUAT* 260–63 • *DAE* 38 • *JEAS* I.7.

LITERATURE
> I. Löw 1907 • L. Freund 1907 • S. Gutesmann 1907, esp. p. 196 • S. Jampel 1907 • T. Nöldeke 1907, esp. pp. 147–48 • J. Barth 1907a • F. Buhl 1908, esp. pp. 22–23 • J. K. Fotheringham 1908–9, esp. pp. 15–16 • N. Herz 1908–9, esp. p. 233 • S. Funk 1909 • M. H. Pognon 1911, esp. pp. 346–48 • E. J. Pilcher 1912, esp. pp. 31–33 • J. K. Fotheringham 1913, esp. p. 571 • S. A. Cook 1915, esp. p. 355 • S. Funk 1924 • G. R. Driver 1932, esp. p. 78 • E. A. Speiser 1934 • E. A. Speiser 1934a • S. H. Horn and L. H. Wood 1954, esp. p. 13 • J. J. Rabinowitz 1957a, esp. pp. 398–99 • R. Yaron 1958b • J. J. Rabinowitz 1959a • R. Yaron 1960, esp. pp. 66–69 • R. Yaron 1961, esp. pp. 22, 32–35, 53–99, 144, 160ff. • A. Verger 1965, esp. pp. 66, 94, 105–30, 176 • Y. Muffs 1969, esp. pp. 51–59, 86, 181 • B. Porten 1971, esp. pp. 244–55 • J. A. Fitzmyer 1971 • J. Naveh 1971c, esp. pp. 23, 32 • S. Segert 1975, esp. pp. 319 • B. Porten 1979, esp. pl. p. 80 • I. Gottlieb 1980, (15–16) • B. Porten 1983, esp. pp. 527–28, 532, 534–36, 542 • B. Porten 1983c, esp. pp. 565, 568 • B. Porten 1984, esp. pp. 381, 384, 394–96, 400 • B. Porten 1985a, esp. pp. 41–43, 49 • J. C. Greenfield 1985a, (6) • B. Porten and H. Z. Szubin 1987a, esp. p. 52 • B. Porten 1987a, esp. pp. 89, 91 • B. Porten 1990, esp. pp. 21–22.

Grant of a House (446)   **TADB2.7**
> Maḥseiah bequeaths another house to Mibtaḥiah. Cairo Museum (J. 37108).

Ed. Pr.   *APA* E, pp. 40–41, 66 +2 pl.

EASY ACCESS
> Editions: *AP* 13.

> Translations: *DAE* 36 • *JEAS* I.5.

LITERATURE
M.-J. Lagrange 1907, esp. pp. 261–63 • S. Gutesmann 1907, esp. p. 196 • T. Nöldeke 1907, esp. p. 147 • J. K. Fotheringham 1908–9, esp. p. 15 • M. H. Pognon 1911, esp. pp. 353–55 • J. K. Fotheringham 1913, esp. p. 571 • J. N. Epstein 1913, esp. p. 235 • S. A. Cook 1915, esp. p. 354 • D. Sidersky 1926, esp. p. 70 • G. R. Driver 1932, esp. pp. 77–78 • L. Borchardt 1932, esp. pp. 300–301 • S. H. Horn and L. H. Wood 1954, esp. pp. 11–12 • R. Yaron 1961, esp. pp. 2, 32–38, 102–27 • E. Volterra 1964 • A. Verger 1965, esp. pp. 84, 99f., 136f., 153 • Y. Muffs 1969, esp. pp. 31, 41, 48 • J. Naveh 1971c, esp. pp. 23, 31 • B. Porten 1979, esp. p. 79 • B. Porten 1981, esp. pp. 169–70, 172–75 • B. Porten and H. Z. Szubin 1982, esp. pp. 124–26 • B. Porten 1983, esp. pp. 528–29, 531–33, 535, 538 • H. Z. Szubin and B. Porten 1983, esp. p. 284 • B. Porten 1983c, esp. p. 565 • B. Porten 1984, esp. pp. 380, 384–86, 394–95, 400 • B. Porten 1985a, esp. pp. 41–42, 49 • B. Porten and H. Z. Szubin 1987, esp. pp. 233, 235–36 • B. Porten and H. Z. Szubin 1987a, esp. p. 56 • B. Porten 1987a, esp. pp. 89, 91 • B. Porten and H. Z. Szubin 1987b, esp. pp. 184–88 • B. Porten 1990, esp. p. 23.

Withdrawal from Goods (440)   **TADB2.8**
Pia b. Paḥi renounces claims to goods held by Mibtaḥiah. Cairo Museum (J. 37112).

Ed. Pr.   *APA* F, p. 42, 67 +1 pl.

EASY ACCESS
Editions: *AP* 14.

Translations: *ANET*^{3} 491 • *DAE* 37 • *JEAS* I.6.

LITERATURE
M.-J. Lagrange 1907, esp. pp. 263–65 • T. Nöldeke 1907, esp. p. 147 • J. K. Fotheringham 1908–9, esp. p. 15 • M. H. Pognon 1911, esp. pp. 339–43 • J. N. Epstein 1913, esp. p. 235 • L. Fischer 1913 • S. A. Cook 1915, esp. pp. 354–55 • D. Sidersky 1926, esp. p. 70 • L. Borchardt 1932, esp. p. 301 • S. H. Horn and L. H. Wood 1954, esp. p. 12 • J. J. Rabinowitz 1961, esp. p. 64 • R. Yaron 1961, esp. pp. 44–47, 55, 62, 80f., 107–26 • A. Verger 1965, esp. pp. 40, 85, 136f., 152, 179, 188, 191 • B. Porten 1968, esp. p. 153 • Y. Muffs 1969, esp. pp. 31f., 44–48, 61, 83 • J. Naveh 1971c, esp. p. 32 • B. Porten 1979, esp. p. 79 • B. Porten and H. Z. Szubin 1982a, esp. p. 652 • B. Porten 1983, esp. pp. 528, 531–32, 534–36 • B. Porten 1983c, esp. p. 565 • B. Porten 1984, esp. pp. 381, 393–96, 400 • B. Porten 1985a, esp. pp. 41–42, 51 • B. Porten and H. Z. Szubin 1987, esp. p. 237 • B. Porten and H. Z. Szubin 1987a, esp. pp. 45, 49, 51, 65–66 • B. Porten 1987a, esp. pp. 89, 91 • B. Porten 1990, esp. p. 21.

Withdrawal from Goods (420)   **TADB2.9**

Menaḥem and Ananiah renounce a claim against Yedaniah and Maḥseiah, sons of Mibtaḥiah. Cairo Museum (J. 37111).

Ed. Pr.   *APA* H, pp. 45–46, 69 +2 pl.

EASY ACCESS
    Editions: *AP* 20.

    Translations: *DAE* 39 • *JEAS* I.8.

LITERATURE
    M.-J. Lagrange 1907, esp. p. 265 • S. Gutesmann 1907, esp. p. 196 • T. Nöldeke 1907, esp. pp. 148–49 • J. K. Fotheringham 1908–9, esp. p. 16 • E. Pritsch 1911 • M. H. Pognon 1911, esp. pp. 348 f. • S. A. Cook 1915, esp. pp. 355–56 • D. Sidersky 1926, esp. pp. 70–71 • G. R. Driver 1932, esp. pp. 78–79 • L. Borchardt 1932, esp. p. 301 • S. H. Horn and L. H. Wood 1954, esp. p. 16 • J. J. Rabinowitz 1958a, esp. pp. 78, 80–82 • R. Yaron 1961, esp. pp. 40–47, 82ff., 107–26, 139 • A. Verger 1965, esp. pp. 40, 68f., 91f., 176, 181 • P. Naster 1968 • Y. Muffs 1969, esp. pp. 30f., 46ff., 71, 83, 119, 122f., 157 • P. Grelot 1970c, esp. pp. 36–38 • J. Naveh 1971c, esp. pp. 23, 32 • B. Porten 1981, esp. p. 169 • H. Z. Szubin and B. Porten 1982, esp. p. 9 • B. Porten and H. Z. Szubin 1982a, esp. p. 652 • B. Porten 1983, esp. pp. 528–29, 531–32, 534–37 • B. Porten 1983c, esp. pp. 565, 569–70 • B. Porten 1984, esp. pp. 380–81, 394–97 • B. Porten 1985a, esp. pp. 41–42, 49–51 • B. Porten and H. Z. Szubin 1987, esp. pp. 234, 237 • B. Porten and H. Z. Szubin 1987a, esp. pp. 45–50, 58–59, 65, 67 • B. Porten 1987a, esp. pp. 89–91 • B. Porten and H. Z. Szubin 1987b, esp. p. 183 • B. Porten 1990, esp. p. 20.

Renunciation of Claim (416)   **TADB2.10**

Yedaniah b. Hoshaiah renounces a claim against a house owned by Yedaniah and Maḥseiah. Cairo Museum (J. 37113).

Ed. Pr.   *APA* J, pp. 46–47, 70 +2 pl.

EASY ACCESS
    Editions: *AaG*Seg 31 • *AP* 25.

    Translations: *DAE* 40 • *JEAS* I.9.

LITERATURE
    M.-J. Lagrange 1907, esp. p. 266 • J. K. Fotheringham 1908–9, esp. p. 16 • M. H. Pognon 1911, esp. pp. 349f. • S. A. Cook 1915, esp. pp. 358–59 • D. Sidersky 1926, esp. p. 71 • L. Borchardt 1932, esp. p. 301 • S. H. Horn and L. H. Wood 1954, esp. p. 17 • J. Hoftijzer 1959, esp. p. 316 • R. Yaron 1961, esp. pp. 40–47, 53, 82–84, 95, 102–23, 139 • A. Verger 1965, esp. pp. 68, 85, 137, 153, 176, 187 • Y. Muffs 1969, esp. pp. 41f., 48, 133, 154 • P. Grelot 1970c, esp. pp. 38–39 • J. Naveh 1971c, esp. pp. 23, 32 • S. Segert 1975, esp. pp. 320, 435 • B. Porten 1979,

esp. p. 79 ● B. Porten 1981, esp. pp. 169–72 ● B. Porten and H. Z. Szubin 1982a, esp. pp. 652, 654 ● B. Porten 1983, esp. pp. 528, 531–32, 535 ● H. Z. Szubin and B. Porten 1983, esp. pp. 281, 284 ● B. Porten 1983c, esp. pp. 565, 569–70 ● B. Porten 1984, esp. pp. 380–81, 385, 394–97, 400 ● B. Porten 1985a, esp. pp. 41–42, 49–50 ● B. Porten and H. Z. Szubin 1987, esp. pp. 232, 235–37 ● B. Porten and H. Z. Szubin 1987a, esp. pp. 59–60 ● B. Porten 1987a, esp. pp. 89–91 ● B. Porten and H. Z. Szubin 1987b, esp. pp. 183, 185–87, 189 ● B. Porten 1990, esp. p. 21.

Assignment of Slaves (410)   TADB2.11

Yedaniah and Maḥseiah divide slaves inherited from Mibtaḥiah. Cairo Museum (J. 37109).

Ed. Pr.   *APA* K, pp. 47–48, 71 +2 pl.

EASY ACCESS
Editions: *AaG* Seg 32 ● *AC* 27 ● *AP* 28.

Translations: *DAE* 41 ● *JEAS* I.10 ● *TUAT* 258–60.

LITERATURE
S. Gutesmann 1907, esp. p. 195 ● T. Nöldeke 1907, esp. p. 149 ● J. K. Fotheringham 1908–9, esp. p. 16 ● M. H. Pognon 1911, esp. pp. 350 f. ● S. A. Cook 1915, esp. pp. 359–61 ● A. Guillaume 1920–21 ● D. Sidersky 1926, esp. p. 72 ● I. Mendelsohn 1949, esp. p. 47 ● S. H. Horn and L. H. Wood 1954, esp. p. 17 ● E. Volterra 1957, esp. pp. 685–86 ● J. J. Rabinowitz 1961, esp. p. 73 ● R. Yaron 1961, esp. pp. 49, 82–84, 101–26 ● A. Verger 1965, esp. pp. 141–58, 176 ● Y. Muffs 1969, esp. pp. 41, 188f. ● J. Naveh 1971c, esp. p. 32 ● S. Segert 1975, esp. pp. 320, 431, 436 ● B. Porten 1981, esp. pp. 169–70, 172, 175 ● H. Z. Szubin and B. Porten 1982, esp. p. 9 ● B. Porten and H. Z. Szubin 1982a, esp. pp. 652–53 ● B. Porten 1983, esp. pp. 528, 531–32, 534–35 ● B. Porten 1983c, esp. pp. 565, 567 ● B. Porten 1984, esp. pp. 394–96, 400 ● B. Porten 1985a, esp. pp. 41–42 ● B. Porten and H. Z. Szubin 1987, esp. pp. 235–37 ● B. Porten and H. Z. Szubin 1987a, esp. p. 61 ● B. Porten 1987a, esp. p. 90 ● B. Porten and H. Z. Szubin 1987b, esp. pp. 185–87 ● B. Porten 1990, esp. p. 21.

B.3.c.8 The Anani Archive (456–402) TADB3

Thirteen documents dealing with two related families.

Loan of Silver (456) TADB3.1

Yehoḥen d. Meshullak borrows from Meshullam b. Zakkur. Berlin, Staatliche Museen (P. 13491).

Ed. Pr. *APO*, pap. 28, pp. 108–12, pls. 28, 29.

EASY ACCESS
Editions: *AaG*Seg 25 • *AC* 23 • *AH* I/1, II.B.3 • *AP* 10 • *APE* 30.

Translations: *DAE* 4 • *JEAS* IV.4.

LITERATURE
H. Torczyner 1912, esp. p. 402 • J. N. Epstein 1913, esp. p. 150 • S. A. Cook 1915, esp. pp. 353–54 • D. Sidersky 1926, esp. pp. 72 f. • L. Borchardt 1932, esp. p. 300 • E. Neufeld 1953–54, esp. pp. 201–2 • S. H. Horn and L. H. Wood 1954, esp. pp. 12–13 • R. A. Parker 1955, esp. pp. 272, 274 • J. Hoftijzer 1959, esp. p. 315 • R. Yaron 1961, esp. pp. 13, 17f., 26, 28, 40, 42, 48–55, 75, 102, 106, 121, 135ff. • A. Verger 1965, esp. pp. 15, 63, 137ff., 148f., 184f. • B. Porten and J. C. Greenfield 1969, esp. pp. 153–54 • Y. Muffs 1969, esp. p. 189 • J. Naveh 1971c, esp. pp. 23, 34 • S. Segert 1975, esp. pp. 320, 431, 438 • B. Porten and H. Z. Szubin 1982a, esp. p. 652 • B. Porten 1983, esp. pp. 528, 531–32, 535–36 • B. Porten 1983c, esp. p. 569 • B. Porten 1984, esp. pp. 383–85, 394–96, 398 • B. Porten 1985a, esp. pp. 41–42, 46, 50–51 • B. Porten 1987a, esp. pp. 89, 91 • B. Porten 1990, esp. p. 25.

Withdrawal from *hyr'* (451) TADB3.2

Mika b. Aḥio acknowledges 5 shekel payment for a *hyr'* from Anani. Brooklyn Museum (47.218.152 + 47.218.155 Frag.4).

Ed. Pr. *BMAP* 1 + 18/4, pp. 131–38, pl. I.

EASY ACCESS

Translations: *DAE* 42 • *JEAS* II.1.

LITERATURE
E. Y. Kutscher 1954, esp. p. 234 • H. L. Ginsberg 1954, esp. p. 156 • S. H. Horn and L. H. Wood 1954, esp. p. 11, pl. 1 • H. Cazelles 1955, esp. pp. 77–78 • R. A. Parker 1955, esp. p. 272 • R. Yaron 1958c, esp. pp. 299–305 • R. Yaron 1961, esp. pp. 10f., 17ff., 26–30, 40, 104–30, 166ff. • A. Verger 1965, esp. pp. 153, 185 • Y. Muffs 1969, esp. p. 33 • J. Naveh 1971c, esp. pp. 24f., 30, 36 • B. Porten 1979, esp. pp. 78–79 • I. Ben-David 1980–81 (1:10) • B. Porten and H. Z. Szubin

1982, esp. p. 123 • B. Porten and H. Z. Szubin 1982a, esp. pp. 652–53 • B. Porten 1983, esp. pp. 527–28 • H. Z. Szubin and B. Porten 1983 • B. Porten 1983c, esp. p. 567 • B. Porten 1984, esp. pp. 394–96 • B. Porten 1985a, esp. pp. 41, 49 • B. Porten and H. Z. Szubin 1987, esp. pp. 232, 237 • B. Porten and H. Z. Szubin 1987a, esp. pp. 50–51 • B. Porten 1987a, esp. p. 89 • B. Porten 1990, esp. p. 21.

Marriage Contract (449)   TADB3.3

Marriage of Ananiah and Tamut. Brooklyn Museum (47.218.89).

Ed. Pr.   *BMAP* 2, pp. 140–50, pl. II, XIX.

EASY ACCESS
Editions: *AaG*Seg 26 • *AC* 24 • *AH* I/1, II.B.4.

Translations: *DAE* 43 • *JEAS* II.2.

LITERATURE
E. Y. Kutscher 1954, esp. p. 234 • H. L. Ginsberg 1954, esp. pp. 156–57 • S. H. Horn and L. H. Wood 1954, esp. p. 11 • H. Cazelles 1955, esp. pp. 78–79 • E. Volterra 1957, esp. pp. 686–70 • R. Yaron 1961, esp. pp. 22, 35, 49–81, 85–99, 163ff. • R. Yaron 1961b, esp. pp. 129–30 • J. Hoftijzer and P. W. Pestman 1962 • A. Verger 1965, esp. pp. 66, 79f., 88, 94, 100, 102, 105–30, 141–78 • Ḥ Farzat 1967 • B. Porten 1968, esp. pp. 205–12 • R. Yaron 1968, esp. pp. 205–9 + 1 pl. • Y. Muffs 1969, esp. pp. 33f. • K. R. Veenhof 1970, pl. 110 • J. Naveh 1971c, esp. pp. 23, 36 • B. Porten 1972 • S. A. Kaufman 1974, esp. p. 53 • S. Segert 1975, esp. p. 431 • B. Porten 1979, esp. pp. 76, 78, 81–84, pl. p. 75 • B. Porten 1981, esp. p. 169 • B. Porten and H. Z. Szubin 1982, esp. p. 123 • B. Porten 1983, esp. pp. 527–28, 531, 534, 536 • B. Porten 1983c, esp. p. 565 • B. Porten 1984, esp. pp. 384, 394–96, 399 • B. Porten 1985a, esp. pp. 41–43 • B. Porten and H. Z. Szubin 1987, esp. pp. 235–37 • B. Porten and H. Z. Szubin 1987a, esp. p. 48 • B. Porten 1987a, esp. pp. 89, 91 • B. Porten and H. Z. Szubin 1987b, esp. p. 188 • B. Porten 1990, esp. pp. 22–23.

Sale of Abandoned Property (437)   TADB3.4

Bagazusht and his wife, Ubil, sell the abandoned house of Apuli to Ananiah. Brooklyn Museum (47.218.95).

Ed. Pr.   *BMAP* 3, pp. 152–64, pl. III.

EASY ACCESS

Translations: *DAE* 44 • *JEAS* II.3.

LITERATURE
C. C. Torrey 1954, esp. pp. 152–53 • E. Y. Kutscher 1954, esp. pp. 234–35 • H. L. Ginsberg 1954, esp. p. 157 • S. H. Horn and L. H. Wood 1954, esp. p. 12 • W.

Eilers 1954–56, esp. p. 330 • H. Cazelles 1955, esp. p. 79 • J. Hoftijzer 1959, esp. pp. 312–14 • J. J. Rabinowitz 1961, esp. p. 69 • R. Yaron 1961, esp. pp. 17–21, 26–28, 46, 55, 64f., 75, 82, 101–32, 166 • A. F. Rainey 1965 • A. Verger 1965, esp. pp. 99, 133ff. • B. Porten 1968, esp. pp. 213–17 • Y. Muffs 1969, esp. pp. 30–35, 41–50, 152 • J. Naveh 1971c, esp. pp. 23, 36 • B. Porten 1979, esp. pp. 78–79 • B. Porten 1981, esp. pp. 169–70, 172–73, 175–76 • B. Porten and H. Z. Szubin 1982 • B. Porten and H. Z. Szubin 1982, esp. pp. 123–31 • H. Z. Szubin and B. Porten 1982, esp. pp. 3–4 • B. Porten and H. Z. Szubin 1982a, esp. pp. 652–53 • H. Z. Szubin and B. Porten 1983, esp. pp. 282–83 • B. Porten 1983, esp. pp. 527–28, 531–32 • B. Porten 1983c, esp. p. 565 • B. Porten 1984, esp. pp. 380, 384–85, 389, 394–97, 399 • B. Porten 1985a, esp. p. 41 • B. Porten and H. Z. Szubin 1987, esp. pp. 233, 235–37 • B. Porten and H. Z. Szubin 1987a, esp. pp. 45, 51, 55, 57, 62, 65–66 • B. Porten 1987a, esp. pp. 89, 91 • B. Porten and H. Z. Szubin 1987b, esp. pp. 179, 183, 185–87, 189 • B. Porten 1990, esp. p. 21.

Deed of Bequest (434)   **TADB3.5**

     Ananiah bequeaths an apartment to his wife Tamut. Brooklyn Museum (47.218.91).

Ed. Pr.   *BMAP* 4, pp. 167–75, pl. IV.

EASY ACCESS
     Editions: *AaG*Seg 27.

     Translations: *DAE* 45 • *JEAS* II.4.

LITERATURE
     E. Y. Kutscher 1954, esp. pp. 235–36 • H. L. Ginsberg 1954, esp. pp. 157–58 • S. H. Horn and L. H. Wood 1954, esp. p. 13 • H. Cazelles 1955, esp. pp. 79–80 • J. Hoftijzer 1959, esp. pp. 314–15 • R. Yaron 1961, esp. pp. 17f., 26–28, 43f., 51, 65, 82–127 • A. Verger 1965, esp. pp. 83, 102, 112, 152, 168 • B. Porten 1968, esp. pp. 217–19 • Y. Muffs 1969, esp. pp. 34, 38, 133 • J. Naveh 1971c, esp. pp. 23, 36 • S. Segert 1975, esp. pp. 320, 432 • B. Porten 1979, esp. pp. 78–79 • B. Porten 1981, esp. pp. 169–70, 172–74 • B. Porten and H. Z. Szubin 1982, esp. pp. 123–24, 131 • H. Z. Szubin and B. Porten 1982, esp. pp. 3–4 • B. Porten and H. Z. Szubin 1982a, esp. p. 652 • B. Porten 1983, esp. pp. 527–28, 531–32 • H. Z. Szubin and B. Porten 1983a, esp. pp. 35–38, 40–41, 44 • B. Porten 1983c, esp. pp. 569–70 • B. Porten 1984, esp. pp. 380, 385, 394–97, 399 • D. Piattelli 1984, esp. pp. 1239–40 • J. W. Wesselius 1984a • B. Porten 1985a, esp. p. 41 • B. Porten and H. Z. Szubin 1987, esp. pp. 233, 235–37 • B. Porten and H. Z. Szubin 1987a, esp. pp. 57–58, 60–61 • B. Porten 1987a, esp. pp. 89, 91 • B. Porten and H. Z. Szubin 1987b, esp. pp. 183–88, 191 • B. Porten 1990, esp. p. 20.

Testamentary Manumission (427) TADB3.6

Meshullam grants freedom to his slave Tamut and her daughter, Yehoyishma, at his death. Brooklyn Museum (47.218.90).

Ed. Pr. *BMAP* 5, pp. 178–87, pl. V.

EASY ACCESS

Editions: *AC* 25.

Translations: *ANESTP* 548 • *DAE* 46 • *JEAS* II.5.

LITERATURE

H. L. Ginsberg 1954, esp. p. 158 • S. H. Horn and L. H. Wood 1954, esp. pp.
13–14 • W. Eilers 1954–56, esp. p. 330, pl. 1 • H. Cazelles 1955, esp. pp. 80–81
• E. Volterra 1957, esp. pp. 687–95 • J. J. Rabinowitz 1958a, esp. p. 79 • R.
Yaron 1961, esp. pp. 12–15, 19f., 26–28, 43f., 49ff., 98–123, 144, 155, 170 • A.
Verger 1965, esp. pp. 84, 94f., 99, 141–78 • B. Porten 1968, esp. pp. 219–21 • H.
L. Ginsberg 1969, esp. p. 548 • Y. Muffs 1969, esp. pp. 39f. • F. E. Deist 1970,
(8–10) • J. Naveh 1971c, esp. pp. 23, 36 • J. C. Greenfield 1977, esp. pp. 113–15
• B. Porten 1979, esp. pp. 78–79 • B. Porten 1981, esp. pp. 169, 176 • B. Porten
and H. Z. Szubin 1982, esp. p. 123 • B. Porten and H. Z. Szubin 1982a, esp. p. 652
• B. Porten 1983, esp. pp. 527–28, 531–32, 536 • H. Z. Szubin and B. Porten
1983, esp. p. 43 • B. Porten 1984, esp. pp. 380, 394–98 • D. Piattelli 1984, esp.
pp. 1239–41, pl. p. 103 • B. Porten and H. Z. Szubin 1987, esp. pp. 232–34 • B.
Porten and H. Z. Szubin 1987a, esp. pp. 45–46, 48, 61–63 • B. Porten 1987a, esp.
p. 89 • J. C. Greenfield 1990a, esp. p. 90 • B. Porten 1990, esp. p. 20 • M. O. Wise
1990, esp. p. 252.

Life Estate of Usufruct (421) TADB3.7

Ananiah grants Yehoyishma rights to part of his house. Brooklyn
Museum (47.218.32).

Ed. Pr. *BMAP* 6, pp. 191–97, pl. VI.

EASY ACCESS

Translations: *DAE* 47 • *JEAS* II.6.

LITERATURE

E. Y. Kutscher 1954, esp. p. 236 • H. L. Ginsberg 1954, esp. p. 158 • S. H. Horn
and L. H. Wood 1954, esp. pp. 14–16 • R. A. Parker 1955, esp. pp. 273–74, pl. 2
• R. Yaron 1960, esp. p. 69 • R. Yaron 1961, esp. pp. 6, 50ff., 64, 97–133, 170 •
A. Verger 1965, esp. pp. 146, 152 • B. Porten 1968, esp. pp. 225–26 • Y. Muffs
1969, esp. p. 133 • J. Naveh 1971c, esp. pp. 23, 36 • B. Porten 1979, esp. pp.
78–79 • B. Porten 1981, esp. p. 169 • B. Porten and H. Z. Szubin 1982, esp. pp.
123–24 • H. Z. Szubin and B. Porten 1982, esp. pp. 3–5 • B. Porten 1983, esp. pp.
527–28, 532 • H. Z. Szubin and B. Porten 1983, esp. pp. 35–36, 38, 41–45 • B.

Porten 1984, esp. pp. 385, 389, 394, 399 • B. Porten 1985a, esp. p. 41 • B. Porten and H. Z. Szubin 1987, esp. pp. 231, 233–38 • B. Porten 1987a, esp. pp. 90–91 • B. Porten and H. Z. Szubin 1987b, esp. pp. 186–88 • H. Z. Szubin and B. Porten 1988 • B. Porten 1990, esp. p. 24.

Marriage Contract (420?)   TADB3.8

Marriage document of Ananiah b. Ḥaggai and Yehoyishma. Brooklyn Museum (47.218.150 + 47.218.97 + fragments of 47.218.155).

Ed. Pr.   *BMAP* 7+15+18, pp. 201–22, 298, pls. VII, XV.

EASY ACCESS
Editions: *AaG*Seg 30.

Translations: *ANESTP* 548 • *DAE* 48 • *JEAS* II.7.

LITERATURE
E. Y. Kutscher 1954, esp. pp. 236–37 • H. L. Ginsberg 1954, esp. pp. 158–59 • S. H. Horn and L. H. Wood 1954, esp. p. 16 • H. Cazelles 1955, esp. pp. 81–84, fig. 1 • J. J. Rabinowitz 1956a • J. J. Rabinowitz 1957, esp. pp. 269–71 • R. Yaron 1960, esp. p. 69 • R. Yaron 1961, esp. pp. 6–12, 35f., 43, 52–95, 122f., 154f., 160ff., 169ff. • A. Verger 1965, esp. pp. 66, 91ff., 94, 105–30, 152f., 169 • B. Porten 1968, esp. pp. 221–25 • B. Porten and J. C. Greenfield 1969, esp. p. 157 • H. L. Ginsberg 1969, esp. pp. 548–49 • Y. Muffs 1969, esp. pp. 3, 42f., 51–56, 133, 195 • B. Porten 1971, esp. pp. 244–55 • J. Naveh 1971c, esp. pp. 23, 36 • B. Porten 1972, esp. pp. 307ff. • M. J. Geller 1977 • B. Porten 1979, esp. pp. 84–85, pls. pp. 84–86 • I. Gottlieb 1980 • B. Porten and H. Z. Szubin 1982, esp. p. 123 • B. Porten 1983, esp. pp. 527, 532, 534 • B. Porten 1983c, esp. pp. 565, 568 • B. Porten 1984, esp. pp. 380, 384, 394–96, 399 • B. Porten 1985a, esp. pp. 41–43 • B. Porten and H. Z. Szubin 1987, esp. pp. 234–38 • B. Porten 1987a, esp. pp. 90–91 • B. Porten and H. Z. Szubin 1987b, esp. p. 188 • B. Porten 1990, esp. p. 21.

Adoption of a Transferred Slave (416)   TADB3.9

Uriah b. Maḥseiah adopts the slave Yedaniah b. Taḥwa. Brooklyn Museum (47.218.96).

Ed. Pr.   *BMAP* 8, pp. 224–31, pl. VIII.

EASY ACCESS
Editions: *AC* 26.

Translations: *DAE* 49 • *JEAS* IV.8.

LITERATURE

E. G. Kraeling 1952, pl. 8 • E. Y. Kutscher 1954, esp. p. 237 • H. L. Ginsberg 1954, esp. p. 159 • S. H. Horn and L. H. Wood 1954, esp. pp. 16–17 • H. Cazelles 1955, esp. p. 84 • R. A. Parker 1955, esp. p. 272 • E. Volterra 1957, esp. p. 696 • Z. W. Falk 1958 • J. J. Rabinowitz 1960, esp. pp. 72–73 • R. Yaron 1961, esp. pp. 15, 40, 49ff., 120ff., 139, 170 • A. Verger 1964b • A. Verger 1965, esp. pp. 23, 68, 88, 95f., 141–74 • B. Porten 1968, esp. p. 212 • W. Henning 1968 • B. Porten and J. C. Greenfield 1969, esp. p. 155 • J. Teixidor 1969, esp. p. 346 • J. Naveh 1971c, esp. p. 36 • S. Segert 1975, esp. p. 431 • B. Porten 1979, esp. pp. 78–79, pl. p. 86 • B. Porten 1981, esp. p. 169 • B. Porten 1983, esp. pp. 527–28, 532 • B. Porten 1983c, esp. p. 565 • B. Porten 1984, esp. pp. 380–81, 394 • D. Piattelli 1984, esp. pp. 1241–44 • B. Porten 1985a, esp. p. 41 • B. Porten and H. Z. Szubin 1987a, esp. pp. 45–46, 48, 58, 60–61, 63, 67 • B. Porten 1987a, esp. p. 90 • B. Porten 1990, esp. pp. 23–24.

Deed of Bequest (404)   **TADB3.10**

Ananiah grants Yehoyishma part of his house on his death. Brooklyn Museum (47.218.92).

Ed. Pr.   *BMAP* 9, pp. 235–44, pl. IX.

EASY ACCESS

Translations: *DAE* 50 • *JEAS* II.8.

LITERATURE

E. G. Kraeling 1952, esp. p. 300, pl. 1 • E. Vogt 1954, esp. p. 267 • E. Y. Kutscher 1954, esp. p. 237 • H. L. Ginsberg 1954, esp. pp. 159–61 • S. H. Horn and L. H. Wood 1954, esp. pp. 17–18 • H. Cazelles 1955, esp. pp. 84–85 • R. Yaron 1957, esp. p. 49 • R. Yaron 1961, esp. pp. 6, 13, 19, 26, 29, 40ff., 48, 50, 98–123, 133, 139f., 151, 168, 175 • A. Verger 1965, esp. pp. 60, 80, 82, 84, 99, 129, 137, 152f., 185 • B. Porten 1979, esp. pp. 226–29 • R. A. Henshaw 1967–68, (19) • B. Porten and J. C. Greenfield 1969, esp. pp. 154–57 • Y. Muffs 1969, esp. pp. 34ff., 133ff. • J. Naveh 1971c, esp. pp. 23, 30, 36 • B. Porten 1979, esp. pp. 78–79 • B. Porten 1981, esp. pp. 169–74 • B. Porten and H. Z. Szubin 1982, esp. pp. 123–24 • H. Z. Szubin and B. Porten 1982, esp. pp. 3–5 • B. Porten and H. Z. Szubin 1982a, esp. p. 652 • B. Porten 1983, esp. pp. 527–28, 531–32, 536 • H. Z. Szubin and B. Porten 1983a, esp. pp. 35–39, 41–45 • B. Porten 1984, esp. pp. 383, 385, 389, 394–97, 399 • J. W. Wesselius 1984a, esp. pp. 127–28 • B. Porten 1985a, esp. p. 41 • J. W. Wesselius 1985a • B. Porten and H. Z. Szubin 1987, esp. pp. 231–38 • B. Porten and H. Z. Szubin 1987a, esp. p. 63 • B. Porten 1987a, esp. p. 91 • B. Porten and H. Z. Szubin 1987b • B. Porten 1990, esp. p. 21.

Dowry Addendum (402)   **TADB3.11**

       Ananiah adds a codicil to the bequest in TADB3.10. Brooklyn Museum (47.218.88).

Ed. Pr.   *BMAP* 10, pp. 247–56, pl. X.

EASY ACCESS

       Translations: *DAE* 51 ● *JEAS* II.9.

LITERATURE

       E. Vogt 1954, esp. pp. 266–67, pl. 1 ● E. Y. Kutscher 1954, esp. p. 237 ● H. L. Ginsberg 1954, esp. p. 161 ● S. H. Horn and L. H. Wood 1954, esp. p. 18 ● H. Cazelles 1955, esp. pp. 85–86 ● R. Yaron 1957, esp. pp. 50–51 ● R. Yaron 1961, esp. pp. 6, 13, 18–20, 26, 29, 40, 43, 50, 98–123, 133, 151, 168, 175 ● A. Verger 1965, esp. pp. 60, 79f., 83, 93f., 99, 137, 152f. ● D. Diringer and R. Regensburger 1968, pl. 2.188a ● R. Yaron 1968, esp. pp. 209–11 ● B. Porten and J. C. Greenfield 1969, esp. pp. 154–57 ● Y. Muffs 1969, esp. pp. 30–38, 182f. ● J. Naveh 1971c, esp. pp. 23, 30, 36 ● B. Porten 1979, esp. pp. 78–79 ● B. Porten 1981, esp. pp. 169–73, 175 ● B. Porten and H. Z. Szubin 1982, esp. pp. 123–24 ● H. Z. Szubin and B. Porten 1982, esp. pp. 3–5 ● B. Porten and H. Z. Szubin 1982a, esp. p. 652 ● B. Porten 1983, esp. pp. 527–28, 531–32 ● H. Z. Szubin and B. Porten 1983, esp. pp. 35–38, 41–45 ● B. Porten 1984, esp. pp. 385, 389, 394–97, 399 ● B. Porten 1985a, esp. p. 41 ● B. Porten and H. Z. Szubin 1987 ● B. Porten and H. Z. Szubin 1987a, esp. p. 64 ● B. Porten 1987a, esp. p. 91 ● B. Porten and H. Z. Szubin 1987b, esp. pp. 179, 183, 185, 187–88 ● B. Porten 1990, esp. p. 20.

Sale of Property (402)   **TADB3.12**

       Ananiah sells house and land to Anani b. Ḥaggai, his son-in-law. Brooklyn Museum (47.218.94).

Ed. Pr.   *BMAP* 12, pp. 268–80, pl. XII.

EASY ACCESS

       Translations: *DAE* 53 ● *JEAS* II.11.

LITERATURE

       E. Vogt 1954, esp. p. 267 ● E. Y. Kutscher 1954, esp. pp. 237–38 ● H. L. Ginsberg 1954, esp. pp. 161–62 ● W. Eilers 1954–56, esp. p. 330 ● R. Yaron 1957, esp. pp. 49–50 ● J. J. Rabinowitz 1958a, esp. pp. 77–78 ● R. Yaron 1958c, esp. pp. 306–10 ● R. Yaron 1961, esp. pp. 6, 11–14, 18–22, 26–34, 40, 44, 49, 52, 75, 98–127, 133, 170, 175 ● A. Verger 1965, esp. pp. 60, 77, 80, 84, 91f., 99, 135ff., 152ff., 168, 185 ● B. Porten 1968, esp. pp. 231–34 ● R. Yaron 1968, esp. p. 211 ● B. Porten and J. C. Greenfield 1969, esp. pp. 154–57 ● Y. Muffs 1969, esp. pp. 34f., 41–50, 76, 133f., 152, 181 ● J. Naveh 1971c, esp. pp. 23, 30, 36 ● B. Porten 1979, esp. pp. 78–79 ● B. Porten 1981, esp. pp. 169–73, 172, 175 ● B. Porten and

H. Z. Szubin 1982, esp. pp. 123–24, 126 ● H. Z. Szubin and B. Porten 1982 ● H. Z. Szubin and B. Porten 1982, esp. pp. 3–5 ● B. Porten and H. Z. Szubin 1982a, esp. pp. 652–53 ● B. Porten 1983, esp. pp. 527–28, 531–32, 535 ● H. Z. Szubin and B. Porten 1983, esp. p. 284 ● H. Z. Szubin and B. Porten 1983a, esp. pp. 35–39, 41–42, 44–45 ● B. Porten 1984, esp. pp. 380–81, 383–85, 389, 394–97, 399 ● J. W. Wesselius 1984a ● B. Porten 1985a, esp. pp. 41, 50–51 ● B. Porten and H. Z. Szubin 1987, esp. pp. 232–37 ● B. Porten and H. Z. Szubin 1987a, esp. pp. 64–65 ● B. Porten 1987a, esp. pp. 89–91 ● B. Porten and H. Z. Szubin 1987b, esp. pp. 179, 183–89 ● B. Porten 1990, esp. p. 19.

Loan of Grain (402)   **TADB3.13**

Anani b. Ḥaggai borrows grain from Pakhnum b. Besa. Brooklyn Museum (47.218.93).

Ed. Pr.   *BMAP* 11, pp. 259–65, pl. XI.

EASY ACCESS

Translations: *DAE* 52 ● *JEAS* II.10.

LITERATURE
E. Y. Kutscher 1954, esp. p. 237 ● H. L. Ginsberg 1954, esp. p. 161 ● J. Hoftijzer 1959, esp. p. 315 ● R. Yaron 1961, esp. pp. 6f., 11–14, 18–32, 44–54, 106f., 123, 135ff., 170 ● R. Yaron 1961b, esp. pp. 127–28 ● A. Verger 1965, esp. pp. 60, 80, 91f., 137ff. ● B. Porten 1968, esp. p. 233 ● R. Yaron 1968, esp. p. 211 ● B. Porten and J. C. Greenfield 1969, esp. pp. 153–55 ● J. Naveh 1971c, esp. pp. 30, 36 ● S. Segert 1975, esp. p. 431 ● B. Porten 1979, esp. pp. 78–79 ● B. Porten and H. Z. Szubin 1982, esp. p. 123 ● B. Porten and H. Z. Szubin 1982a, esp. p. 652 ● B. Porten 1983, esp. pp. 527–29, 531–32, 537 ● B. Porten 1983c, esp. pp. 565, 568–69 ● B. Porten 1984, esp. pp. 380, 383, 385, 394, 396, 399 ● B. Porten 1985a, esp. pp. 41, 51 ● B. Porten and H. Z. Szubin 1987, esp. p. 232 ● B. Porten and H. Z. Szubin 1987a, esp. pp. 62–64 ● B. Porten 1987a, esp. pp. 89–91 ● B. Porten and H. Z. Szubin 1987b, esp. pp. 183, 186 ● B. Porten 1990, esp. p. 19.

B.3.c.9   Elephantine: Miscellaneous Contracts   TADB4

Fragmentary Debt Cancellation (early 5th c.)   **TADB4.1**

> Sumki b. Shasher cancels the debt of Shelomam b. Galgal. Cairo
> Museum (J. 43497) + Ägyptisches Museum, Berlin (P. 23104).

Ed. Pr.   *APO*, pap. 44, p. 139, pl. 38.

EASY ACCESS
  Editions: *AP* 49 • *APE* 45 • *NESE* 3. 16–28 (additional fragment).

  Illustrations: *NESE* 3. 17.

LITERATURE
  R. Yaron 1961, esp. pp. 2, 14, 26, 41, 135–36 • P. Swiggers 1981b • B. Porten
  1983, esp. p. 528 • B. Porten 1984, esp. pp. 383, 394 • B. Porten 1985a, esp. pp.
  42, 49–51.

Loan of Silver (ca. 487)   **TADB4.2**

> Gemariah b. Aḥio borrows silver from X b. Yatama. Bodleian Library
> (MS. Heb. c. 59[P]).

Ed. Pr.   A. Cowley and G. B. Gray 1903, esp. pp. 202–8, 259–63 + pl. [photo].

EASY ACCESS
  Editions: *AP* 11 • *APA* L • *APE* 88 • *ESE* 2. 224–28 • *NSI* app. 2 (p. 404) •
                  RAO 6. 147–58, 260–67 • *RES* 491, 1799.

  Translations: *DAE* 3 • *JEAS* IV.3.

  Illustrations: *APA* L.

LITERATURE
  A. H. Sayce 1903, esp. pp. 315–16 • J. Halévy 1903 • G. B. Gray 1903 • C. H. W.
  Johns 1905 • S. de Ricci 1906, esp. pp. 29–30 • M.-J. Lagrange 1907, esp. pp.
  266–67 • E. Meyer 1911, esp. p. 1032 • G. R. Driver 1932, esp. p. 77 • E. Neufeld
  1953–54, esp. pp. 201–2 • R. Yaron 1961, esp. pp. 10–17, 23–29, 32, 42, 54, 75,
  135ff. • A. Verger 1965, esp. pp. 62f., 91, 103, 137ff., 153 • Y. Muffs 1969, esp.
  pp. 35f., 184ff., 202 • B. Porten 1979, esp. pl. p. 81 • B. Porten and H. Z. Szubin
  1982a, esp. pp. 651, 652 • B. Porten 1983, esp. p. 532 • B. Porten 1983c, esp. pp.
  568–69 • B. Porten 1984, esp. pp. 383–84, 394–95 • B. Porten 1985a, esp. pp.
  42–49, 51 • B. Porten 1987a, esp. p. 91 • B. Porten 1990, esp. p. 18.

Obligation to Deliver Grain (483)   **TADB4.4**

Hoshea b. Hoduiah and Ahiab b. Gemariah accept an obligation to deliver grain to Syene. Staatliche Museen, Berlin (P. 13493).

Ed. Pr.   *APO*, pap. 25, pp. 99–102, pls. 25, 26.

EASY ACCESS
Editions: *AP* 2 • *APE* 27.

Translations: *DAE* 54.

LITERATURE
F. Perles 1911–12, esp. p. 14:500 • J. N. Epstein 1912, esp. pp. 131–32 • P. Volz 1912 • J. N. Epstein 1913, esp. pp. 148–50 • R. Yaron 1961, esp. pp. 2, 6, 10, 13–14, 17, 23–27, 29–30, 38, 123, 140, 169 • A. Verger 1965, esp. pp. 67, 86, 91, 98, 150 • Y. Muffs 1969, esp. pp. 52, 56–58, 86–89, 167 • R. Schmitt 1972 • B. Porten 1981, esp. p. 169 • B. Porten 1983, esp. pp. 528, 532–33, 540 • B. Porten 1984, esp. pp. 383, 394–95 • B. Porten 1985a, esp. pp. 41–42 • B. Porten 1987a, esp. p. 89 • B. Porten 1990, esp. p. 18.

Obligation to Deliver Grain (483)   **TADB4.3**

A duplicate (or first draft) of TADB4.4. Cairo Museum (J. 43485).

Ed. Pr.   *APO*, pap. 26, pp. 106–7, pl. 27.

EASY ACCESS
Editions: *AP* 3 • *APE* 29.

LITERATURE
J. N. Epstein 1912, esp. pp. 131–32 • J. N. Epstein 1913, esp. p. 150 • S. A. Cook 1915, esp. pp. 350–51 • R. Yaron 1961, esp. pp. 2, 10, 13–14, 17, 23–24, 26–27, 29 • A. Verger 1965, esp. pp. 67, 86, 150 • B. Porten 1983, esp. pp. 528, 532–33, 536, 540 • B. Porten 1984, esp. pp. 394–95 • B. Porten 1985a, esp. pp. 41–42 • B. Porten 1987a, esp. p. 89.

Papryus Fragments related to TADB4.3–4 (484)   **AP.4**

Fragments apparently concerning the same transaction as the previous two documents. Staatliche Museen, Berlin (P. 13455).

Ed. Pr.   *APO*, pap. 41, p. 136, pl. 36.

EASY ACCESS
Editions: *AP* 4 • *APE* 42.

LITERATURE
F. Perles 1911–12, esp. p. 14:500.

Fragmentary Loan of Silver (407)   **TADB4.5**
Cairo Museum (J. 43487).

Ed. Pr.   *APO*, pap. 29, pp. 61–62, pl. 15.

EASY ACCESS
Editions: *AP* 29 ● *APE* 15.

Translations: *DAE* 6.

LITERATURE
S. A. Cook 1915, esp. p. 364 ● R. Yaron 1961, esp. pp. 3–11, 25, 135, 139 ● A. Verger 1965, esp. pp. 91, 140, 149 ● B. Porten 1983, esp. pp. 528–29, 532, 535–36, 543 ● B. Porten 1984, esp. pp. 380, 383, 394 ● B. Porten 1985a, esp. pp. 41–42, 50 ● B. Porten 1987a, esp. pp. 89–90 ● B. Porten 1990, esp. p. 18.

Loan of Silver (400)   **TADB4.6**
Staatliche Museen, Berlin (P. 13476).

Ed. Pr.   *APO*, pap. 35, pp. 128–30, pl. 34.

EASY ACCESS
Editions: *AP* 35 ● *APE* 37.

Translations: *DAE* 7.

LITERATURE
J. N. Epstein 1912, esp. pp. 131–32 ● J. N. Epstein 1913, esp. p. 225 ● S. A. Cook 1915, esp. p. 365 ● R. Yaron 1961, esp. pp. 2, 11, 13–14, 25, 55, 106, 135, 139, 170, 175 ● A. Verger 1965, esp. pp. 60, 78, 92, 136, 140 ● B. Porten and J. C. Greenfield 1969, esp. pp. 153–57 ● B. Porten 1979, esp. pp. 90–92, pl. p. 87 ● B. Porten 1983, esp. pp. 528, 532, 535 ● B. Porten 1984, esp. pp. 380, 383, 394–95, 400 ● B. Porten 1985a, esp. pp. 42, 50 ● B. Porten 1987a, esp. pp. 89–90 ● B. Porten 1990, esp. p. 19.

B.3.c.10 Elephantine: Conveyances   **TADB5**

Deed of Exchange of Property (495)   **TADB5.1**

> Two pairs of sisters exchange half a share of property. Staatliche
> Museen, Berlin (P. 13489).

Ed. Pr.   *APO*, pap. 30, pp. 113–15, pl. 30.

EASY ACCESS
    Editions: *AP* 1 • *APE* 31.

    Translations: *DAE* 2 • *JEAS* IV.2.

LITERATURE
    J. N. Epstein 1913, esp. p. 222 • S. A. Cook 1915, esp. p. 364 • R. Yaron 1961,
    esp. pp. 10, 13f., 17, 23, 29, 32, 37, 40, 48, 55, 84, 104, 115–25 • A. Verger 1965,
    esp. pp. 15f., 68, 91, 99, 179f. • B. Porten 1968, esp. pp. 22–23 • J. Naveh 1971c,
    esp. p. 34 • B. Porten 1979, esp. pl. p.81 • B. Porten and H. Z. Szubin 1982a • B.
    Porten 1983, esp. pp. 528–29, 531–32, 536, 539 • H. Z. Szubin and B. Porten
    1983, esp. p. 284 • B. Porten 1984, esp. pp. 380, 382, 394, 400 • B. Porten 1985a,
    esp. pp. 41–42, 46–51 • B. Porten and H. Z. Szubin 1987a, esp. pp. 45, 49 • B.
    Porten 1987a, esp. p. 89 • B. Porten and H. Z. Szubin 1987b, esp. p. 187 • B. Por-
    ten 1990, esp. p. 18.

Fragment of Legal Text (end 5th c.)   **TADB5.2**

> Document of withdrawal of Mattan b. Yashobiah. Staatliche Museen,
> Berlin (P. 13444,3 + 13448,3,5).

Ed. Pr.   *APO*, p. 213, pl. 58/3 + pp. 220–21, pl. 60/3, 5.

EASY ACCESS
    Editions: *AP* 65+67 • *APE* 71+73.

LITERATURE
    J. N. Epstein 1912, esp. pp. 137 f. • J. N. Epstein 1913, esp. p. 234 • B. Porten and
    H. Z. Szubin 1982a, esp. pp. 653–54 • B. Porten 1985a, esp. p. 42 • B. Porten
    1990, esp. p. 25.

Conveyance (end 5th c.)   **TADB5.3**

> Fragment from the end of a conveyance. Staatliche Museen, Berlin (P.
> 13607).

Ed. Pr.   B. Porten and A. Yardeni 1989 (*TADB*), no. 5.3.

Conveyance (end 5th c.)   **TADB5.4**

     Fragments from a contract. Cairo Museum (J. 43491).

Ed. Pr.   *APO*, pap. 37, p. 131, pl. 35.

EASY ACCESS
     Editions: *AP* 47 • *APE* 38.

LITERATURE
     J. N. Epstein 1913, esp. p. 225 • A. Dupont-Sommer 1946–47(a) • R. Yaron 1961, esp. pp. 40, 121 • J. Naveh 1971c, esp. p. 35 • B. Porten 1983, esp. p. 528 • B. Porten 1984, esp. pp. 394–96.

Mutual Quitclaim (end 5th c.)   **TADB5.5**

     Miptaḥiah d. Gemariah and Isweri, her sister. Cairo Museum (J. 43489).

Ed. Pr.   *APO*, pap. 33, pp. 122–25, pl. 33 + 74/4, pl. 61/4.

EASY ACCESS
     Editions: *AP* 43 • *APE* 35.

     Translations: *DAE* 8.

LITERATURE
     F. Perles 1911–12, esp. p. 14:500 • J. N. Epstein 1913, esp. pp. 224–25 • G. R. Driver 1932, esp. p. 82 • R. Yaron 1961, esp. pp. 2, 11, 13, 19–20, 26, 29–30, 32, 55, 106–7, 110, 120, 123–25, 170 • B. Porten 1968, esp. pp. 271–72 • B. Porten and H. Z. Szubin 1982a, esp. p. 652 • B. Porten 1983, esp. pp. 528, 532 • B. Porten 1984, esp. pp. 383, 394, 396 • B. Porten 1985a, esp. p. 42 • B. Porten and H. Z. Szubin 1987a, esp. pp. 445, 62, 64–65 • B. Porten 1987a, esp. pp. 89–90 • B. Porten and H. Z. Szubin 1987b, esp. p. 183 • B. Porten 1990, esp. p. 19.

B.3.c.11 Elephantine: Marriage Contracts   TADB6

Marriage Contract (446)   TADB6.1
            Brooklyn Museum (47.218.12).

Ed. Pr.   *BMAP* 14, pp. 293–96, pl. XIV.

        Translations: *JEAS* IV.5.

LITERATURE
        B. Porten 1971, esp. pp. 243–55 • B. Porten 1981, esp. p. 41 • B. Porten 1989.

Marriage Contract (end 5th c.)   TADB6.2
            Fragments. Cairo Museum (J. 43470).

Ed. Pr.   *APO*, pap. 9, pp. 49–50, pl. 10.

EASY ACCESS
        Editions: *AP* 36 • *APE* 9.

        Translations: *JEAS* IV.7.

LITERATURE
        D. S. Margoliouth 1912, esp. pp. 71–72 • R. Yaron 1961, esp. p. 2 • A. Verger
        1965, esp. p. 106 • B. Porten 1971, esp. pp. 257–61 • J. Naveh 1971c, esp. p. 33 •
        J. C. Greenfield 1975, esp. p. 312 • B. Porten 1984, esp. p. 394 • B. Porten 1989.

Marriage Contract (end 5th c.)   TADB6.3
            Cairo Museum (J. 43488).

Ed. Pr.   *APO*, pap. 31, pp. 116–17, pl. 31.

EASY ACCESS
        Editions: *AP* 46 • *APE* 32.

LITERATURE
        J. N. Epstein 1912, esp. p. 132 • R. Yaron 1960, esp. p. 69 • R. Yaron 1961, esp.
        pp. 2, 10, 13–14, 16–17, 23, 26, 29, 33, 69 • B. Porten and H. Z. Szubin 1982a,
        esp. p. 652 • B. Porten 1983, esp. pp. 528, 532 • B. Porten 1984, esp. p. 394 • B.
        Porten 1985a, esp. p. 50 • B. Porten 1989.

Marriage Contract (425?)   **TADB6.4**
         Staatliche Museen, Berlin (P. 13465).

Ed. Pr.   *APO*, pap. 34, pp. 126–27, pl. 33.

EASY ACCESS
     Editions: *AP* 18 ● *APE* 36.

     Translations: *DAE* 5 ● *JEAS* IV.6.

LITERATURE
     R. Yaron 1961, esp. pp. 16, 18, 21f., 26ff., 32, 43, 53–57, 64, 122, 160, 169 ● B. Porten 1971, esp. pp. 255–56 ● J. Naveh 1971c, esp. pp. 23, 35 ● B. Porten 1983c, esp. p. 569 ● B. Porten 1984, esp. pp. 394–95 ● B. Porten and H. Z. Szubin 1987, esp. pp. 235–36 ● B. Porten and H. Z. Szubin 1987b, esp. p. 188 ● B. Porten 1989.

B.3.c.12 Elephantine: Affidavits and Legal Records   TADB7

Affidavit about Fish (413?)   TADB7.1

>   Oath concerning the theft of fish. Cairo Museum (J. 43490).

Ed. Pr.   *APO*, pap. 36, pp. 120–21, pl. 32.

EASY ACCESS
>   Editions: *AP* 45 ● *APE* 34.

>   Translations: *DAE* 11.

LITERATURE
>   J. N. Epstein 1913, esp. pp. 223–24 ● G. R. Driver 1932, esp. p. 82 ● R. Yaron
>   1958c ● R. Yaron 1961, esp. pp. 2, 11, 13, 18, 45–46, 135, 157 ● B. Porten 1968,
>   esp. p. 153 ● A. Verger 1965, esp. pp. 40, 188, 190–91 ● B. Porten 1983, esp. p.
>   528 ● B. Porten 1983c ● B. Porten 1984, esp. pp. 383, 394–95 ● B. Porten 1985a,
>   esp. pp. 41–42 ● B. Porten 1987a, esp. pp. 89–90 ● B. Porten and H. Z. Szubin
>   1987b, esp. p. 183 ● B. Porten 1990, esp. p. 18.

Record of Challenge and Oath (401)   TADB7.2

>   Malchiah agrees to swear to his innocence (of theft and rape) before
>   Ḥerembethel. Cairo Museum (J. 43486).

Ed. Pr.   *APO*, pap. 27, pp. 103–5, pl. 26.

EASY ACCESS
>   Editions: *AP* 7 ● *APE* 28.

>   Translations: *DAE* 9 ● *JEAS* IV.10.

LITERATURE
>   M.-J. Lagrange 1907, esp. pp. 261–63 ● S. Gutesmann 1907, esp. p. 196 ● T.
>   Nöldeke 1907, esp. p. 147 ● J. K. Fotheringham 1908–9, esp. p. 15 ● M. H. Pog-
>   non 1911, esp. pp. 353–55 ● J. K. Fotheringham 1913, esp. p. 571 ● J. N. Epstein
>   1913, esp. p. 235 ● S. A. Cook 1915, esp. p. 354 ● D. Sidersky 1926, esp. p. 70 ●
>   G. R. Driver 1932, esp. pp. 77–78 ● L. Borchardt 1932, esp. pp. 300–301 ● S. H.
>   Horn and L. H. Wood 1954, esp. pp. 11–12 ● R. Yaron 1961, esp. pp. 2, 32–38,
>   102–27 ● E. Volterra 1964 ● A. Verger 1965, esp. pp. 84, 99f., 136f., 153 ● B.
>   Porten 1968, esp. pp. 156, 295, 315–17 + plate ● Y. Muffs 1969, esp. pp. 31, 41,
>   48 ● J. Naveh 1971c, esp. pp. 23, 31 ● B. Porten 1979, esp. p. 79 ● B. Porten 1981,
>   esp. pp. 169–70, 172–75 ● B. Porten and H. Z. Szubin 1982, esp. pp. 124–26 ● B.
>   Porten 1983, esp. pp. 528–29, 531–33, 535, 538 ● H. Z. Szubin and B. Porten
>   1983, esp. p. 284 ● B. Porten 1983c, esp. p. 565 ● B. Porten 1984, esp. pp. 380,
>   384–86, 394–95, 400 ● B. Porten 1985a, esp. pp. 41–42, 49 ● B. Porten and H. Z.
>   Szubin 1987, esp. pp. 233, 235–36 ● B. Porten and H. Z. Szubin 1987a, esp. p. 56
>   ● B. Porten 1987a, esp. pp. 89, 91 ● B. Porten and H. Z. Szubin 1987b, esp. pp.

184–88 • B. Porten 1990, esp. p. 23.

Affidavit (416?) TADB7.3

Oath concerning a donkey. Staatliche Museen, Berlin (P. 13485).

Ed. Pr. *APO*, pap. 32, pp. 118–19, pl. 32.

EASY ACCESS
Editions: *AP* 44 • *APE* 33.

Translations: *DAE* 10 • *JEAS* IV.9.

LITERATURE
J. N. Epstein 1912, esp. p. 132 • J. N. Epstein 1913, esp. pp. 222–23 • R. Yaron 1961, esp. pp. 2, 10, 41, 45 • A. Verger 1965, esp. pp. 186ff. • B. Porten 1968, esp. pp. 154, 317–18 + photo • J. Naveh 1971c, esp. p. 34 • B. Porten 1979, esp. pp. 101–2, pl. p. 103 • H. Z. Szubin and B. Porten 1982, esp. p. 9 • B. Porten 1983c, esp. pp. 563, 567 • B. Porten 1984, esp. pp. 391, 393–94 • B. Porten 1987a, esp. p. 89.

Affidavit (end 5th c.) TADB7.4

Endorsement of an oath. Cairo Museum (J. 43501).

Ed. Pr. *APO*, pap. 47, p. 143, pl. 39.

EASY ACCESS
Editions: *AP* 59 • *APE* 49.

LITERATURE
P. Swiggers 1981b, esp. pp. 127–28 • J. Teixidor 1985, esp. p. 733 • J. Naveh 1985c, esp. p. 211 • R. Zadok 1985c, esp. p. 175 • J. A. Fitzmyer 1986, esp. p. 543.

B.3.c.13 Legal Document (300?) AP.82

Fragmentary deposition (?). Bodleian Library (Aram. e.2 [P]).

Ed. Pr. A. E. Cowley 1915b.

EASY ACCESS
Editions: *AP* 82.

LITERATURE
G. R. Driver 1932, esp. pp. 86–87.

B.3.c.14 Elephantine: Miscellaneous and Fragmentary Legal Texts

Lepsius Fragments (end 5th c.)   **TADB8.5**

> Court record concerning rent, imprisonment, and payment. Staatliche Museen, Berlin (P. 3206).

Ed. Pr.   R. Lepsius 1849–59, pl. 124.

EASY ACCESS
    Editions: *AP* 69 • *APE* 64 • *APO* 60 • *CIS* 149.

    Illustrations: *APO* pl. 51 • *CIS* pl. 19.

LITERATURE
    C. Clermont-Ganneau 1879, esp. p. 27 • S. de Ricci 1906, esp. p. 27.

AP 50 (end 5th c.) (Cairo Museum)   **AP.50**

Ed. Pr.   *APO*, pap. 46, p. 141, pl. 38.

EASY ACCESS
    Editions: *AP* 50 • *APE* 47.

AP 64 (end 5th c.)   **AP.64**

Ed. Pr.   *APO*, frags. 17–29, pp. 208–10, pl. 57.

EASY ACCESS
    Editions: *AP* 64 • *APE* 70B.

LITERATURE
    B. Porten 1990, esp. p. 20.

AP 68 (end 5th c.)   **AP.68**

Ed. Pr.   *APO*, frags. 1–12, pp. 223–26, pl. 61.

EASY ACCESS
    Editions: *AP* 68 • *APE* 74.

LITERATURE
    B. Porten 1980, esp. pp. 49–51, pl. p. 103 • B. Porten 1990, esp. pp. 18, 25.

BMAP 16 (end 5th c.)   **BMAP.16**

       Brooklyn Museum (47.218.13).

Ed. Pr.   *BMAP* 16, pp. 300–302, pl. XVIa, b.

B.3.c.15 Elephantine: Lists and Accounts

de Vogüé Papyrus Fragment (5th c.?)   TADC3.25
> Fragmentary account of substitutions; income. Cairo Museum.

Ed. Pr.   *CIS* II 153, pl. 20, 21.

EASY ACCESS
>   Editions: *AP* 78.

LITERATURE
>   S. de Ricci 1906, esp. p. 28.

Inventory (end 5th c.)   AP.79
> Fragment giving dimensions of some objects. Present location unknown.

Ed. Pr.   C. J. M. de Vogüé 1902a.

EASY ACCESS
>   Editions: *AP* 79 • *APE* 89 • *ESE* 2.217–19 • *RAO* 6.246–48 • *RES* 246.

LITERATURE
>   S. de Ricci 1906, esp. p. 30.

Fragmentary Account (end 5th c.)   TADC3.16
> Concerning grain. Brooklyn Museum (47.218.153).

Ed. Pr.   *BMAP* 17, p. 304, pl. XVII.

List of Names (end 5th c.)   TADC3.3
> Two fragments with two columns of names. Cairo Museum

Ed. Pr.   *APO*, pap. 22, pp. 94–95, pl. 24.

EASY ACCESS
>   Editions: *AP* 52 • *APE* 25.

LITERATURE
>   J. N. Epstein 1913, esp. p. 148.

Ahiqar Palimpsest **TADC3.9**
>
> Undertext of TADC1.1; previously unpublished document containing port duty lists for incoming and outgoing cargo ships.

LITERATURE
 B. Porten 1990, esp. p. 17.

List (end 5th c.) **TADC3.13**
>
> Fragmentary list of memoranda. Staatliche Museen, Berlin (P. 13447.B, C).

Ed. Pr. *APO*, pap 62, rev. col 2, p. 199; frags. 1 and 3, pp. 204–5; pap. 61, rev., pp. 205–6, pl. 55; pl. 56r; pl. 53r.

EASY ACCESS
 Editions: *AP* 61 + 62 + 63 • *APE* 67ii + 68E + 69.

LITERATURE
 J. N. Epstein 1913, esp. p. 234 • B. Porten 1990, esp. p. 17.

Account (end 5th c.) **TADC3.14**
>
> Disbursement of barley to Syenian garrison. Cairo Museum

Ed. Pr. *APO*, pap. 19, pp. 86–89, pls. 21–22.

EASY ACCESS
 Editions: *AP* 24 • *APE* 20.

 Translations: *DAE* 55.

LITERATURE
 J. N. Epstein 1913, esp. pp. 147–48 • B. Porten 1990, esp. pp. 26–27.

Donor List (end 5th c.) **TADC3.15**
>
> List of donors to the temple of YHW. Staatliche Museen, Berlin (P. 13488).

Ed. Pr. *APO*, pap.18, pp. 73–85, pls. 17–20.

EASY ACCESS
 Editions: *AaG*Seg 29 • *AP* 22 • *APE* 19.

 Translations: *ANET*[3] 491 • *ATAT* 453–54 • *DAE* 89 • *JEAS* V.4.

LITERATURE
> F. Perles 1911–12, esp. p. 14:500 ● I. Lévi 1912, esp. pp. 175–84 ● J. N. Epstein 1912, esp. p. 131 ● J. N. Epstein 1912a, esp. pp. 139–42 ● J. N. Epstein 1913, esp. pp. 145–47 ● S. A. Cook 1915, esp. p. 356 ● M. D. Cassuto 1942 ● W. F. Albright 1943 ● B. Porten 1968, esp. pp. 320–27 ● R. Degen 1974b, esp. pp. 72–73, pl. 21 ● B. Porten 1986, esp. pp. 8–13 ● B. Porten 1990, esp. p. 18.

List of Names (440–50)   TADC4.4

> List of nine names. Cairo Museum

Ed. Pr.   *APO*, pap. 17, pp. 71–72, pl. 17.

EASY ACCESS
> Editions: *AP* 12 ● *APE* 18.

> Translations: *DAE* 56 ● *JEAS* V.1.

LITERATURE
> F. Perles 1911–12, esp. pp. 14:499–500 ● J. N. Epstein 1912, esp. pp. 130 f. ● E. Lipiński 1975, esp. pp. 268–69 ● E. Lipiński 1978a, esp. pp. 252–53 ● B. Porten 1987.

List of Names (end 5th c.)   TADC4.5

> Fragment containing list of nine names of men. Cairo Museum

Ed. Pr.   *APO*, pap. 21, p. 92, pl. 23.

EASY ACCESS
> Editions: *AP* 19 ● *APE* 23.

> Translations: *DAE* 57 ● *JEAS* V.2.

LITERATURE
> B. Porten 1987, esp. p. 77.

List of Names (end 5th c.)   TADC4.6

> Fragment with fifteen names. Cairo Museum

Ed. Pr.   *APO*, pap. 20, pp. 90–91, pl. 23.

EASY ACCESS
> Editions: *AP* 23 ● *APE* 22.

> Translations: *DAE* 58 ● *JEAS* V.3.

LITERATURE
> H. Torczyner 1912, esp. p. 402 • B. Porten 1987, esp. p. 78.

List of Names (end 5th c.)   TADC4.7
>   Fragmentary. Staatliche Museen, Berlin (P. 13482).

Ed. Pr.   *APO*, pap. 23, p. 93, pl. 23.

EASY ACCESS
> Editions: *AP* 51 • *APE* 24.

LITERATURE
> B. Porten 1987, esp. pp. 77–78.

List of Names (end 5th c.)   TADC4.8
>   Fragmentary. Cairo Museum (J. 13481).

Ed. Pr.   *APO*, pap. 24, pp. 95–96, pl. 24.

EASY ACCESS
> Editions: *AP* 53 • *APE* 26.

> Translations: *DAE* 59.

List of Names [Pap. Borgianus] (end 5th c.)   TADC4.9
>   Fragmentary. Rome, Sacra Congregatio de Propaganda Fide.

Ed. Pr.   J. Euting 1885a, p. 671.

EASY ACCESS
> Editions: *AP* 74 • *CIS* 148.

> Illustrations: *CIS* pl. 15.

LITERATURE
> E. Ledrain 1884b, esp. pp. 30–32 • S. de Ricci 1906, esp. p. 27.

B.3.c.16 Papyrus Luparensis (422?)   TADC3.12
>   Fragmentary log book of wine rations. Louvre.

Ed. Pr. J. J. L. Bargès 1862.

EASY ACCESS
Editions: *AP* 72 • *CIS* 146 • *NSI* 77.

Illustrations: *CIS* pl. 17.

Translations: *DAE* 12.

LITERATURE
C. Clermont-Ganneau 1879, esp. pp. 24–25 • F. Praetorius 1881, esp. p. 444 • W. Groff 1888 • W. Groff 1889 • C. J. M. de Vogüé 1889 • S. de Ricci 1906, esp. p. 26 • B. Porten 1990, esp. pp. 30–31.

B.3.c.17 Account (300?) TADC3.28

A merchant's register of accounts. Bodleian Library (Aram. a.1[P]).

Ed. Pr. A. H. Sayce and A. E. Cowley 1907 + 6 pls.

EASY ACCESS
Editions: *AaG*Seg 47 • *AP* 81.

Translations: *DAE* 13.

B.3.c.18 Harrow School Papyrus (300?) TADC3.27

A column of accounts. England, Harrow School Museum.

Ed. Pr. A. E. Cowley 1923 (*AP* 83), pp. 202–203.

LITERATURE
B. Porten 1990, esp. p. 27.

Elephantine: Ostraca

B.3.c.19 Vienna Ostracon I (475?) ViennaOstr.1

Fragmentary letter concerning bread. Vienna, National Museum (A. O. 2).

Ed. Pr.   R. Degen 1978b (*NESE* 3), pp. 34–39 + drawing, photo.

B.3.c.20 Passover Ostracon (end 5th c.) PassOst

Letter concerning the care of children and arrangements for the Passover. Bodleian Museum (44030).

Ed. Pr.   A. H. Sayce 1911b.

EASY ACCESS
   Editions: *RES* 1793.

   Translations: *DAE* 94.

LITERATURE
   A. H. Sayce 1912 • A. Schollmeyer 1912 • S. Daiches 1912 • J. Halévy 1912d • A. Cowley 1915a, esp. pp. 222–23 • G. R. Driver 1935, esp. p. 56 • E. L. Sukenik and J. [E.Y.] Kutscher 1942 • A. Dupont-Sommer 1946–47(b) • S. Talmon 1958, esp. p. 73.

B.3.c.21 Passover Ostracon 2 (end 5th c.) APO77.2

Fragmentary letter mentioning Passover and an exchange of letters. Staatliche Museen, Berlin (P. 10679).

Ed. Pr.   *ESE* 2.229–34 + photo.

EASY ACCESS
   Editions: *APE* 77/2 • *APO* 77/2 • *ESE* 3. 257, n. 1 • *RAO* 8. 133 • *RES* 1792.

   Illustrations: *APO* 64/2.

   Translations: *DAE* 93.

LITERATURE
   J. Halévy 1911a, esp. pp. 487–88 • S. A. Cook 1915, esp. p. 357 • G. R. Driver 1935, esp. p. 58 • A. Vincent 1937, esp. pp. 267–69 • A. Dupont-Sommer 1946–47(b).

B.3.c.22 Ostracon to Uriah and Aḥutab (end 5th c.)   APO76.1

Letter to Uriah concerning the shearing of a sheep and to Aḥutab concerning bread. Cairo Museum

Ed. Pr.   *APO* 76/1, pp. 233–34, pl. 63/1.

EASY ACCESS
Editions: *AC* 36 • *APE* 76/1.

Translations: *DAE* 95.

LITERATURE
F. Perles 1911–12, esp. p. 14:503 • J. C. Greenfield 1960 • M. Dahood 1960a.

B.3.c.23 Aḥuṭab Ostracon (end 5th c.)   APO78.2

A fragmentary letter to Aḥuṭab. Staatliche Museen, Berlin (P. 10680).

Ed. Pr.   *ESE* 2.234–36 + photo.

EASY ACCESS
Editions: *APE* 78/2 • *APO* 78/2 • *ESE* 3.257, n. 1 • *RAO* 8.135 • *RES* 1795.

Illustrations: *APO* pl. 65/2.

LITERATURE
J. N. Epstein 1913, esp. p. 234 • R. Weill 1913.

B.3.c.24 Munich Ostracon 1 (end 5th c.)   MunichOstr.1

Fragmentary letter to Yirpeiah requesting news (?). Munich Museum
(898)

Ed. Pr.   *ESE* 3.21–22 (+ photo).

EASY ACCESS
Editions: *RES* 1298.

B.3.c.25 Munich Ostracon 2   MunichOstr.2

Fragmentary letter concerning a cup, oil, and wood. Munich Museum
(899).

Ed. Pr.   M. Lidzbarski 1915, pp. 20–21 (+ plate).

EASY ACCESS
Editions: *RES* 1299.

B.3.c.26 ABC Ostracon (end 5th c.)   **ABCOstr**
Ostracon with alphabet on one side (52 x 40 mm.). Pontifical Biblical
Institute, Jerusalem.

Ed. Pr.   A. Lemaire and H. Lozachmeur 1977 (+ drawing).

LITERATURE
J. Teixidor 1979, esp. p. 389.

B.3.c.27 Aimé-Giron Ostracon 1 (end 5th c.)   **AGironOstr.1**
Cairo Museum (J. 49635).

Ed. Pr.   N. Aimé-Giron 1926, pp. 23–27.

LITERATURE
G. R. Driver 1945, esp. p. 12 • J. B. Segal 1987, esp. pp. 70–71, pl. 2.

B.3.c.28 Aimé-Giron Ostracon 2 (end 5th c.)   **AGironOstr.2**
Fragmentary letter to Salluwa about a tunic left in the temple of YHW.
Cairo Museum (J. 49624).

Ed. Pr.   N. Aimé-Giron 1926, pp. 27–29.

EASY ACCESS

Translations: *DAE* 90.

LITERATURE
A. Dupont-Sommer 1946–47(a) • A. Dupont-Sommer 1947a.

B.3.c.29 Bodleian Ostracon (end 5th c.)   **BodOstr.1**
Fragmentary letter mentioning the house of El'aqab. Bodleian Library
(Aram. Insc. 4).

Ed. Pr.   A. Cowley and G. B. Gray 1903.

EASY ACCESS
Editions: *APA* Q • *ESE* 2. 243, 402 • *RES* 497 = 1805.

B.3.c.30 Cairo Ostracon 1 (end 5th c.)   **CairoOstr.1**
Letter to Ḥaggai concerning the *marzeaḥ*. Cairo Museum (J. 35468a).

Ed. Pr.   A. H. Sayce 1909a.

EASY ACCESS
      Editions: *AC* 34 ● *ESE* 3.119–21 [facs.] ● *RES* 1295

      Translations: *DAE* 92.

LITERATURE
      J. Starcky 1952 ● J. C. Greenfield 1974b, esp. p. 454 ● J. Naveh 1982, pl. 10A.

B.3.c.31 Cairo Ostracon 2 (end 5th c.)   CairoOstr.2

Anonymous letter requesting that barley and a small cup be sent. Cairo
Museum (J. 35468b).

Ed. Pr.   M. Lidzbarski 1915, p. 122 (+ drawing).

EASY ACCESS
      Editions: *AC* 35 ● *RES* 1296 ● *TA* 3.

      Translations: *DAE* 20.

LITERATURE
      J. Naveh 1982, Fig. 79, p. 86.

B.3.c.32 Cairo Ostracon 3 (end 5th c.)   CairoOstr.3

Incomplete list of names. Cairo Museum (J. 35468c).

1 [...חא רב רוגח
     םלשמ רב היכ
     [....נ]ב בהנ

Ed. Pr.   M. Lidzbarski 1915, p. 122 (+ drawing).

EASY ACCESS
      Editions: *RES* 1297 ● *TA* 4.

B.3.c.33 Clermont-Ganneau Elephantine Ostraca (end 5th c.) ClGan

A collection of about 300 ostraca and fragments originally in the possession of Ch. Clermont-Ganneau. A few have been published; the rest are
due to be published by M. Snyzcer.

Ed. Pr.   16) A. Dupont-Sommer 1948.
                 44) A. Dupont-Sommer 1963.
                 70) A. Dupont-Sommer 1945a.
                 125) H. Lozachmeur 1990.

130, 136, 137) A. Dupont-Sommer 1964 (quotations only).
152) A. Dupont-Sommer 1949b.
167, 175) A. Dupont Sommer 1947a.
169) A. Dupont-Sommer 1941–45.
186) A. Dupont-Sommer 1957.
204) A. Dupont-Sommer 1960a.
228) H. Lozachmeur 1971.
277) A. Dupont-Sommer 1944a.

EASY ACCESS
Editions:　　　70) *AaGSeg* 36.
　　　　　　　152) *AaGSeg* 35 • *AC* 33a • *AH* I/1, II.A.5.
　　　　　　　186) *AC* 33b.

Translations:　70) *ANET* 491 • *DAE* 87.
　　　　　　　44) *DAE* 99.
　　　　　　　152) *DAE* 91.
　　　　　　　169) *DAE* 19.
　　　　　　　277) *ANET* 491 • *DAE* 88.

LITERATURE
44) J. Naveh 1965–66, esp. pp. 157–58 • J. Naveh 1966, esp. pp. 24–25 • K. R. Veenhof 1968, esp. p. 134.

70) A. Dupont-Sommer 1947a, esp. p. 4 • J. C. Greenfield 1971b, esp. p. 266.

152) A. Dupont-Sommer 1945 • A. Dupont-Sommer 1946–47 • A. Dupont-Sommer 1960a, esp. pp. 71–75 • J. Teixidor 1971, esp. p. 480 • S. Segert 1975, esp. pp. 440, 441.

186) A. Dupont-Sommer 1947a, esp. pp. 178–81 • A. Dupont-Sommer 1957.

228) J. Teixidor 1973, esp. p. 430.

B.3.c.34　Cowley Ostracon 1 (end 5th c.)　　　　　CowleyOstr

Letter to the writer's mother, קוליה. Cambridge University Library (131–33).

Ed. Pr.　　　A. Cowley 1929.

EASY ACCESS

Translations:　*DAE* 23.

LITERATURE
S. Daiches 1929 • J. Teixidor 1973, esp. pp. 430–31.

B.3.c.35 Segal Ostracon   **SegalOstr**
British Museum (133028).

Ed. Pr.   J. B. Segal 1969.

LITERATURE
J. Teixidor 1970a, esp. p. 373.

B.3.c.36 Uriah Ostracon (end 5th c.)   **APE.91**
Letter concerning salary, *qpr'*, *ḥnt'*, and marking a runaway slave.
Bodleian Library (Aram. Insc. 1).

Ed. Pr.   A. Cowley and G. B. Gray 1903, pp. 264–66.

EASY ACCESS
Editions: *APA* M • *APE* 91 • *ESE* 2.236–41 • *RAO* 6.158–62, 7:240, 8:141,
133 • *RES* 492 = 1800.

Translations: *DAE* 22.

LITERATURE
A. H. Sayce 1903, esp. p. 316 • J. Halévy 1904 • A. H. Sayce 1908 • N. Herz
1908–9, esp. p. 233.

B.3.c.37 Cucumber Ostracon (end 5th c.)   **APE.92**
Broken letter mentioning cucumber seed. Bodleian (Aram. Insc. 2).

Ed. Pr.   A. Cowley and G. B. Gray 1903, pp. 311–12.

EASY ACCESS
Editions: *APA* N • *APE* 92 • *ESE* 2. 241, 401 • *RAO* 8. 141 • *RES* 493 =
1801.

LITERATURE
A. H. Sayce 1903 • A. Cowley 1915a, esp. p. 221.

B.3.c.38 Ismun-Ṣeḥo Ostracon (end 5th c.)   **APE.94**
Fragmentary ostracon, possibly containing a deposition. British Museum
(14219).

Ed. Pr.   *CIS* II pp. 139–40 (No. 138), pl. 12.

EASY ACCESS
Editions: *APE* 94 • *ESE* 2. 242 • *KAI* 271 • *NESE* 1. 23–37 • *NSI* 74 • *RES*
495 = 1803.

Illustrations: *NESE* 1, pl. 2.

LITERATURE
A. Cowley and G. B. Gray 1903, esp. p. 313 • S. de Ricci 1906, esp. p. 33 • J. Teixidor 1973, esp. p. 430.

B.3.c.39 Golenischeff Ostracon I (end 5th c.)   APE.96
Fragmentary list of names. Golenischeff Collection. Leningrad.

Ed. Pr.   *CIS* II pp. 176–77 (No. 155), pl. 20.

EASY ACCESS
Editions: *APE* 96.

LITERATURE
S. de Ricci 1906, esp. p. 34.

B.3.c.40 Golenischeff Ostracon II (end 5th c.)   APE.97
List of names. Golenischeff Collection. Leningrad.

Ed. Pr.   *CIS* II pp. 175–76 (No. 154), pl. 20.

EASY ACCESS
Editions: *APE* 97.

LITERATURE
S. de Ricci 1906, esp. p. 34.

B.3.c.41 ḤWNY Ostracon (end 5th c.)   APO76.2
Fragmentary letter mentioning *ḥwny* and *rtwny*. Cairo Museum.

Ed. Pr.   *APO* 76/2, pp. 234–35, pl. 63/2.

EASY ACCESS
Editions: *APE* 76/2.

B.3.c.42 Maḥseiah Ostracon (end 5th c.)   APO77.1
Fragmentary letter mentioning oil for Maḥseiah. Staatliche Museen, Berlin (P. 8763).

Ed. Pr.   A. Cowley and G. B. Gray 1903, p. 314.

EASY ACCESS
Editions: *APA* P • *APO* 77/1 • *ESE* 2. 243 • *RES* 496(A), 1804(B).

Illustrations: *APO* pl. 64/1.

B.3.c.43 Meshullak Ostracon (end 5th c.)   APO84.7

Fragmentary letter mentioning *mšlk*. Staatliche Museen, Berlin (P. 11379).

Ed. Pr. *APO* 84/7, p. 250, pl. 71/7.

B.3.c.44 Strasbourg Ostracon 1 (end 5th c.)   StrasbourgOstr.1

A letter to Leptines from Abiytay. Strasbourg Library.

Ed. Pr. *ESE* 3.23–25 + plate.

EASY ACCESS
Editions: *AaG*Seg 46 • *AC* 37 • *RES* 1300.

Translations: *DAE* 24.

B.3.c.45 Strasbourg Ostracon 2 (end 5th c.)   StrasbourgOstr.2

A broken list of names and numbers. Strasbourg Library.

Ed. Pr. *ESE* 3.25–26.

EASY ACCESS
Editions: *RES* 1301.

B.3.c.46 Strasbourg Ostracon 3 (end 4th c.)   StrasbourgOstr.3

Fragmentary list or receipt (?). Strasbourg Library.

Ed. Pr. *ESE* 3.299–301 + drawing.

B.3.c.47 Dream Ostracon (ca. 300)   DreamOstr

Enigmatic letter concerning a dream. Staatliche Museen, Berlin (P. 1137).

Ed. Pr. J. Euting 1887.

EASY ACCESS
Editions: *AC* 51 • *APE* 78/3 • *APO* 78/3 • *CIS* 137 • *KAI* 270 • *NSI* 73 • *TSSI* 26.

Translations: *DAE* 21.

Illustrations:　　*CIS* pl. 12 ● *KAI* pl. 25 ● *TSSI* pl. 8/2.

LITERATURE
G. Hoffmann 1896, esp. pp. 223–24 ● S. de Ricci 1906, esp. p. 33 ● A. Dupont-Sommer 1948, esp. pp. 117–30 ● B. A. Levine 1964 ● J. Teixidor 1967, esp. p. 178 ● B. Porten 1968, esp. p. 275.

B.3.c.48　Fragmentary Ostraca (5th c.)

Ostraca too fragmentary or illegible to yield a connected context.

Aimé-Giron Ostracon 3　　　　　　　　　　　　　　　　　AGironOstr.3

Ed. Pr.　　　　N. Aimé-Giron 1926, pp. 29–31.

APE 93　　　　　　　　　　　　　　　　　　　　　　　　　APE.93
Bodleian Library (Aram. Insc. 3).

Ed. Pr.　　　　A. Cowley and G. B. Gray 1903, p. 312.

EASY ACCESS
Editions:　　　*APA* O ● *APE* 93 ● *ESE* 2.241, 402 ● *RES* 494 = 1802.

APE 95　　　　　　　　　　　　　　　　　　　　　　　　　APE.95
Fragment of a letter. British Museum (14220).

Ed. Pr.　　　　*CIS* II, pp. 141–42 (No. 139), pl. 12.

EASY ACCESS
Editions:　　　*APE* 95.

LITERATURE
S. de Ricci 1906, esp. p. 34.

APO 76/3　　　　　　　　　　　　　　　　　　　　　　　APO76.3
Staatliche Museen, Berlin (P. 11369).

Ed. Pr.　　　　*APO* 76/3, p. 235, pl. 63/3.

EASY ACCESS
Editions:　　　*APE* 76/3.

LITERATURE
J. N. Epstein 1912, esp. p. 138.

APO 76/4   APO76.4
Cairo Museum

Ed. Pr.   *APO* 76/4, pp. 235–36, pl. 63/4.

EASY ACCESS
Editions: *APE* 76/4.

LITERATURE
J. N. Epstein 1913, esp. p. 234.

APO 76/5   APO76.5
                Staatliche Museen, Berlin (P. 11377).

Ed. Pr.   *APO* 76/5, p. 36, pl. 63/5.

EASY ACCESS
Editions: *APE* 76/5.

APO 78/1   APO78.1
                Staatliche Museen, Berlin (P. 11380).

Ed. Pr.   *APO* 78/1, pp. 238–39, pl. 65/1.

EASY ACCESS
Editions: *APE* 78/1.

APO 79/3   APO79.3
                Staatliche Museen, Berlin (P. 11363).

Ed. Pr.   *APO* 79/3, p. 241, pl. 66/3.

APO 79/4   APO79.4
                Staatliche Museen, Berlin (P. 11453).

Ed. Pr.   *APO* 79/4, p. 241, pl. 66/4.

APO 79/5   **APO79.5**

           Staatliche Museen, Berlin (P. 11374).

Ed. Pr.   *APO* 79/5, p. 241, pl. 66/5.

APO 80/1   **APO80.1**

           Staatliche Museen, Berlin (P. 11382).

Ed. Pr.   *APO* 80/1, p. 241, pl. 67/1.

APO 80/2   **APO80.2**

           Staatliche Museen, Berlin (P. 11375).

Ed. Pr.   *APO* 80/2, pp. 241–42, pl. 67/2.

APO 80/3   **APO80.3**

           Staatliche Museen, Berlin (P. 11378).

Ed. Pr.   *APO* 80/3, p. 242, pl. 67/3.

APO 80/6   **APO80.6**

           Cairo Museum

Ed. Pr.   *APO* 80/6, p. 242, pl. 67/6.

APO 80/7   **APO80.7**

           Staatliche Museen, Berlin (P. 11368).

Ed. Pr.   *APO* 80/7, p. 242, pl. 67/7.

EASY ACCESS
      Editions: *APE* 80.

APO 84/5   **APO84.5**

           Staatliche Museen, Berlin (P. 11376).

Ed. Pr.   *APO* 84/5, p. 250, pl. 71/5.

APO 77/1   **APO77.1**

Staatliche Museen, Berlin (P. 8763).

Ed. Pr.   A. Cowley and G. B. Gray 1903, p. 314.

EASY ACCESS
Editions: *APA* P • *APO* 77/1 • *ESE* 2. 243 • *RES* 496 = 1804.

Illustrations: *APO* pl. 64/1.

Elephantine: Miscellaneous Texts

B.3.c.49 Elephantine Jar Inscriptions (end 5th c.)   ElJarI

Sixty-five inscriptions on jars or pieces of jars; 12 are Aramaic, the rest Phoenician. Staatliche Museen, Berlin.

Ed. Pr.   M. Lidzbarski 1912 (+ 6 plates).

EASY ACCESS
Editions: *APO* 82/6, 14c, 15a, 83/4, 84/4, 6, 8b–c, 9a, 11, 85/19, 86/10, 14.

Illustrations: *APO* pls. 70–73.

B.3.c.50 Elephantine Stone 1 (end 5th c.)   ElSt.1

Stone with a list of names. Staatliche Museen, Berlin (P. 11385).

Ed. Pr.   *APO* 79/2, pp. 240–41, pl. 66/2.

(A
ישביה בר מיכיה
אושע בר נתן [....]
חנן בר זכור
שמעיה בר זכור
(B
גמריה בר ישב [...]
מיכיה בר נתן בר אוש[...]

B.3.c.51 Elephantine Stone 2 (end 5th c.)   ElSt.2

Staatliche Museen, Berlin (No. 18502).

לנסנו ברת פחנום

Ed. Pr.   *APO* 87/4, p. 257, pl. 74/4.

EASY ACCESS
Editions: *APE* 87.

B.3.c.52 Elephantine Mummy Label (end 5th c.)   ElMumLab

Wooden mummy label. Staatliche Museen, Berlin (No. 18464).

שבה בר 1
הושע

Ed. Pr.   *APO* 84/13, p. 251, pl. 71/13.

EASY ACCESS
  Editions: *APE* 84/13.

B.3.c.53 Elephantine Wooden Stamp (end 5th c.)   ElWoStamp
Staatliche Museen, Berlin (No. 18462).

להושע 1
בעלידגל

Ed. Pr.   *APO* 84/12, p. 251, pl. 71/12.

EASY ACCESS
  Editions: *APE* 84/12.

LITERATURE
  R. Dussaud 1911, esp. p. 352.

B.3.c.54 Elephantine Wooden Strip (end 5th c.)   ElWoStrip
Object of unknown purpose bearing a proper name. Staatliche Museen, Berlin (No. 19435).

Ed. Pr.   *APO* 81/3, p. 244, pl. 68/3.

B.3.c.55 Papyrus Fragments (5th c.)
28 papyrus fragments of letters, contracts, accounts, and lists in the Staatliche Museen, Berlin.

Papyrus Fragment 1   DegenPapFrag.1

Ed. Pr.   R. Degen 1974b (*NESE* 2), pp. 72–73, pl. 6/21.

LITERATURE
  B. Porten 1988, esp. pp. 23–26 + drawing.

Papyrus Fragment 2   DegenPapFrag.2

Ed. Pr.   R. Degen 1974b (*NESE* 2), pp. 73–74, pl. 6/22.

LITERATURE
  B. Porten 1988, esp. pp. 19–21 + drawing.

Berlin 23103   **TADC3.4**
  Fragmentary account concerning land. Staatliche Museen, Berlin (P. 23103).

Ed. Pr.   R. Degen 1974b (*NESE* 2), pp. 74–78, pl. 6/22.

LITERATURE
  B. Porten 1988, esp. pp. 26–29 + drawing.

Papyrus Fragment 4   **DegenPapFrag.4**

Ed. Pr.   R. Degen 1978c (*NESE* 3), pp. 15–28, pl. 2/5.

LITERATURE
  B. Porten 1988, esp. p. 21.

Papyrus Fragment 5   **DegenPapFrag.5**

Ed. Pr.   R. Degen 1978c (*NESE* 3), p. 28, pl. 2/6.

LITERATURE
  B. Porten 1988, esp. pp. 49–50.

Papyrus Fragment 6   **DegenPapFrag.6**

Ed. Pr.   R. Degen 1978c (*NESE* 3), p. 29, pl. 2/6.

LITERATURE
  B. Porten 1988, esp. p. 52 + drawing.

Papyrus Fragment 7   **DegenPapFrag.7**

Ed. Pr.   R. Degen 1978c (*NESE* 3), pp. 29–31, pl. 2/7.

LITERATURE
  B. Porten 1988, esp. pp. 21–22 + drawing.

Papyrus Fragment 8   **DegenPapFrag.8**

Ed. Pr.   R. Degen 1978c (*NESE* 3), p. 31, pl. 2/8.

LITERATURE
    B. Porten 1988, esp. p. 43 + drawing.

Papyrus Fragments 1–2, 6, 9–13, 15–20, 22–25, 27–28   **MiscPapFrags**

Ed. Pr.   B. Porten 1988.

B.3.d The Arsames Letters

B.3.d.1   The Arsames Letters   TADA6

> Sixteen documents dealing with the affairs of the Persian satrap Arsames
> (Arsham).

LITERATURE

> L. Borchardt 1933 • E. Mittwoch 1939 • G. R. Driver 1949 • J. T. Milik 1954a •
> G. R. Driver 1955 • H. Petschow 1956 • E. Y. Kutscher 1957 • W. Eilers
> 1957–58 • E. Benveniste 1958 • G. Cardascia 1958 • S. Segert 1958c • W. Eilers
> 1962 • J. Harmatta 1963 • F. Altheim and R. Stiehl 1964–69, esp. pp. 2:562–67;
> 4:23, 62–63 • A. Díez Macho 1965 • J. C. Greenfield 1970 • J. D. Whitehead
> 1974 • J. C. Greenfield 1975 • J. D. Whitehead 1978 • J. C. Greenfield 1981a, esp.
> pp. 126–27 • J. C. Greenfield 1982b • M. W. Stolper 1989.

Arsames Papyrus Letter (427)   TADA6.1

> A fragmentary letter from Achaemenes to Arsames. Cairo Museum (J.
> 43466).

Ed. Pr.   *APO*, pap. 4, pp. 34–35, pl. 5.

EASY ACCESS
> Editions: *AP* 17 • *APE* 5.

> Translations: *DAE* 60.

LITERATURE

> E. Meyer 1911, esp. pp. 1042–43 • H. Torczyner 1912, esp. p. 399 • J. N. Epstein
> 1912, esp. p. 128 • S. A. Cook 1915, esp. p. 355 • G. R. Driver 1932, esp. p. 78 •
> B. Porten 1968, esp. pp. 51–52 • J. Naveh 1971c, esp. p. 33 • B. Porten 1980, esp.
> p. 46 • P.-E. Dion 1982b, esp. pp. 529–33, 539, 547–54 • B. Porten 1983b • B.
> Porten 1990, esp. p. 19.

Arsames Boat Repair Letter (411)   TADA6.2

> Arsames authorizes Waḥpremaḥi to have a boat repaired. Cairo
> Museum (J. 43469).

Ed. Pr.   *APO*, pap. 8, pp. 44–49, pl. 8–9.

EASY ACCESS
> Editions: *AP* 26 • *APE* 8.

> Translations: *DAE* 61.

LITERATURE

E. Meyer 1911, esp. pp. 1035–39 • F. Perles 1911–12, esp. pp. 14:498–99, 15:54–55 • A. Büchler 1912 • A. S. Lewis 1912, esp. pp. 210–11 • D. S. Margoliouth 1912, esp. pp. 71–72 • H. Torczyner 1912, esp. pp. 399–400 • J. N. Epstein 1912, esp. p. 128 • D. S. Margoliouth 1912a, esp. pp. 351–53 • J. N. Epstein 1913, esp. pp. 140–43 • J. N. Epstein 1913a, esp. p. 310 • S. A. Cook 1915, esp. p. 360 • G. R. Driver 1932, esp. pp. 79–80 • L. Borchardt 1932, esp. p. 301 • E. Hammershaimb 1955 • B. Porten 1968, esp. p. 57 • P. Grelot 1970b • M. N. Bogolyubov 1971 • J. Naveh 1971c, esp. p. 33, Fig. 6/1 • P. S. Alexander 1978, esp. pp. 158–59, 166–68 • B. Porten 1980, esp. pp. 47–48, pl. p. 103 • P.-E. Dion 1982b, esp. pp. 538, 549, 554, 563 • B. Porten 1990, esp. p. 20.

Arsames Letter 3 (end 5th c.)   TADA6.3

Arsames orders Artavant to have runaway slaves punished. Bodleian Library, Oxford (Pell. Aram. VII).

Ed. Pr.   G. R. Driver 1954, pp. 13–15, no. 3.

EASY ACCESS

Translations: *DAE* 64.

LITERATURE

J. Naveh 1971c, esp. pp. 28–29, Fig. 6/2 • P. S. Alexander 1978, esp. pp. 158–59, 162–64, 167 • P.-E. Dion 1982b, esp. pp. 538, 549–51, 554.

Arsames Letter 2 (end 5th c.)   TADA6.4

Arsames orders Artavant to allow Psamshek to administer a grant of land. Bodleian Library, Oxford (Pell. Aram. XII and part of IV).

Ed. Pr.   G. R. Driver 1954, pp. 12–13, no. 2.

EASY ACCESS

Translations: *DAE* 62.

LITERATURE

H. Cazelles 1955, esp. pp. 90–91 • J. Naveh 1971c, esp. pp. 28–29 • P. S. Alexander 1978, esp. pp. 164, 167 • P.-E. Dion 1982b, esp. pp. 538, 554 • B. Porten and H. Z. Szubin 1985, esp. p. 286 • H. Z. Szubin and B. Porten 1987.

Arsames Letter 1 (end 5th c.) **TADA6.5**

A fragment from Arsames to Artavant concerning his domains. Bodleian Library, Oxford (Pell. Aram. VI).

Ed. Pr. G. R. Driver 1954, pp. 10–12, no. 1.

EASY ACCESS

Translations: *DAE* 63.

LITERATURE
H. Cazelles 1955, esp. p. 90 ● J. Naveh 1971c, esp. pp. 28–29 ● P. S. Alexander 1978, esp. pp. 158–59, 167 ● B. Porten 1979, esp. pl. p. 94 ● P.-E. Dion 1982b, esp. p. 538.

Arsames Letter 5frg (end 5th c.) **TADA6.6**

A fragment from Arsames concerning his domains. Bodleian Library, Oxford (Pell. Aram. fragment V).

Ed. Pr. G. R. Driver 1954, pp. 17–20, 12–13, nos. 3.1 + 2.5.

LITERATURE
B. Porten 1979, esp. p. 96.

Arsames Letter 5 (end 5th c.) **TADA6.7**

Arsames instructs Artahant to have certain Cilician slaves released. Bodleian Library, Oxford (Pell. Aram. IV).

Ed. Pr. G. R. Driver 1954, pp. 17–20, no. 5.

EASY ACCESS
Editions: *AH* I/1, II.A.2.

Translations: *DAE* 66.

LITERATURE
W. Eilers 1954–56, esp. p. 330 ● H. Cazelles 1955, esp. pp. 91–93, fig. 2 ● J. Naveh 1971c, esp. pp. 28–29, Fig. 6/3 ● S. Segert 1975, esp. p. 439 ● P. S. Alexander 1978, esp. pp. 158–59, 162–63, 167 ● B. Porten 1979, esp. p. 94 ● P.-E. Dion 1982b, esp. pp. 538, 550, 552, 554, 563 ● J. Naveh 1982, pl. 9.

Arsames Letter 4 (end 5th c.)   **TADA6.8**

Arsames commands Armapiya to comply with Psamshek's orders. Bodleian Library, Oxford (Pell. Aram. II).

Ed. Pr.   G. R. Driver 1954, pp. 16–17, no. 4.

EASY ACCESS
Editions: *AaG*Seg 38.

Translations: *DAE* 65.

LITERATURE
H. Cazelles 1955, esp. p. 91 • J. J. Rabinowitz 1960, esp. pp. 73–74 • J. Naveh 1971c, esp. pp. 28–29, Fig. 6/2 • P. S. Alexander 1978, esp. pp. 164, 166–67 • J. Teixidor 1979, esp. pp. 356–57 • P.-E. Dion 1982b, esp. pp. 538, 549–54.

Arsames Letter 6 (end 5th c.)   **TADA6.9**

Arsames commands various officials to supply rations for Nakhthor and his party. Bodleian Library, Oxford (Pell. Aram. VIII).

Ed. Pr.   G. R. Driver 1954, pp. 20–23, no. 6.

EASY ACCESS
Editions: *AaG*Seg 37.

Translations: *DAE* 67.

LITERATURE
W. Eilers 1954–56, esp. pp. 330–31, pl. 1 • H. Cazelles 1955, esp. pp. 93–94 • J. Naveh 1971c, esp. pp. 28–29 • P. S. Alexander 1978, esp. p. 164 • P.-E. Dion 1982b, esp. pp. 538, 554, 566.

Arsames Letter 7 (end 5th c.)   **TADA6.10**

Arsames admonishes Nakhthor to preserve and augment his Egyptian estates. Bodleian Library, Oxford (Pell. Aram. I).

Ed. Pr.   G. R. Driver 1954, pp. 25–28, no. 8.

EASY ACCESS
Editions: *AH* I/1, II.A.3.

Translations: *DAE* 68.

LITERATURE
E. Y. Kutscher 1945 ● H. Cazelles 1955, esp. p. 94 ● D. Diringer and R. Regensburger 1968, pl. 2.187c ● J. Naveh 1971c, esp. pp. 28–29, Fig. 6/4 ● S. A. Kaufman 1974, esp. p. 101 ● S. Segert 1975, esp. pp. 437, 439 ● P. S. Alexander 1978, esp. pp. 158–59, 164, 166–67 ● P.-E. Dion 1982b, esp. pp. 538, 550, 554.

Arsames Letter 8 (end 5th c.) TADA6.11

Arsames instructs his officials to respect the hereditary lease of land of Petosiri. Bodleian Library, Oxford (Pell. Aram. XIII).

Ed. Pr. G. R. Driver 1954, pp. 25–28, no. 8.

EASY ACCESS
Editions: *AC* 30.

Translations: *ANET* 633 ● *DAE* 69.

LITERATURE
M. Kamil 1948 ● H. Cazelles 1955, esp. p. 94 ● K. A. Kitchen 1965a ● H. L. Ginsberg 1969, esp. p. 633 ● J. Naveh 1971c, esp. pp. 28–29 ● S. A. Kaufman 1974, esp. pp. 54–55, 78 ● S. Segert 1975, esp. p. 439 ● P. S. Alexander 1978, esp. pp. 158–59, 164, 166–67 ● P.-E. Dion 1982b, esp. pp. 538, 549, 552, 554, 563 ● B. Porten and H. Z. Szubin 1985, esp. pp. 284–87.

Arsames Letter 9 (end 5th c.) TADA6.12

Arsames instructs his officials to have certain statues made and sent to him. Bodleian Library, Oxford (Pell. Aram. III).

Ed. Pr. G. R. Driver 1954, pp. 28–29, no. 9.

EASY ACCESS
Editions: *AaG*Seg 39 ● *AH* I/1, II.A.4.

Translations: *DAE* 70.

LITERATURE
H. Cazelles 1955, esp. p. 95 ● K. A. Kitchen 1965a, esp. pp. 158–60 ● J. Naveh 1971c, esp. pp. 28–29 ● S. A. Kaufman 1974, esp. p. 78 ● S. Segert 1975, esp. p. 439 ● P. S. Alexander 1978, esp. pp. 158–59, 166–67 ● P.-E. Dion 1982b, esp. pp. 538, 552.

Arsames Letter 10 (end 5th c.) TADA6.13

Arsames instructs his representatives to see to it that the income from Varuvahya's estates is forwarded. Bodleian Library, Oxford (Pell. Aram. IX).

Ed. Pr.   G. R. Driver 1954, pp. 29–31, no. 10.

EASY ACCESS

Translations: *DAE* 71.

LITERATURE
H. Cazelles 1955, esp. p. 95 • K. A. Kitchen 1965a, esp. pp. 160–61 • J. Naveh 1971c, esp. pp. 28–29 • S. Segert 1975, esp. p. 438 • P. S. Alexander 1978, esp. pp. 158–59, 166–67 • P.-E. Dion 1982b, esp. pp. 538, 549–51.

Arsames Letter 11 (end 5th c.)   **TADA6.14**
Varuvahya asks Arsames' representatives to send the income from his estates (see 6.13). Bodleian Library, Oxford (Pell. Aram. V).

Ed. Pr.   G. R. Driver 1954, pp. 31–33, no. 11.

EASY ACCESS

Translations: *DAE* 72.

LITERATURE
W. Eilers 1954–56, esp. p. 331 • H. Cazelles 1955, esp. p. 95 • J. Naveh 1971c, esp. pp. 28–29 • P. S. Alexander 1978, esp. pp. 158–59, 167 • P.-E. Dion 1982b, esp. p. 538.

Arsames Letter 12 (end 5th c.)   **TADA6.15**
Varpish orders Nakhthor to release certain detained Cilicians and to return misappropriated property. Bodleian Library, Oxford (Pell. Aram. XIV).

Ed. Pr.   G. R. Driver 1954, pp. 33–35, no. 12.

EASY ACCESS

Translations: *DAE* 73.

LITERATURE
H. Cazelles 1955, esp. pp. 95–96 • J. Naveh 1971c, esp. pp. 28–29 • J. C. Greenfield 1975, esp. pp. 312–13 • P. S. Alexander 1978, esp. pp. 158–59, 167 • B. Porten 1979, esp. pl. p. 93 • P.-E. Dion 1982b, esp. p. 538.

Arsames Letter 13 (end 5th c.)   **TADA6.16**

> Artaḥaya complains to Nakhthor that the wrong goods were sent. Bodleian Library, Oxford (Pell. Aram. X).

Ed. Pr.   G. R. Driver 1954, pp. 35–36, no. 13.

EASY ACCESS
> Editions: *AaG*Seg 40.

> Translations: *DAE* 74.

LITERATURE
> H. Cazelles 1955, esp. pp. 96–97 • J. Naveh 1971c, esp. pp. 28–29 • S. Segert 1975, esp. p. 439 • P. S. Alexander 1978, esp. pp. 164, 167 • B. Porten 1979, esp. pl. p. 94–95 • P.-E. Dion 1982b, esp. p. 538 • M. O. Wise 1990, esp. p. 253.

B.3.e Memphis/Saqqarah

B.3.e.1 Saqqarah Ostracon (6th c.)   SaqOstr
Ostracon in two fragments (13 x 12 mm).

1 לפסמשך בר [...]
רב כצרא

Ed. Pr.   N. Aimé-Giron 1931 (*TA* 2), pp. 4–5, pl. 1.

LITERATURE
J. B. Segal 1987, esp. p. 70, pl. 1.

B.3.e.2 Saqqarah Baal Stele (end 6th c.)   SaqBaalStel
Limestone block (20 x 16 cm.).

1 לאנן בר אליש
כמרא זי
בעל בעל ענות

Ed. Pr.   A. Dupont-Sommer 1956.

EASY ACCESS
Editions: *TA* 110*bis*.

Translations: *DAE* 77.

B.3.e.3 Memphis Name List (5th c.)   TADC4.3
List of names. Cairo Museum (J. 50056).

Ed. Pr.   N. Aimé-Giron 1931 (*TA* 46, 50, 25, 47, 26, 30, 33, 61, 75), pp. 37–40,
43–44, 48–49, 51, 54, pls. 6–8.

B.3.e.4 Memphis Papyrus 3 (5th c.)   MemPap.3
List of names. Cairo Museum (J. 50056).

Ed. Pr.   N. Aimé-Giron 1931 (*TA* 27), pp. 40–41, pl. 6.

B.3.e.5 Memphis Papyrus 4 (5th c.)   MemPap.4
List of names. Cairo Museum (J. 50056).

Ed. Pr.   N. Aimé-Giron 1931 (*TA* 28), p. 42, pl. 6.

B.3.e.6   Memphis Shipyard Journal (472–71)   TADC3.7
Papyrus journal fragments from the Memphis dockyard.

Ed. Pr.   N. Aimé-Giron 1931 (*TA* 5–24), pp. 12–37, pl. 2–5.

LITERATURE
R. A. Bowman 1941a • B. Porten 1990, esp. pp. 28–30.

B.3.e.7   Memphis Ointment Jar (451)   MemOJar
Alabaster vase. British Museum.

ב 3 לפחנס שנת 13 ארתחששש מלכא

Ed. Pr.   E. Bresciani 1958a.

LITERATURE
J. Naveh 1967–68 • J. Naveh 1968a, esp. p. 317 + Fig. 2 • M. Silverman 1969a •
M. Silverman 1969b.

B.3.e.8   Memphis Libation Altar (5th–4th c.)   MemLibAlt
Limestone altar with votive inscription (30 x 59 cm.). Louvre.

Ed. Pr.   M. le duc de Luynes 1855.

EASY ACCESS
Editions: *CIS* 123 • *HNE* 448 • *KAI* 268 • *NSI* 72.

Illustrations: *CIS* pl. 12 • *HNE* pl. 28/2.

Translations: *DAE* 84.

LITERATURE
E. Renan 1856 • H. Ewald 1856 • J. Bargès 1856 • H. Ewald 1856–57, esp. p. 57
• H. Ewald 1856a, esp. pp. 134–37 • M. A. Levy 1857a, esp. pp. 65–73 • A.-C.
Judas 1858–59 • A. Merx 1868, esp. pp. 693–96 • [J.] Lauth 1878, esp. pp.
131–38 • C. Clermont-Ganneau 1879, esp. pp. 37–39 • F. Praetorius 1881, esp. p.
442 • C. Clermont-Ganneau 1883, esp. pp. 415–18 • E. Ledrain 1884a, esp. pp.
21–22 • P. Berger 1891, esp. pp. 213–14 • S. de Ricci 1906, esp. pp. 30–31 • E.
Lipiński 1977, esp. p. 111.

B.3.e.9   Ptah Stele (5th c.)   MemStel

Painted stela bearing an Egyptian text and a short Aramaic inscription.
Cairo, Michaelidis Collection.

חרמן
וכנוהי פטאסי
בר אשע אתה
למנפי קדם פתח

Ed. Pr.   Y. Leibovitz 1956 + photo.

LITERATURE
   J. Naveh 1968, esp. p. 317 + Fig. 1.

B.3.e.10   Memphis Wooden Jar (5th–4th c.)   MemWoJar

משחאל כמרא זי ענת

Ed. Pr.   E. Bresciani 1958.

B.3.e.11   Memphis Plaque (403?)   MemPlaque

A triangular plaque bearing two identical lines, one in ink, the other
incised. Ashmolean Museum (Aram. O. 1).

ב 20+3+1 לאב שנת 2 ארתחשסס

Ed. Pr.   A. Cowley 1909.

LITERATURE
   A. Lemaire 1987a, esp. pp. 52–55 + photo.

B.3.e.12   Memphis Wooden Tablet (4th c.)   MemWoTab

Wooden account tablet with lists of names and commodities. Michaelidis Collection.

Ed. Pr.   E. Bresciani 1958.

LITERATURE
   J. T. Milik 1958–59, esp. p. 335, n. 7 ● G. Garbini 1967a, esp. pp. 95–96 ● J.
   Naveh 1968, esp. p. 321 + Fig. 6 ● M. Silverman 1969a ● M. Silverman 1969b.

B.3.e.13 Family List (?)   TADC3.10
Fragmentary list of family units. Staatliche Museen, Berlin (P. 23128–34).

Ed. Pr.   B. Porten 1988.

B.3.e.14 Papyrus Fragment 1 (5th c.)   TADC4.1
Fragmentary list of names.

Ed. Pr.   N. Aimé-Giron 1921.

EASY ACCESS
    Editions: *AP* App. A.

B.3.e.15 Papyrus Fragment 2 (5th c.)   TADC3.5
Fragmentary government accounts.

Ed. Pr.   N. Aimé-Giron 1921.

EASY ACCESS
    Editions: *AP* App. B–C.

B.3.e.16 Saqqarah Papyrus Letter (436–35)   TADA5.1
Fragmentary semi-official letter composed of three fragments. Académie des Inscriptions, Paris.

Ed. Pr.   M. Sznycer 1971, pl. 1–2.

EASY ACCESS
    Editions: *RAO* 6. 255–57 • *RES* 1808 + 1809 + 1810.

LITERATURE
    B. Porten 1983a.

B.3.e.17 Saqqarah Papyrus Fragment 4 (436)   SaqPapFrag.4
Fragment

Ed. Pr.   Ch. Clermont-Ganneau 1905 (*RAO* 6), esp. p. 256.

EASY ACCESS
    Editions: *RES* 1807.

B.3.3.18　Saqqarah Papyrus Fragment 5 (mid 5th c.)　　SaqPapFrag.5
Fragment containing part of the greeting formula of a letter.

Ed. Pr.　　　　　N. Aimé-Giron 1939a (No. 122), pp. 339–43 + photo.

B.3.3.19　Saqqarah Ptah Tomb Papyrus (mid 5th c.)　　SaqPtahTomb
Papyrus fragment with administrative text found in a grave. Cairo Museum (J. 36449).

Ed. Pr.　　　　　A. H. Sayce and A. E. Cowley 1906.

EASY ACCESS
　　Editions:　　　*ESE* 3.128–29 • *RES* 1791.

B.3.3.20　Saqqarah Plate (mid–5th c.)　　　　　　　SaqPlt
Stone plate found with a mummy.

לתאשר

Ed. Pr.　　　　　N. Aimé-Giron 1939 (No. 118), pp. 46–47 + drawing.

LITERATURE
　　E. Lipiński 1977, esp. pp. 104–10.

B.3.3.21　Saqqarah Wooden Fragment (mid 5th c.)　　SaqWoodFrag
Fragmentary wooden cross-bar (21.5 x 8.5 cm.). Cairo Museum (J. 63380).

עבד רֹ[......]

Ed. Pr.　　　　　N. Aimé-Giron 1939 (No. 115), p. 43, pl. 3.

B.3.3.22　Saqqarah Funerary Stele (482)　　　　　　SaqStel
Limestone stele with funerary text and reliefs. Formerly in the Staatliche Museen, Berlin; now destroyed.

Ed. Pr.　　　　　R. Lepsius and J. Euting 1877.

EASY ACCESS
　　Editions:　　　*AC* 21 • *CIS* 122 • *HNE* 448 • *KAI* 267 • *NSI* 71 • *TSSI* 23.

　　Translations:　*DAE* 85.

　　Illustrations:　*CIS* pl. 11 • *HNE* pl. 28/1.

LITERATURE
>
> W. Wright 1875–83, pl. LXIII (photo) • [J.] Lauth 1878, esp. pp. 97–115 • A. Mariette 1880 • F. Praetorius 1881, esp. pp. 442–44 • S. de Ricci 1906, esp. p. 30 • M. Burchardt 1911, esp. pp. 73–74 • S. A. Cook 1915, esp. p. 251 • B. Porten 1990, esp. p. 28.

B.3.e.23　Saqqarah Mummy Labels (5th c.)　　　　　　SaqMumLab

> Three wooden mummy labels. Michaelidis Collection.

Ed. Pr.　　　　E. Bresciani 1958.

LITERATURE
>
> J. Naveh 1967–68 • J. Naveh 1968a, esp. p. 321 + Figs. 3–5 • M. Silverman 1969a • M. Silverman 1969b, esp. p. 193.

B.3.e.24　North Saqqarah Papyri (5th–4th c.)　　　　　NSaqPap

> A collection of 202 fragmentary papyri. Of the texts that yield a connected context, most deal with legal or commercial matters. The larger papyri that have been re-edited and re-published in *TADB* and *TADC* are listed separately below.

Ed. Pr.　　　　J. B. Segal 1983a (+ 38 plates).

North Saqqarah Papyrus 35　　　　　　　　　　　　TADB4.7

> Cairo Museum (No. 1565).

Ed. Pr.　　　　J. B. Segal 1983a, pp. 53–54, pl. 8.

LITERATURE
>
> P. Swiggers 1981b, esp. pp. 127–28 • J. Teixidor 1985, esp. p. 733 • J. Naveh 1985c, esp. p. 211 • R. Zadok 1985c, esp. p. 175 • J. A. Fitzmyer 1986, esp. p. 543.

Sale of Slaves　　　　　　　　　　　　　　　　　TADB5.6

> Cairo Museum (No. 1576).

Ed. Pr.　　　　J. B. Segal 1983a, pp. 22–25, pl. 2.

LITERATURE
>
> J. Teixidor 1985, esp. p. 733 • J. Blau 1985–86, esp. p. 217 • J. Naveh 1985c, esp. p. 211 • R. Zadok 1985c, esp. p. 174 • S. Shaked 1987, esp. p. 409.

North Saqqarah Papyrus 29   **TADB8.1**
>   Report or court record. Cairo Museum (No. 1592).

Ed. Pr.   J. B. Segal 1983a, pp. 48–49, pl. 6.

LITERATURE
>   R. Zadok 1985c, esp. pp. 174–75 • R. Zadok 1986, esp. p. 42.

North Saqqarah Papyrus 10+44   **TADB8.2**
>   Court record regarding slaves. Cairo Museum (Nos. 1567 + 1566).

Ed. Pr.   J. B. Segal 1983a, pp. 27–29, pl. 2 + pp. 62–64, pl. 11.

LITERATURE
>   J. W. Wesselius 1984b, esp. p. 703 • E. Ullendorff 1985 • J. Teixidor 1985, esp. p.
>   733 • R. Zadok 1985c, esp. p. 175 • J. Oelsner 1988, esp. p. 182 • B. Porten 1990,
>   esp. p. 28.

North Saqqarah Papyrus 5   **TADB8.3**
>   Court record regarding slaves. Cairo Museum (No. 1564).

Ed. Pr.   J. B. Segal 1983a, pp. 19–20, pl. 2.

LITERATURE
>   K. T. Zauzich 1985, esp. p. 115 • R. Zadok 1985c, esp. p. 174 • R. Zadok 1986,
>   esp. p. 43 • S. Shaked 1987, esp. p. 409.

North Saqqarah Papyrus 28+30+61 (431)   **TADB8.4**
>   Court record regarding assault. Cairo Museum (Nos. 1581 + 5926 +
>   5927).

Ed. Pr.   J. B. Segal 1983a, pp. 45–48, pl. 6 + pp. 49–50, pl. 7 + pp. 83–84, pl.
                   15.

LITERATURE
>   J. W. Wesselius 1984b, esp. p. 703 • J. Teixidor 1985, esp. pp. 732–33 • R. Zadok
>   1985c, esp. pp. 174–75 • R. Zadok 1986, esp. p. 42 • B. Porten 1990, esp. p. 27 •
>   S. Shaked 1987, esp. p. 409.

North Saqqarah Papyrus 9   **TADB8.6**
>   Three court decisions concerning slave(s), reclaiming valuables, and
>   assault. Cairo Museum (No. 1578).

Ed. Pr.   J. B. Segal 1983a, pp. 25–26, pl. 2.

LITERATURE
   E. Ullendorff 1985 • K. T. Zauzich 1985, esp. p. 116 • J. Naveh 1985c, esp. p. 211
   • R. Zadok 1985c, esp. p. 174 • R. Zadok 1986, esp. pp. 42–43 • S. Shaked 1987,
   esp. pp. 409, 411.

North Saqqarah Papyrus 4   **TADB8.7**
   Court record of interrogation concerning slaves. Cairo Museum (No.
   1577).

Ed. Pr.   J. B. Segal 1983a, pp. 17–19, pl. 1.

LITERATURE
   E. Ullendorff 1985 • J. Teixidor 1985, esp. p. 732 • J. Blau 1985–86, esp. p. 216 •
   J. Naveh 1985c, esp. p. 211 • R. Zadok 1985c, esp. p. 174 • J. A. Fitzmyer 1986,
   esp. pp. 543–44 • S. Shaked 1987, esp. pp. 408–09.

North Saqqarah Papyrus 1   **TADB8.8**
   Record of interrogation. Cairo Museum (No. 1591).

Ed. Pr.   J. B. Segal 1983a, pp. 13–14, pl. 1.

LITERATURE
   J. Teixidor 1985, esp. p. 732 • S. Shaked 1987, esp. pp. 408, 410–11.

North Saqqarah Papyrus 2   **TADB8.9**
   Court record concerning slave, suit, and oath. Cairo Museum (No.
   2203).

Ed. Pr.   J. B. Segal 1983a, pp. 14–15, pl. 1.

LITERATURE
   J. W. Wesselius 1984b, esp. p. 703 • E. Ullendorff 1985 • J. Teixidor 1985, esp. p.
   732 • J. Blau 1985–86, esp. p. 216 • S. Shaked 1987, esp. pp. 408, 412.

North Saqqarah Papyrus 3+16   **TADB8.10**
   Court record concerning a document and fields. Cairo Museum (Nos.
   2200 + 5883).

Ed. Pr.   J. B. Segal 1983a, pp. 15–17, pl. 1 + p. 32, pl. 3.

LITERATURE

J. W. Wesselius 1984b, esp. p. 703 • J. Teixidor 1985, esp. p. 732 • S. Shaked 1987, esp. p. 412.

North Saqqarah Papyrus 21   **TADB8.11**

Court record concerning rent and a blind man (?). Cairo Museum (No. 1911).

Ed. Pr.   J. B. Segal 1983a, pp. 36–37, pl. 5.

LITERATURE

J. W. Wesselius 1984b, esp. p. 703 • J. Naveh 1985c, esp. p. 211 • R. Zadok 1985c, esp. p. 174.

North Saqqarah Papyrus 6   **TADB8.12**

Court record. Cairo Museum (No. 1583).

Ed. Pr.   J. B. Segal 1983a, pp. 20–22, pl. 2.

LITERATURE

E. Ullendorff 1985 • K. T. Zauzich 1985, esp. p. 116.

North Saqqarah Papyrus 47   **TADC3.6**

Fragmentary account of land. Cairo Museum (No. 5881).

Ed. Pr.   J. B. Segal 1983a, pp. 66–67, pl. 11.

North Saqqarah Papyrus 20+19   **TADC3.8**

Fragmentary account of silver. Cairo Museum (Nos. 2212 + 2195).

Ed. Pr.   J. B. Segal 1983a, pp. 35–36, pl. 4 + pp. 34–35, pl. 4.

North Saqqarah Papyrus 45   **TADC3.18**

Fragmentary account of grain and oil. Cairo Museum (No. 2201).

Ed. Pr.   J. B. Segal 1983a, pp. 64–65, pl. 11.

North Saqqarah Papyrus 57   TADC3.20
            Fragment of land registry. Cairo Museum (No. 2215).

Ed. Pr.   J. B. Segal 1983a, p. 81, pl. 14.

LITERATURE
    J. Bargès 1862 ● B. Porten 1990, esp. pp. 30–31.

North Saqqarah Papyrus 48   TADC3.22
            Fragment of land registry. Cairo Museum (No. 1560).

Ed. Pr.   J. B. Segal 1983a, pp. 67–68, pl. 12.

North Saqqarah Papyrus 87   TADC3.23
            Fragment of land registry. Cairo Museum (No. 5891).

Ed. Pr.   J. B. Segal 1983a, p. 102, pl. 23.

North Saqqarah Papyrus 106   TADC3.24
            Fragment of land registry. Cairo Museum (No. 5666).

Ed. Pr.   J. B. Segal 1983a, p. 111, pl. 27.

North Saqqarah Papyrus 53   TADC4.2

Ed. Pr.   J. B. Segal 1983a, pp. 76–77, pl. 13.

B.3.e.25 North Saqqarah Ostraca (5th–4th c.)   NSaqOstr
            Twenty-six inscribed ostraca. Five are Aramaic; the rest Phoenician.

Ed. Pr.   J. B. Segal 1983a, pp. 139–45, pls. 36–38.

B.3.e.26 Bar Pawenesh (Saqqarah, ?)   TADC1.2
            Two large papyrus fragments (now joined!) relating the story of Ḥor bar
            Pawenesh. British Museum.

Ed. Pr.   M. A. Lanci 1827, tab. I–II.

EASY ACCESS
    Editions: *AP* 71 ● *CIS* 145 ● *NSI* 76.

LITERATURE

W. Gesenius 1837, pp. 236–45, pls. 31–33 ● A. Merx 1868, pp. 695–96 ● C. Clermont-Ganneau 1879, pp. 26–27 ● W. Wright 1875–83, pls. XXV–XXVI ● S. R. Driver 1890, pl. III ● S. de Ricci 1906, esp. pp. 25–26 ● G. R. Driver 1932, esp. p. 83 ● B. Porten 1986, esp. pp. 14–16 + photo, drawing ● B. Zuckerman 1987, esp. pp. 31–35 + photo.

B.3.e.27 Saqqarah Sarcophagi (5th–4th c.)   SaqSarcI

Fourteen inscriptions on lids of sarcophagi or other funerary objects.

Ed. Pr.   N. Aimé-Giron 1931 (*TA* 95–106, 108, 112).

EASY ACCESS

Translations: *DAE* 76 (= *TA* 99).

B.3.e.28 Saqqarah Stele Fragment (4th c.)   SaqSteleFrag

Fragment of limestone stele (13.2 x 11 cm.).

גֹרך פטאסיׄ בר יהא]...[

Ed. Pr.   N. Aimè-Giron 1939 (No. 117).

B.3.e.29 Tumma Stele (Saqqarah, 4th c.)   TumStel

Stele with bas-relief and funerary inscription.

ברכה תמא ברת בכרנף לוסרי

Ed. Pr.   C. Clermont-Ganneau 1909.

EASY ACCESS

Editions: *RES* 1788.

LITERATURE

E. de Knevett 1909 ● I. Lévy 1927 ● E. Lipiński 1975c.

B.3.f Varia and of Unknown Egyptian Origin

B.3.f.1 Graffiti   TA.91–4

Graffiti from various locations in Egypt.
1) Rock surface, Abu Simbel.
2–3) Rock surface, between Tomâs and 'Afieh.
4) Flagstone, temple of Karnak.

שמ[...] / רו[...] / שרדלה (1
וע[.]פי בר לוי (2
אכי בר חרזבד (3
קף [.....] (4

Ed. Pr.   N. Aimé-Giron 1931 (*TA* 91–93), pp. 84–89, pl. 12.

B.3.f.2 Sheikh Fadl Tomb (near Oxyrhynchus, 475–450)   ShFTI

Several very fragmentary inscriptions. In situ.

Ed. Pr.   N. Aimé-Giron 1923.

EASY ACCESS
  Editions: *AC* 15.

LITERATURE
  R. Weill 1913 • E. Y. Kutscher 1954, esp. p. 246 • M. E. Sherman 1966 • B. Porten 1968, esp. pp. 16–17 • J. Naveh 1971c, esp. pp. 40–41.

B.3.f.3 Aswan Stele (458)   AswStel

Fragment of a sandstone orthostat (26 x 45 cm.).

Ed. Pr.   C. J. M. de Vogüé 1903.

EASY ACCESS
  Editions: *AC* 22 • *APE* 98 • *ESE* 2.221–23 • *RES* 438 = 1806.

  Translations: *DAE* 75.

LITERATURE
  S. de Ricci 1906, esp. p. 32 • M. H. Pognon 1911, esp. pp. 351 f. • R. A. Parker 1941 • S. H. Horn and L. H. Wood 1954, esp. pp. 10–11 • M. N. Bogolyubov 1966 • J. Teixidor 1969, esp. p. 346 • E. Lipiński 1985a.

B.3.f.4   Aswan Sarcophagi (5th c.)   AswSarc

Three anthropoidal sandstone sarcophagi. Aswan Museum.

(1 שבתי
(2 חור
(3 אברתי ברת שמשנורי

Ed. Pr.   W. Kornfeld 1967 (+ 8 plates).

LITERATURE
K. R. Veenhof 1968, esp. pp. 134–35 • B. Porten 1969, esp. p. 121 • J. Teixidor
1971, esp. p. 480.

B.3.f.5   Mariette Papyrus Fragments (5th c)   TADC3.21

Fragmentary account of land. Cairo Museum.

Ed. Pr.   J. Euting 1887, pp. 408–9, pl. 7.

EASY ACCESS
Editions: *AP* 75 • *CIS* 150.

Illustrations: *CIS* pl. 20.

LITERATURE
C. J. M. de Vogüé 1868, esp. p. 132 • S. de Ricci 1906, esp. p. 27.

B.3.f.6   Abusir Papyri (near Saqqarah, 5th c.)   AbuPapFrag.1–2

Two papyrus fragments with lists. Cairo Museum.

Ed. Pr.   S. de Ricci 1906, p. 28 + drawings.

EASY ACCESS
Editions: *ESE* 3.127–28 • *RES* 1789–90.

B.3.f.7   Serapium Papyrus (5th c.)   SerapiumPap

Small letter fragment. Cairo Museum.

1 [...] שלם מראי
[...ה]עלים חד תמ

Ed. Pr.   J. Euting 1885a.

EASY ACCESS
Editions: *AP* 77 • *CIS* 152.

Illustrations: *CIS* pl. 20.

LITERATURE
S. de Ricci 1906, esp. p. 28.

B.3.f.8   Pontifical Biblical Institute Papyrus (5th c.)   PIBPap

Papyrus fragment (23 x 23 mm.). Pontifical Biblical Institute, Jerusalem.

[...]לאמֹ[...] 1
[...] פֹ[...]
[...]דֹמֹ /// /[...]

Ed. Pr.   A. Lemaire and H. Lozachmeur 1977.

B.3.f.9   Bakenrenef Fragment (5th c.)   BakFrag

Jar fragment found in tomb complex.

מגלת

Ed. Pr.   E. Bresciani 1980.

B.3.f.10   Wadi Hammamath Alphabet (5th c.)   HamAl

West Semitic alphabet incised as a graffito. In situ.

Ed. Pr.   A. Dupont-Sommer 1947.

EASY ACCESS
Editions: *AC* 43 • *NESE* 3. 1–2 (+ drawing).

LITERATURE
G. Goyon 1957, esp. pp. 116–17, pl. XXXV • W. K. Simpson 1959, esp. pp. 35–36 • G. Goyon 1985.

B.3.f.11   Mellawi Mummy Wrapper (mid-5th c.)   MelMWr

Piece of linen mummy bandage. Michaelidis Collection.

חרמנתן בר עשתרנתן

Ed. Pr.   E. Bresciani 1958.

LITERATURE
J. Naveh 1967–68 • J. Naveh 1968a, esp. p. 321, n. 3 + Fig. 2a • M. Silverman 1969a • M. Silverman 1969b.

B.3.f.12 Maskhûṭa Bowls (450–400) Maskh

Four silver bowls bearing votive inscriptions to the goddess Han-'Ilat. Brooklyn Museum.

Ed. Pr.   1–3) I. Rabinowitz 1956.
                   4) I. Rabinowitz 1959.

EASY ACCESS
    Editions: 1) *AC* 44A • *TSSI* 25.
                    2) *AC* 44B.
                    3) *AC* 44C • *AaG*Seg 45.

    Translations: 1) *ANET* 657.
                    2) *DAE* 79.
                    3) *DAE* 78.

LITERATURE
    A. J. Wensinck 1931 • F. M. Cross 1955 • W. F. Albright 1955 • A. M. Honeyman 1960 • J. M. Miller 1969 • W. J. Dumbrell 1971 • J. Teixidor 1972a, esp. p. 439 • A. Lemaire 1989a, esp. p. 102 • E. A. Knauf 1990, esp. p. 207.

B.3.f.13 Cairo Papyrus 3484 (mid 5th c.) TADC3.11

Ed. Pr.   TADC3.

B.3.f.14 Abydos Papyrus (418–7) AbydPap

Papyrus fragment. National Archaeological Museum, Madrid. The authenticity of this papyrus has been questioned; see the discussion in J. Naveh 1968a and J. Teixidor 1972.

Ed. Pr.   J. Teixidor 1964.

EASY ACCESS
    Editions: *TSSI* 29.

    Translations: *DAE* 83.

    Illustrations: *TSSI* fig. 14.

LITERATURE
    J. Teixidor 1964a • F. Vattioni 1965b • J. Naveh 1964–65, esp. p. 191 • J. Naveh 1966, esp. pp. 30–31 • J. Naveh 1967–68 • K. R. Veenhof 1968, esp. pp. 136–37 • J. Naveh 1968a, esp. pp. 321–35 • M. Silverman 1969a • M. Silverman 1969b • J. Teixidor 1972.

B.3.f.15 Turin Papyrus (end 5th c.)   TADA5.3

Fragment containing address and greetings. Turin Museum (Prov. 645).

Ed. Pr.   H. A. Hamaker 1828, tab. III, no. 3.

EASY ACCESS
   Editions: *AC* 52 • *AP* 70 • *CIS* 144 • *RAO* 6. 227, no. 1 • *RES* 1820.

   Illustrations: *CIS* pl. 15.

LITERATURE
   E. F. F. Beer 1833, pl. 1 • W. Gesenius 1837, esp. pp. 233–36, pl. 30 • A. Merx
   1868, pp. 696–97 • C. Clermont-Ganneau 1878 • S. de Ricci 1906, esp. p. 25 • A.
   Dupont-Sommer 1949a, esp. p. 90 • J. Naveh 1971c, esp. p. 36 • P. S. Alexander
   1978, esp. pp. 162 • P.-E. Dion 1982b, esp. pp. 529–32, 547–54.

B.3.f.16 Fragmentary Letter (end 5th c.)   TADA5.4

Four lines mentioning an interrogation and an Egyptian priest. Cairo
Museum (J. 59204).

Ed. Pr.   J. Euting 1885a, p. 670, no. 2a, pl. 6.

EASY ACCESS
   Editions: *AP* 76 • *CIS* 151.

   Illustrations: *CIS* pl. 20, 21.

LITERATURE
   S. de Ricci 1906, esp. p. 28 • J. Naveh 1971c, esp. p. 36.

B.3.f.17 Salt Stele (5th–4th c.)   SaltSt

A single name on a limestone funerary stele acquired by Henry Salt (39
x 31 cm.). Sold at auction in 1902, its present location is unknown.

Ed. Pr.   W. Gesenius 1837, pp. 232–33, pl. 29 (facsimile).

שמיתי

EASY ACCESS
   Editions: *CIS* 143 • *RES* 490.

   Illustrations: *CIS* pl. 14.

LITERATURE
   C. Clermont-Ganneau 1879, esp. pp. 34–37 • S. A. Cook 1904, + photo • S. de
   Ricci 1906, esp. p. 33.

B.3.f.18   Carpentras Stele (5th–4th c.)   Carp

Broken limestone stele with funerary inscription (35 x 33 cm.). Carpentras, France, Municipal Library.

Ed. Pr.   M. Rigord 1704.

EASY ACCESS

Editions: *AaG* Seg 44 • *AC* 49 • *AH* I/1, II.C.2 • *CIS* 141 • *HNE* 448 • *KAI* 269 • *NSI* 75 • *TSSI* 24.

Illustrations: *CIS* pl. 13 • *HNE* pl. 28/3 • *KAI* pl. 34 • *TSSI* fig. 13.

Translations: *DAE* 86.

LITERATURE

B. de Montfaucon 1724, esp. pp. 207–8, LIV • A. C. P. Caylus 1752, pp. 1:74–75 • M. l'abbé [J. J.]? Barthélemy 1768 • G. Fabricy 1803 • O. G. Tychsen 1815, esp. pp. 91–93 • U. F. Kopp 1821, esp. pp. 227–41 • H. A. Hamaker 1822, esp. p. 69 • A. Mai 1825, esp. pp. 31–70 • M. A. Lanci 1825 • E. Rödiger 1828 • F. F. Beer 1833 • J. Fürst 1835, esp. pp. 22–23 • W. Gesenius 1837, esp. pp. 226–32, pls. 28–29 • A.-C. Judas 1847, esp. pp. 86–88 • F. Lenormant 1867, esp. pp. 514–15 • A. Geiger 1868 • A. Merx 1868, esp. pp. 697–99 • J. Derenbourg 1868 • M. A. Levy 1868 • J. Halévy 1874, esp. p. 152 • J. Halévy 1878 • K. Schlottmann 1878 • P. de Lagarde 1878 • [J.] Lauth 1878, esp. pp. 115–31 • C. Clermont-Ganneau 1879, esp. pp. 31–33 • H. V. Lund 1879–80 • E. Ledrain 1884a, esp. p. 1 • S. R. Driver 1890, esp. pp. xviii–xxi. • S. de Ricci 1906, esp. pp. 32–33 • C. C. Torrey 1926 • M. E. Sherman 1966 • P. Grelot 1967 • J. Teixidor 1969, esp. p. 346 • B. Couroyer 1970 • P. Grelot 1970 • J. Teixidor 1972a, esp. p. 438 • E. Lipiński 1977, esp. pp. 112–15 • B. Couroyer 1980 • W. H. Shea 1981.

B.3.f.19   Gizeh Graffito (Cairo, 5th–4th c.)   GizGr

Fragmentary column found in the temple of the Sphinx (17 x 31 cm. diameter). Cairo Museum (29-12-28-1).

1   [מר]דֹכשֹׁמכֹן כן אמר מצֹׁי[ת...]
[...] הו עמי סוסא 5 [ ] כדונן אף 2 גמלן [...]
[....]מֹו[...]

Ed. Pr.   N. Aimé-Giron 1931 (*TA* 90), pp. 78–83, pls. 5, 11.

B.3.f.20   Wadi El-Hudi Horus Stele Graffiti (5th–4th c.)   WHudiGr

Seven graffiti of from one to nine lines each incised on the front and back of a stele bearing images of Horus. Cairo Museum.

Ed. Pr.   N. Aimé-Giron 1939 (No. 124), pp. 351–63, pls. 51–56.

B.3.f.21 Aimé-Giron Papyrus Fragments   TA

Numerous papyrus fragments with little or no clear context. Some of them have been joined into identifiable texts (see TADC3.7, TADC3.17, TADC4.3). The ones gathered here remain unidentified.

Ed. Pr.   N. Aimé-Giron 1931 (*TA* 29, 31, 32, 34–45, 48–49, 51–60, 62–74, 76, 79–86, 88– 89), pls. 5–8.

LITERATURE
67) S. A. Kaufman 1974, esp. p. 37.

B.3.f.22 Fragmentary Account of Grain (5th–4th c.)   TADC3.17

Ed. Pr.   N. Aimé-Giron 1931 (*TA* 78+77), pp. 65–66, pl. 8.

LITERATURE
E. G. Kraeling 1953, esp. p. 304, pl. XVII.

B.3.f.23 Abydos Inscriptions (5th–3d c.)   AbydI

Sixty-odd graffiti lightly incised on the pillars, staircase chamber, and inner rooms of the Seti and Ramses temples in Abydos; 16 are Aramaic.

Ed. Pr.   H. Zotenberg 1868.

EASY ACCESS
Editions: *AC* 40 ● *CIS* 125–133 ● *ESE* 3.93–116 ● *RES* 607–610, 1363–77.

Translations: *DAE* 80–82.

Illustrations: *CIS* pls. 16–18 ● *ESE* 3, pls. 7–11.

LITERATURE
C. Ricque 1869 ● M. A. Levy 1870 ● M. A. Murray 1904, pl. XXIV/21–22 ● S. de Ricci 1906, esp. p. 31 ● N. Aimé-Giron 1931, esp. p. 79 ● J. Naveh 1964–65, esp. p. 191 ● J. Naveh 1966, esp. pp. 30–31 ● W. Kornfeld 1978a.

B.3.f.24 El-Hibeh Papyrus Letter (end 5th c.)   TADA3.11

Fragmentary letter to Yashobiah. Archeological Museum, Florence (Inv. no. 11913).

Ed. Pr.   E.Bresciani 1959 + plate.

LITERATURE
> J. T. Milik 1960 ● J. Hoftijzer 1962 ● B. Porten 1980, esp. p. 49 ● P. Swiggers 1980 ● P.-E. Dion 1982b, esp. pp. 530, 541, 560–65.

B.3.f.25 Vatican Papyrus (4th c.)   TADC3.19
> Seven papyrus fragments of a treasury account. Vatican Museum.

Ed. Pr.   C. J. M. de Vogüé 1868, pp. 125–31, pl. 16.

EASY ACCESS
> Editions: *AP* 73 ● *CIS* 147.

> Illustrations: *CIS* pl. 18.

LITERATURE
> W. Gesenius 1837, esp. p. 245 ● C. Clermont-Ganneau 1879, esp. p. 24 ● F. Praetorius 1881, esp. p. 444 ● E. Ledrain 1884b, esp. pp. 23–30 ● S. de Ricci 1906, esp. pp. 26–27 ● B. Porten 1990, esp. p. 28.

B.3.f.26 An Endorsement (390)   TA.86bis
> Aramaic endorsement on a Demotic Egyptian contract. Cairo Museum (J. 50103)

כתב פסי בר פֿמאֿ

Ed. Pr.   N. Aimé-Giron 1931 (*TA* 86*bis*), pp. 67–69 + photo.

B.3.f.27 Amherst Demotic Papyrus (4th c.)   PapAmherst
> A scroll (Papyrus Amherst "63") with 23 columns of Aramaic religious and narrative texts in Demotic script. The greater part of the scroll is in the J. Pierpont Morgan Library (New York); some fragments are at the University of Michigan.

Ed. Pr.   R. A. Bowman 1944 (initial description and tentative translation of a few lines). See also C. F. Nims and R. C. Steiner 1983, R. C. Steiner and C. F. Nims 1984, 1985, S. P. Vleeming and J. W. Wesselius 1985.

EASY ACCESS
> Editions: *AC* 55.

LITERATURE
> A. Dupont-Sommer 1943–45 ● A. Dupont-Sommer 1945a ● W. F. Albright 1950, esp. pp. 9–10 ● S. P. Vleeming and J. W. Wesselius 1982 ● C. F. Nims and R. C. Steiner 1983 ● K. A. D. Smelik 1983 ● S. P. Vleeming and J. W. Wesselius 1983–84 ● R. C. Steiner and C. F. Nims 1984 ● Anon. 1985 ● K. T. Zauzich 1985a

• K. A. D. Smelik 1985 • R. C. Steiner and C. F. Nims 1985 • S. P. Vleeming and J. W. Wesselius 1985 • S. P. Vleeming and J. W. Wesselius 1985a • S. Segert 1986 • I. Kottsieper 1988 • Z. Zevit 1990.

B.3.f.28　Vatican Funerary Stele (4th c.)　　　　　VatFunStel
Limestone stele (39 x 30 cm.).　Vatican Museum.

ענחחפי בר תחבס מנחה זי אוסרי אלהא

Ed. Pr.　　　　F. Lenormant 1867.

EASY ACCESS
Editions:　　　*CIS* 142 • *HNE* 448 • *KAI* 272.

Illustrations:　*HNE* pl. 28/4.

LITERATURE
C. Clermont-Ganneau 1879, esp. pp. 33–34 • E. Ledrain 1884a, esp. pp. 22–23 • P. Berger 1891, esp. p. 218 • S. de Ricci 1906, esp. p. 33.

B.3.f.29　Wadi Sheikh Sheikhun Graffito (Akhmim, 4th c.)　　WaSh
In situ.

1　ברך [פט]פתח קדם [...]
אלהא שנת 3 מלכא

Ed. Pr.　　　*CIS* II, p. 135 (No. 134).

EASY ACCESS
Editions:　　　*RAO* 6: 267–70 (+ drawing) • *RES* 1817.

LITERATURE
A. H. Sayce 1904 • U. Bouriant 1889, esp. pp. 147, 149 • S. de Ricci 1906, esp. p. 31.

B.3.f.30　Jequier Papyrus (late 4th c.)　　　　　TADC3.26
Fragmentary administrative text.　Cairo Museum (J. 50052).

Ed. Pr.　　　N. Aimé-Giron 1931 (*TA* 87), pp. 70–75, pl. 10.

B.3.f.31　Egyptian Aramaic Statuette (4th–3rd c.)　　　EgAramStat
Clay statuette, possibly a forgery.　Private collection.

אוי לי

Ed. Pr.   E. Bresciani 1971a.

LITERATURE
> J. Teixidor 1972a, esp. pp. 438–39.

B.3.f.32 Luxor Ostracon (4th–3d c.)   LuxorOstr

> Ostracon acquired by W. Spiegelberg.

יהב ש[מ]ע[ו]ן בר פ[..].[ש]ודת 1
ואנתתה כסף ר 3 בשם כסף
מלחא כתב יוסֿף ספרא
ב 30 לתעבנ[י] שנת 33

Ed. Pr.   M. Lidzbarski 1927 (no photo or drawing).

LITERATURE
> B. Porten 1990, esp. p. 28.

B.3.f.33 Edfu Ostraca (4th–3d c.)   EdfuOstr

> Seven ostraca from the Ptolemaic period in Egypt.

Ed. Pr.   1) *ESE* 2.243–49 (+ drawing).
2) *APO* 75/2, pl. 62.
3) *APO* 81/1, pl. 68.
4) *APO* 81/2, pl. 68.
5) N. Aimé-Giron 1931 (*TA 4bis*), pp. 8–11, pl. 1.
6) N. Aimé-Giron 1939 (No. 113, pl. III).
7) N. Aimé-Giron 1939 (No. 120, pl. IV).

EASY ACCESS
> Editions: 1) *APO* 75/1 • *RES* 1794.

> Illustrations: 1) APO pl. 62.

LITERATURE
> 1) E. Meyer 1911, esp. p. 1027.
> 2) H. Torczyner 1912, esp. p. 403 • J. N. Epstein 1912, esp. p. 138.
> 4) J. Naveh 1982, pl. 10C.
> 6) J. B. Segal 1987.

B.3.f.34 Fayum Wooden Panel (Rubaiyat, ca. 300)   **Rub**

A wooden panel with a portrait on one side and inscription on the other.
Theodor Graf Collection, Vienna.

בעלעדר

Ed. Pr.   S. de Ricci 1906 (No. 14), p. 33 + drawing.

LITERATURE
F. Rosenthal 1939, esp. p. 297.

B.3.f.35 Louvre Palette (ca. 300)   **LouvPal**

Wooden scribal palette bearing list of accounts. Louvre (L16811).

Ed. Pr.   A. Lemaire 1987a + photo.

B.3.f.36 Dahshur Graffiti (Memphis, ca. 300)   **DahshurGr**

Fragmentary columns bearing graffiti. Private collection.

[..]רת[...] (1
חרמש (2
[...]זב[חרמש (3

Ed. Pr.   A. H. Sayce 1904.

EASY ACCESS
Editions: *RES* 1818.

LITERATURE
S. de Ricci 1906, esp. p. 31 ● N. Aimé-Giron 1931, esp. p. 97, n. 1.

B.3.f.37 Ma'sârah Quarry Inscription (ca. 300)   **Masarah**

Graffito. In situ.

פטי בר שמן בבלי

Ed. Pr.   A. H. Sayce 1904.

EASY ACCESS
Editions: *RES* 1819.

LITERATURE
S. de Ricci 1906, esp. p. 31 ● A. H. Sayce 1924.

B.3.f.38 Rosette Phialê (ca. 300)   RosPh

Silver libation bowl. London, R. Erskine Collection.

תריפרן

Ed. Pr.   A. D. H. Bivar 1961 (+ photos).

B.3.f.39 Alexandrian Necropolis Texts (ca. 300)   AlexNecr

Three grave stela with painted texts; the second consists of isolated
letters yielding no connected text.

(1
עקביה
בר אליוענ֗
י
(3
בים 10 [...]
אפלונ[.....]

Ed. Pr.   C. Clermont-Ganneau *RAO* 8: 59–65.

B.3.f.40 Vienna Ostraca (3d c., Edfu?)   ViennaOstr.2–4

Three ostraca of uncertain provenience; R. Degen suggests Edfu.
National Museum, Vienna (A.O. 2–4).

Ed. Pr.   R. Degen 1978b (*NESE* 3), pp. 39–47 + drawings, photos.

B.3.f.41 Edfu Tomb Inscriptions (3rd c.)   EdfuTomb

Nine gravestones, some broken, with Aramaic names.

עזגד בר מדי (1
שלמצין ברת עזגד
עזג[ד ב]ר מדי
זבדיה ב[ר] עזגד
משלם ב[ר] עזגד
עבדיהו בר (2
שמעון
אורי (3
נתני בר שמען (4
חרה בר ג[...] (5
פחא בר[...] (6
זבי (7
פחי קצן (8
[...]ד[...] (9

Ed. Pr. W. Kornfeld 1973.

LITERATURE
R. Degen 1978d ● W. Kornfeld 1979.

B.3.f.42 Levi della Vida Papyrus (3d–2d c.) TADC3.29

Name list with quantities of oil. Istituto di Studi del Vicino Oriente, University of Rome.

Ed. Pr. E. Bresciani 1962 (+ tab. 1).

LITERATURE
J. Naveh 1965–66, esp. pp. 159–60 ● J. Naveh 1966, esp. pp. 35–36 ● K. R. Veenhof 1968, esp. p. 137 ● R.Degen 1978d ● B. Porten 1990, esp. p. 28.

B.4 Arabia

B.4.1   Teima Inscriptions General Information

LITERATURE

C. Clermont-Ganneau 1884 • C. Huber 1884, esp. p. 291 n. 85 • D. H. Müller 1884 • J. Halévy 1884 • E. Renan 1884–85 • A. Neubauer 1885, esp. pp. 209–14 • A. Neubauer 1885a • S. A. Rashid 1974, esp. pp. 155–60 • R. Degen 1974a • E. A. Knauf 1990.

B.4.2   Teima Funerary Stele VII (6th c.)   Teima.7
Brown-gray grave stone (68.5 x 43 cm.)

1 נפש רם
ל... בֹּרת
...דִֹּי

Ed. Pr.   F. Altheim and R. Stiehl 1970, pp. 141–42, pls. 5, 6.

EASY ACCESS
    Editions: *NESE* 2: 88–89.

    Illustrations: *NESE* 2: 89, pl. 8/29.

B.4.3   Teima Funerary Stele VIII (6th c.)   Teima.8
Brown-gray grave stone (82 x 30 cm.)

1 נפֹש .מרא
ל בר אדנשי

Ed. Pr.   F. Altheim and R. Stiehl 1970, pp. 23–26, pls. 7, 8.

EASY ACCESS
    Editions: *NESE* 2: 90–91.

    Illustrations: *NESE* 2: 90, pl. 8/30.

LITERATURE   J. Teixidor 1977, esp. p. 271.

B.4.4   Teima Stele I (5th c.)   Teima.1
Sandstone stele with 23-line inscription in relief (1 m. x 42 cm.). Louvre.

Ed. Pr.   T. Nöldeke 1884, pp. 813–19, pls. 6–7.

EASY ACCESS
   Editions: *CIS* 113 • *NSI* 69 • *KAI* 228 • *HNE* 447 • *AC* 45 • *RES* 1816 •
                TSSI 30 • *AaG* Seg 49.

   Illustrations: *CIS* pl. 9 • *HNE* pl. 27.

LITERATURE
   J. P. Peters 1884–85, esp. pp. 115–16 • J. Halévy 1884a, esp. pp. 2–8 • J. Halévy
   1885 • P. Berger 1885 • J. Halévy 1886 • R. Duval 1888 • H. Winckler 1894 • H.
   Winckler 1898 • F. Hommel 1899, esp. pp. 135–36 • W. Spiegelberg 1906, esp. p.
   1103 • J. Euting 1914, esp. pp. 157–61 • G. R. Driver 1945, esp. p. 11 • G. R.
   Driver 1948, esp. p. 121 • A. Caquot 1951–52, esp. p. 58, n. 5 • S. Gevirtz 1961,
   esp. p. 145 • S. A. Kaufman 1974, esp. p. 38 • E. Lipiński 1977, esp. pp. 116–17 •
   B. Aggoula 1985, esp. pp. 61–65 • C. H. Gordon 1985 • E. A. Knauf 1990, esp.
   pp. 203, n. 11, 206, 212–13.

B.4.5   Teima Inscription V (5th c.)   Teima.5
   Fragment of stele reused in construction of a house. In situ.

1 [סמראֹ
  [במראֹ
  [.זידן ל
  [אלהתא [לחיֹ
5 י נפש]ה ונפֹ]
  ש אחר]תה
  [לעלם דֹ
  [ר׳ שנת

Ed. Pr.   F. Altheim and R. Stiehl 1964–69, pp. 5/1:74–75, pl. 27.

EASY ACCESS
   Editions: *NESE* 2: 83–87.

   Illustrations: *NESE* 2, pl. 8/27.

LITERATURE
   J. B. Segal 1969, esp. pp. 170–73 • J. Teixidor 1970a, esp. pp. 372–73 • F.
   Altheim and R. Stiehl 1971, esp. pp. 2:243–46 • R. Degen 1974a.

B.4.6   Teima Funerary Stele VI (5th c.)   Teima.6
   Much weathered stele.

1 לוחנר זי
מֹשה

Ed. Pr.   F. Altheim and R. Stiehl 1964–69, pp. 5/1:75–77, pl. 28.

EASY ACCESS
   Editions: *NESE* 2:87–88.

   Illustrations: *NESE* 2, pl. 8/28.

LITERATURE   J. Teixidor 1970a, esp. p. 373.

B.4.7   Teima Plaque (5th c.)   Teima.9

Two fragments of a limestone plaque (13 x 15.2 cm. and 16 x 10.5 cm.).
Riyadh Museum 35.

1 קבר .[ ]
   [   ]
   [נתֹ]
   בֹ.[.]ו[.]

Ed. Pr.   A. Jamme and J. Starcky 1970, pp. 133, 139, pl. 35a.

EASY ACCESS
   Editions: *NESE* 2: 91.

   Illustrations: *NESE* 2: 91

B.4.8   Khubu el-Gharbi Funerary Stele (ca. 400)   Teima.12

Grave stone (56 x 27 cm.).   Riyadh Museum 36.

1 מחרמני
   בר נתם

Ed. Pr.   A. van den Branden 1956, p. 2:61, nr. 290, pl. 12.

EASY ACCESS
   Editions: *NESE* 2: 92–93.

   Illustrations: *NESE* 2: 93. J. M. Sola-Solé 1967 ● J. Starcky and A. Jamme 1970,
                    esp. pp. 133–35, 139, nr. 36 ● R. Degen 1974a.

B.4.9   Jebel ed-Dighš Funerary Stele (?)   Teima.13

רמלן

Ed. Pr.   A. J. Jaussen and R. Savignac 1909, 1914, 1922, p. 2/1:223, nr. 342, pl.
                28.

EASY ACCESS
     Editions: *NESE* 2: 93.

B.4.10   Hejra Grave Marker (ca. 400)   Teima.15

[ ] מיתב זי רמננתן בר [

Ed. Pr.   Ch. Doughty 1891, pp. 1–60, pl. 3 fol. 1.

EASY ACCESS
     Editions: *CIS* 117 • *NESE* 2: 94– 95.

     Illustrations: *CIS* pl. 10.

LITERATURE
     A. J. Jaussen and R. Savignac 1909, 1914, 1922, esp. p. 2/1:236, nr. 146, pls. 27, 9.

B.4.11   Engraver's Block (Hejra, ca. 400)   Teima.16

1 בר ד.ד.ר
[......]
שמתאלש.
למרפרדהת.

Ed. Pr.   A. J. Jaussen and R. Savignac 1909,1914,1922, p. 2/1:233, nr. 127.

EASY ACCESS
     Editions: *RES* 1139 • *NESE* 2: 95.

B.4.12   Teima Ostracon XVII (Hejra, ca. 400)   Teima.17

1 מענאלהי
נעמה

Ed. Pr.   J. Euting 1885, pp. 13–14, nr. 5, p.12, pl. 1.

EASY ACCESS
     Editions: *CIS* 118 • *NESE* 2: 95–96.

Illustrations: *CIS* pl. 10.

LITERATURE
A. J. Jaussen and R. Savignac 1909, 1914, 1922, esp. p. 2:203, nr 268, pl. 115 • J.
Euting 1914, esp. p. 247.

B.4.13   El-'Ula Stele (near Hejra, ca. 400)   Teima.18

מאן

Ed. Pr.   Ch. Doughty 1891, pl. 17 fol. 31.

EASY ACCESS
Editions: *CIS* 119 • *NESE* 2: 96.

Illustrations: *CIS* pl. 10.

B.4.14   Teima Stele XX (ca. 400)   Teima.20

1 [שנת . . . בביר]ת תימא
[ה]קִים פצגו שהרו בר
[מ]לכי לחין העלי בין[ת]
[צ]לם זי רב ומֹרחבה ו
5 [ה]קים כרסאא זנה קדם
צלם זי רב למיתב שנגלא
ואשימא אלהי תימא
לחיי נפש פצגו
שהרו וזרעה מרא[י]א
10 [ו] ל[ח]יי נפשה זי [לה]

Ed. Pr.   A. Livingstone 1983 et al., pp. 108–11, pl. 96.

LITERATURE
G. Bawden et al. 1980 • B. Aggoula 1985, esp. pp. 66–68 • F. M. Cross 1986 • K.
Beyer and A. Livingstone 1987, esp. pp. 286–88 • E. A. Knauf 1990, esp. pp. 206,
210–11, 214.

B.4.15   Teima Funerary Stele XXI (ca. 400)   Teima.21
Grave stone (130 x 28 cm.).

1 נפש חטלח בר
ת מענתן

Ed. Pr.   A. Livingstone et al. 1983, pp. 106–7, pls. 87, 94b.

LITERATURE   K. Beyer and A. Livingstone 1987, esp. p. 288.

B.4.16   Teima Funerary Stele XXII (ca. 400)   Teima.22
Grave stone (55 x 30 cm.).

1 נפש שיע
א בר גרמן
בירח אב זי
שנת 16

Ed. Pr.   A. Livingstone et al. 1983, p. 107, pl. 94b.

LITERATURE
B. Aggoula 1985, esp. pp. 68–69 • K. Beyer and A. Livingstone 1987, esp. pp. 288–89.

B.4.17   Teima Funerary Stele XXIII (ca. 400)   Teima.23
Grave stone (72 x 26 cm.).

1 נפש תים
בר זיד

Ed. Pr.   A. Livingstone et al. 1983, p. 107, pl. 94c.

LITERATURE   K. Beyer and A. Livingstone 1987, esp. p. 289.

B.4.18   Teima Funerary Stele XXIV (ca. 400)   Teima.24
Grave stone (48 x 18 cm.).

1 נפש
גרמא
להי
בר זי
5 דן

Ed. Pr.   A. Livingstone et al. 1983, p. 107, pl. 95a.

LITERATURE   K. Beyer and A. Livingstone 1987, esp. pp. 289–90.

B.4.19   Teima Funerary Stele XXV (ca. 400)   Teima.25
Grave stone with two inscriptions (23 x 29 cm.).

A

נֿפש גֿרמן בר מ

תֿמנן גדא

B

נפש בצֿרֿ ברת

מו

Ed. Pr.   A. Livingstone et al. 1983, p. 108, pl. 95b.

LITERATURE   K. Beyer and A. Livingstone 1987, esp. p. 290.

B.4.20   Teima Stele XXVII (Qaṣr al-Ḥamrā, ca. 400)   Teima.27
(30 x 50 cm.).

1 זי קרב תימו בר אֿלהֿו

לדרעא לחיי נפשה

ונפשהום זי פרקמננ>ו<

בר ועדו >ו<כרימו בֿרה זי

5 [פֿר]קֿחיו

Ed. Pr.   K. Beyer and A. Livingstone 1990.

LITERATURE
E. A. Knauf 1990, esp. p. 207.

B.4.21   Teima Votive II (4th c.)   Teima.2
Stone pedestal (28 x 30 cm.). Louvre.

1 [מֿ]יתבא זי קר

[נ] מענן בר עמ

[ר]ן לצלם אלה

א לחיי נפשה

Ed. Pr.   T. Nöldeke 1884, pp. 819–20.

EASY ACCESS
     Editions: *CIS* 114 • *KAI* 229 • *AC* 50 • *NSI* 70 • *HNE* 447 • *NESE* 2: 81–82.

     Illustrations: *CIS* pl. 10 • *HNE* pl. 26/5.

LITERATURE
J. Halévy 1884a, esp. pp. 2–8 • P. Berger 1885, esp. p. 77 • C. Doughty 1888, esp. pp. 291, 296 • P. Berger 1891, esp. pp. 216–17 • G. R. Driver 1938, esp. pp. 188–89.

B.4.22   Teima Votive II Draft (4th c.)   Teima.2a
Squeeze, apparently of a poor preliminary draft of Teima.2.

מענן <ב>ר עמרן 1
מיתבא זי קרב
א לחיי נפשה
לצלמ אלה

Ed. Pr.   G. R. Driver 1938, pp. 188–89.

EASY ACCESS
     Editions: *NESE* 2: 81–82, pl. 7.

B.4.23   Teima Funerary Stele III (4th c.)   Teima.3
Grave stone (65 x 15 cm.).   Louvre.

נפש עלן ברת שבען

Ed. Pr.   T. Nöldeke 1884, p. 819.

EASY ACCESS
     Editions: *CIS* 115 ● *KAI* 230 ● *HNE* 447.

     Illustrations: *CIS* pl. 10.

LITERATURE   J. Halévy 1884a, esp. pp. 2–8 ● P. Berger 1885, esp. p. 78.

B.4.24   Teima Funerary Stele IV (4th c.)   Teima.4
Grave stone.   In situ.

[...]נפש פצי 1
[...]בר במת
בר [י]ת[נ]דן

Ed. Pr.   C. Doughty 1891, p. 59, pl. 27 fol. 52.

EASY ACCESS
     Editions: *CIS* 116 ● *NESE* 2: 82–83.

     Illustrations: *CIS* pl. 10.

LITERATURE
     J. Halévy 1884a, esp. pp. 2–8 ● J. Euting 1885, esp. pp. 9–10 ● P. Berger 1885, esp. pp. 77–78 ● C. Doughty 1888, esp. pp. 65–66 ● F. A Winnett and W. L. Reed 1970, esp. p. 28 ● R. Degen 1974a.

B.4.25   Teima Funerary Stele X (4th c.)   Teima.10
Sandstone grave marker (29 x 28 cm.). Riyadh Museum.

[נפ]ש חד

Ed. Pr.   A. Jamme and J. Starcky 1970, pp. 135, 139, pl. 37.

EASY ACCESS
Editions: *NESE* 2: 91–92.

B.4.26   Teima Ostracon XXVI (?)   Teima.26

[...] חמר קדר [...]

Ed. Pr.   A. Livingstone et al. 1983, p. 108 pl. 88.

LITERATURE
K. Beyer and A. Livingstone 1987, esp. p. 292.

B.4.27   Bahrain Vase Inscription (3d c.?)   BahrVase
Restored vase (20.5 x 16.5 cm.).   National Museum of Bahrain.

קבעא זנה יהב ברך לנבר

Ed. Pr.   M. Sznycer 1984.

B.4.28   Wadi Madhbaḥ Grave Marker (Hejra, ca. 200)   Teima.14

ש[לם] ברהם בר נחשטב

Ed. Pr.   J. Euting 1885, p. 13 nr. 42.

EASY ACCESS
Editions: *CIS* 120 • *NESE* 2: 94 (+ drawing).

Illustrations: *CIS* pl. 10.

LITERATURE
J. Halévy 1884a, esp. pp. 8–16 • G. R. Driver 1957a, esp. p. 52 • J. Teixidor 1977,
esp. p. 271.

B.4.29　El-'Ula Stele (near Hejra, ca. 200)　　　Teima.19

אלנפיו בר עבד[ו]

Ed. Pr.　　　J. Euting 1885, p. 13, nr. 44; p. 12, pl. 1.

EASY ACCESS
　　Editions:　　*CIS* 121 • *NESE* 2: 96–97.

　　Illustrations:　*CIS* pl. 10 • *NESE* 2, pl. 7/26.

LITERATURE
　　J. Euting 1914, esp. p. 241, n. 1.

B.4.30　Teima Stone Basin (2d c.)　　　Teima.11

תימן עתעקב בר י[.]ו

Ed. Pr.　　　A. J. Jaussen and R. Savignac 1909, 1914, 1922, p. 2/1:222, nr. 336, pl. 119.

EASY ACCESS
　　Editions:　　*NESE* 2: 92 (+ drawing).

LITERATURE
　　R. Degen 1974a, esp. p. 92.

B.5 Asia Minor

B.5.1   Caucasus Silver Bowl (6th–5th c.)   CaucSilBo
Bowl decorated with pictures in relief. Moscow.

דכביר

Ed. Pr.   K. Schlottmann 1878.

EASY ACCESS
  Editions: *CIS* 110.

  Illustrations: *CIS* pl. 8.

B.5.2   Meydancikkale Inscriptions (Cilicia, mid-6th c.)   Meyd
1) Mostly illegible 15-line inscription on a block set in a city wall. In situ.
2) Mostly illegible 13-line funerary inscription. In situ.

Ed. Pr.   A. Lemaire and H. Lozachmeur 1987.

B.5.3   Abydos Lion Weight (Mysia, ca. 500)   AbydLiW
Iron weight in shape of a lion (ca. 26 kg.). British Museum.

אספרן לקבל סתריא זי כספא

Ed. Pr.   Ch. J. M. de Vogüé 1862.

EASY ACCESS
  Editions: *AC* 20 ● *CIS* 108 ● *NSI* 67 ● *HNE* 446 ● *KAI* 263 ● *AAG*Seg 56.

  Illustrations: *CIS* pl. 7 ● *HNE* pl. 26/1.

LITERATURE
  M. A. Levy 1862a, esp. pp. 203–5 ● M. A. Levy 1862a, esp. pp. 203–5 ● J. Brandis 1866, esp. p. 54, n. 2 ● A. Geiger 1867 ● C. J. M de Vogüé 1868b ● M. J. Oppert 1874, esp. p. 477, 484 ● E. Ledrain 1882a ● E. Ledrain 1884d, esp. p. 67 ● G. Hoffmann 1896, esp. pp. 235–36 ● W. L. Bevan 1896, esp. p. 1731 ● C. C. Torrey 1912, esp. pp. 91–92 ● H. H. Schaeder 1929–30, esp. p. 267 ● F. Rosenthal 1939, esp. pp. 24–25.

B.5.4   Kesecek Köyü Votive (Cilicia, end 5th c.)   Kesecek

Votive inscription originally carved on a cliff (30.5 x 45.7 cm.) Yale Babylonian Collection (YBC 2435).

Ed. Pr.   C. C. Torrey 1915a.

EASY ACCESS
   Editions: *AC* 48 • *AaG*Seg 52 • *KAI* 258 • *TSSI* 33.

   Translations: *TUAT* 2:578.

LITERATURE
   S. Gevirtz 1961, esp. p. 146 • R. S. Hanson 1968, esp. pp. 3–5 + photo, drawing • J. Teixidor 1970a, esp. pp. 373–74 • E. Lipiński 1975a, esp. pp. 146–71 • J. Teixidor 1979, esp. pp. 392–93.

B.5.5   Daskyleion Funerary Stele (450–400)   Daskyleion

Stele decorated with relief.   Archaeological Museum, Istanbul.

1 אלה צלמה זי אלנף בר אשי
  הו עבד לנפשה הומיתך
  בל ונבו זי ארחא זנה
  יהוה עדה איש אל יעמל

Ed. Pr.   A. Dupont-Sommer 1966.

EASY ACCESS
   Editions: *TSSI* 37.

   Illustrations: *TSSI* fig. 12.

LITERATURE
   E. Akurgal 1956 • F. Altheim and R. Stiehl 1964–69, esp. pp. 5/1: 72–74 • M. Mellink 1965, esp. p. 148 • E. Akurgal 1966 • F. M. Cross 1966 • G. M. A. Hanfmann 1966 • A. Dupont-Sommer 1966a • M. Delcor 1967 • N. Dolunay 1967 • K. R. Veenhof 1968, esp. pp. 139–40 • R. S. Hanson 1968, esp. p. 3 • P. Bernard 1969 • E. Lipiński 1973, esp. p. 369 • J. Teixidor 1974, esp. p. 329 • E. Lipiński 1975a, esp. pp. 146–71 • E. Lipiński 1975a, esp. pp. 150–53 • E. Lipiński 1977, esp. p. 117 • F. Altheim, R. Stiehl, and M. Cremer 1985.

B.5.6   Sultaniye Köy Stele (Helvatepe, 5th c.)   SultStel

Marble funerary stele found in two pieces.   Archaeological Museum, Bursa, Turkey.

1 זנה סמלא זי אדה א[מ]רדוש זי אריבם
כזי הו טב עבד וכן עבד לה במיתא
[ו]כן אריבם טב והמר זילה

Ed. Pr. F. Altheim, R. Stiehl, D. Metzler and E. Schwertheim, 1983.

B.5.7 Gözneh Boundary Stone (Cilicia, 5th–4th c.) GozBdSt
Boundary inscription on a cliff. In situ.

Ed. Pr. J. A. Montgomery 1907.

EASY ACCESS
Editions: *AC* 42 • *KAI* 259 • *TSSI* 34.

LITERATURE
J. R. Metheny 1907, esp. pp. 156–57, 163 • J. Halévy 1908b • C. C. Torrey 1912, esp. pp. 90–91 • G. R. Driver 1935, esp. pp. 50–52 • S. Gevirtz 1961, esp. p. 145 • R. S. Hanson 1968, esp. pp. 9–10 + photo, drawing • J. Teixidor 1970a, esp. p. 374 • E. Lipiński 1975a, esp. pp. 146–71 • J. Naveh 1982, Fig. 77, p. 84 • G. M. A., ed. Hanfmann 1983, esp. p. 106.

B.5.8 Saraidin Graffito (Cilicia, 5th–4th c.) SarGr
Rock inscription (also known as the "Jagdinschrift") in a square frame. In situ.

Ed. Pr. D. H. Müller 1892.

EASY ACCESS
Editions: *AC* 47 • *HNE* 446 • *KAI* 261 • *NSI* 68 • *RES* 955 • *TSSI* 35.

Illustrations: *HNE* pl. 26 • *KAI* pl. 21 • Diringer 1968, fig. 153b.

LITERATURE
T. Nöldeke 1892 • J. Halévy 1893a • A. Poebel 1932, 52–53 • J. Friedrich 1957a • H. Jensen 1958, esp. pp. 284, 263 (facs.) • D. Diringer and R. Regensburger 1968, pl. 2.187b.

B.5.9 Arebsun Stelae (Cappadocia, 5th–4th c.) Arebsun
Three stelae decorated with reliefs.
1) Basalt stele with reliefs (1.3 m. x 57 cm.) Text unpublished. Istanbul.
2) Basalt stele with reliefs and text on three surfaces. Istanbul.
3) Stele with reliefs and unpublished (non-Aramaic?) text. Istanbul.

Ed. Pr.   Y. I. Smirnov 1896.

EASY ACCESS
     Editions: 2) *AC* 58 • *AagSeg* 57 • *ESE* 1:59–74, 319–26 • *KAI* 264 • *RES* 1785.

LITERATURE
     C. Clermont-Ganneau 1898 • J. Halévy 1898 • H. Reichelt 1901 • J. Marquart 1907, esp. pp. 118–21 • C. C. Torrey 1917–18, esp. p. 194 • A. Dupont-Sommer 1949a, esp. p. 98 • A. Catastini 1987, esp. pp. 273–74.

B.5.10   Bahadirli Inscriptions (near Karatepe, 5th–4th c.)   Bahad

     1) Boundary inscription on a basalt stele (53 x 44 cm.)
     2) Black basalt fragment (26 x 19 x 18 cm.)

(1
1 זנה תחום כרביל
וכרשי קריתא
זי מהחסן כבבה
זי פושר זי בכשתבלי
5 ואיש זי יחגה
לתחומא זנה קדם
כבבה זי פושר
או איש אחרא
[....]

(2
1 [...]..א
[...]ה. לה
[...]למתא

Ed. Pr.   1) A. Dupont-Sommer 1961.
              2) A. Dupont-Sommer 1950–51a.

EASY ACCESS
     Editions: 1) *KAI* 278 • *TSSI* 36.

     Illustrations: 1) *TSSI* pl. 7, 2.

LITERATURE
     A. Dupont-Sommer 1962 • A. Dupont-Sommer and L. Robert 1964 • A. Dupont-Sommer 1965 • G. Garbini 1965 • G. Levi della Vida 1965 • G. Ryckmans 1965 • J. Naveh 1964–65, esp. pp. 193–94 • J. Naveh 1966, esp. pp. 32–33 • J. Teixidor 1967, esp. pp. 180–81 • K. R. Veenhof 1968, esp. pp. 138–39 • R. S. Hanson 1968, esp. p. 11 + drawing.

B.5.11 Hemite Inscription (near Karatepe, 5th–4th c.) **Hem**
Small marble fragment (18 x 22 cm.)

[...] 1
[...].ן עמד שפקא ואת.]
[...]ה סנמפי חשתר.]
[.....].נגז וא]

Ed. Pr.   A. Dupont-Sommer 1950–51, pp. 45–47.

B.5.12 Limyra Bilingual (Lycia, 5th–4th c.) **LimBil**
Greek-Aramaic tomb inscription. In situ.

[א]סתודנה זנה [א]רתים בר ארזפי עבד אחר מן זי מ[...]

Ed. Pr.   C. Fellows 1841, pp. 209, 468, p. 36/1.

EASY ACCESS
   Editions: *CIS* 109 • *KAI* 262 • *HNE* 446.

   Illustrations: *CIS* pl. 7.

LITERATURE
   E. Sachau 1887 • J. Darmesteter 1888 • F. Perles 1926 • A. D. H. Bivar 1961a •
   R. S. Hanson 1968, esp. pp. 5–7 + drawing • E. Lipiński 1975a, esp. pp. 146–71.

B.5.13 Lydian (Sardis) Bilingual (5th–4th c.) **LydBil**
Lydian-Aramaic bilingual funerary text on broken marble stele. In situ.

Ed. Pr.   E. Littmann 1916, pp. 23–38, pl. 14.

EASY ACCESS
   Editions: *AaG*Seg 54 • *AC* 46 • *KAI* 260.

   Translations: *TUAT* 2:574–75.

LITERATURE
   O. A. Danielsson 1917 • S. A. Cook 1917 • C. C. Torrey 1917–18 • M. Lidzbarski 1917–18 • A. Cuny 1920–21 • A. Cowley 1921 • F. Bilabel 1921 • A. Mentz
   1922 • A. Cuny 1923 • J. Fraser 1923 • W. Buckler 1924 • W. Brandenstein 1929
   • F. Sommer 1930 • L. H. Gray 1930 • P. Kahle and F. Sommer 1930 • W. Brandenstein 1931–32 • J. Friedrich 1932, esp. pp. 108–10 • W. Brandenstein 1932 •
   P. Meriggi 1934–36 • G. R. Driver 1935, esp. p. esp4 • W. F. Albright 1949, esp.
   p. 1:63 • S. Gevirtz 1961, esp. p. 148 • J. Teixidor 1970a, esp. p. 374 • M. N.
   Bogolyubov 1974 • E. Badian 1978 • J. Naveh 1982, pl. 11A.

B.5.14   Xanthos Inscriptions (4th c.)   **Xanthos**

1) Limestone orthostat with Lydian, Greek, and Aramaic inscriptions on three sides (1.35 x .58 m.) In situ.
2) Limestone fragment (16 x 12 cm.)
3) Limestone fragment (12 x 12 cm.)

Ed. Pr.   1) A. Dupont-Sommer 1974.
2–3) A. Dupont-Sommer 1979.

LITERATURE

C. Llinas 1974 • E. Laroche 1974 • H. Metzger 1974 • R. Gusmani 1975 • H. Lozachmeur 1975 • A. R. Millard 1975 • J. Teixidor 1975, esp. pp. 287–89 • J. Teixidor 1976, esp. pp. 310, 335 • P. Frei 1976–77 • G. Garbini 1977 • O. Carruba 1977 • R. Gusmani 1977 • J. Teixidor 1978 • O. Carruba et al. 1978 • P. Frei and V. Shevoroshkin 1978 • J. Teixidor 1979, esp. pp. 393–94 • M. Mayrhofer 1979 • R. Gusmani 1979 • A. Dupont-Sommer 1979a • H. Metzger, ed. 1980 • H. Humbach 1981 • I. Hahn 1981 • P. Frei 1981 • R. Contini 1981 • W. A. P. Childs 1981, esp. pp. 77–78 • J. Blomqvist 1982 • H. Eichner 1983 • J. Bousquet 1986 • C. Le Roy 1987 • A. Faber 1988, esp. pp. 223–24.

B.5.15   Agaca Kale Bilingual (late 4th c.)   **AgacaKale**

Greek-Aramaic funerary (?) text inscribed in a niche on a rock. In situ.

בגנתא [...] מ[.]א 1
די רמן ב[.....]
כאל[....] בראה
הרי[...] ברא די רמן
חשת[.....]מן 5

Ed. Pr.   F. Cumont 1905.

EASY ACCESS
Editions: *ESE* 2:249–50 • *RES* 954.

LITERATURE

H. N. Fowler 1905 • H. Schenkl 1905 • T. Reinach 1905 • T. Reinach 1905a • H. H. von der Osten 1928–29 • M. Sprengling 1928–29 • H. H. von der Osten 1929, esp. pp. 122–27 • H. Lozachmeur 1975 • E. Lipiński 1975a, esp. pp. 197–208 • E. Lipiński 1978b.

B.6 Iran and the East

B.6.1   Luristan Bronze Vessels (8th-7th c.)   LurBr

1 Bronze juglet (15 cm. ht.), 2 bronze cups. Fouroughi Collection, Teheran.

1) [...]א זי עבדת פראתן אלסתר
לעתרמצרן נגש
2) לכמראלה בר אלסמך עבד עזר
3) ל[.....] כתב אבאצר כסא זנה לחיי נבשה

Ed. Pr.   A. Dupont-Sommer 1964a.

EASY ACCESS
    Editions: 1) *TSSI* 11.
                     2) *TSSI* 12.

LITERATURE
General
R. Dussaud 1949b • O. M. Dalton 1964 • J. Naveh 1964–65, esp. pp. 194–95 • J. Naveh 1966, esp. pp. 20–22 • J. Teixidor 1967, esp. pp. 183–85 • C. Nylander 1968 • K. R. Veenhof 1968, esp. pp. 137–38.
1) G. Garbini 1967a, esp. pp. 92–94 • R. Degen 1969, esp. p. 23 • E. Lipiński 1977, esp. pp. 98–99.

B.6.2   Persepolis Tablets (500)   PersepTab

Ca. 700 (!?) as yet unpublished Aramaic clay tablet fragments plus 44 Elamite tablets with unpublished Aramaic endorsements from the Persepolis Fortification archive. The Aramaic tablets are mostly records of wine (חמר) rations. Oriental Institute, Chicago.

LITERATURE
R. Dussaud 1934 • R. T. Hallock 1950 • W. Hinz 1960–61 • R. T. Hallock 1969, esp. p. 82 • M. Dandamaev and V. G. Lukonin 1989, esp. p. 379.
See also the literature for the following entry.

B.6.3   Persepolis Inscriptions (5th c.)   Persep

Administrative notations on 163 ritual vessels found in the Persepolis Treasury. Oriental Institute, Chicago.

Ed. Pr.   R. A. Bowman 1970.

LITERATURE
Anon. 1934, esp. p. 232 • E. Herzfeld 1938 • E. F. Schmidt 1939 • M. Sprengling 1940 • G. G. Cameron 1948, esp. pp. 6, 23 • M. Sprengling 1953, esp. pp. 1–35 •

E. F. Schmidt 1953, 1957, 1970 • A. Maricq 1958 • M. L. Chaumont 1963 • G. G. Cameron 1965 • J. Z. Smith 1971 • B. A. Levine 1972 • J. Naveh and S. Shaked 1973 • J. R. Hinnells 1973 • J. Teixidor 1973, esp. pp. 431–32 • M. N. Bogolyubov 1973 • J. A. Delaunay 1974 • J. Teixidor 1974, esp. pp. 331–32 • S. A. Kaufman 1974, esp. p. 59 • J. Oelsner 1975 • W. Hinz 1975 • J. A. Delaunay 1976 • E. Lipiński 1977a • M. Mayrhofer 1978 • J. M. Fennelly 1980 • J. C. Greenfield 1984–86, esp. p. 154.

B.6.4   Silver Label (Iran [?], 250)   IranSilLab

Inscription on a silver plaquette. Foroughi Collection, Teheran.

שקרתא זי עבד חנבנדך ושבור [......] 1
לגדי אלהא
לחיוהי ולחיי אחוהי ודודהי

Ed. Pr.   A. Dupont-Sommer 1964.

LITERATURE   J. Naveh 1964–65, esp. pp. 196–97 • J. Naveh 1966, esp. pp. 34–35 • K. R. Veenhof 1968, esp. p. 138.

B.6.5   Asoka Inscriptions General Information

LITERATURE
E. Senart 1881–86 • V. A. Smith 1904, esp. pp. 150–54 • E. Hultzsch 1925 • A. Cunningham 1961 • E. Benveniste 1964 • D. Schlumberger 1964 • P. H. L. Eggermont 1965–66 • M. C. Joshi and B. M. Pande 1967 • P. H. L. Eggermont 1969 • D. Schlumberger 1972 • K. R. Norman 1972 • J. Teixidor 1975, esp. p. 289 • M. N. Bogolyubov 1977 • L. García Daris 1980 • B. Brentjes 1981, esp. p. 141 • G. D. Davary 1981 • L. Schober 1981, esp. pp. 160–69 • G. Itō 1981a • B. N. Mukherjee 1984.

B.6.6   Asoka I (Taxila-Sirkap) (Pakistan, 3d c.)   Asok.1

Fragmentary marble pillar. In situ.

Ed. Pr.   L. D. Barnett 1915 and A. Cowley 1915.

EASY ACCESS
Editions: *AC* 54 • *KAI* 273.

LITERATURE
E. Herzfeld 1927–28 • H. H. Schaeder 1929–30 • F. C. Andreas 1932 • H. Birkeland 1938 • F. Altheim 1947, esp. p. 29, n. 3 • F. Altheim 1948–50, esp. p. 2:178–88, 204–5 • F. Altheim 1949, esp. pp. 5–17 • J. Marshall 1951, esp. pp. 15, 164–66 • G. M. Bongard-Levin 1956 • F. Altheim and R. Stiehl 1957, esp. pp. 9–20 • R. Choudhary 1958 • F. Altheim and R. Stiehl 1963, esp. pp. 12–14 • F.

Altheim and R. Stiehl 1964–69, esp. pp. 4:39–40, 214 • H. Humbach 1969 • E. Y. Kutscher, J. Naveh, and S. Shaked 1969–70, esp. pp. 125–26 • R. Degen 1969–70 • H. Humbach 1969a • F. Altheim and R. Stiehl 1970, esp. pp. 338–43 • W. T. In der Smitten 1971a • J. Teixidor 1973, esp. p. 433 • M. N. Bogolyubov 1976 • G. Itō 1977 • H. Humbach 1979, esp. pp. 190–92 • F. R. Allchin 1982.

B.6.7 Asoka II (Pul-i Darunta, Afghanistan, 3d c.) Asok.2

Fragmentary monument. Kabul Museum.

Ed. Pr. H. Birkeland 1938.

EASY ACCESS
Editions: *AC* 53A.

LITERATURE
F. Rosenthal 1939, esp. pp. 33–34 • F. Altheim 1947, esp. pp. 27–43 • F. Altheim 1947–48 • W. B. Henning 1949–51 • F. Altheim and R. Stiehl 1963, esp. p. 73 • F. Altheim and R. Stiehl 1964–69, esp. pp. 5/2: 285 • C. Caillat 1966 • E. Y. Kutscher, J. Naveh, and S. Shaked 1969–70, esp. pp. 126–28 • J. Teixidor 1979, esp. pp. 394–95.

B.6.8 Asoka III (Kandahar, Afghanistan, 3d c.) Asok.3

Greek-Aramaic bilingual set in a panel cut into a rock. In situ.

Ed. Pr. G. Pugliese-Carratelli et al. 1958.

EASY ACCESS
Editions: *AC* 53B • *KAI* 279 • *Aag*Seg 59.

LITERATURE
J. Bloch 1950 • P. H. L. Eggermont 1956, esp. pp. 90–96 • F. Altheim and R. Stiehl 1958 • É. Lamotte 1958 • A. Pohl 1958, esp. p. 420 • U. Scerrato 1958 • U. Scerrato 1958a • U. Scerrato 1958b • D. Schlumberger, L. Robert, A. Dupont-Sommer and E. Benveniste 1958 • C. Gallavotti 1959 • D. D. Kosambi 1959 • P. Nober 1959 • C. Picard 1959 • A. Pohl 1959 • F. Zucker 1959 • A. Dupont-Sommer 1959a • C. Gallavotti 1959a • F. Altheim and R. Stiehl 1959 • F. Altheim and R. Stiehl 1959a • P. Nober 1959b • F. Altheim and R. Stiehl 1959–62 • A. Dupont-Sommer 1960 • G. Pugliese-Carratelli 1960 • J. Robert and L. Robert 1960, esp. pp. 204–5 • R. Thapar 1961, esp. pp. 260–61 • H. Filliozat 1961–62 • P. H. L. Eggermont and J. Hoftijzer 1962 • F. Altheim and R. Stiehl 1963, esp. pp. 21–32 • G. Garbini 1964 • G. Pugliese-Carratelli and G. Garbini 1964 • D. Schlumberger 1964 • F. Altheim and R. Stiehl 1964–69, esp. pp. 4:39–40, 214 • G. Itō 1967 • F. Altheim and R. Stiehl 1969, esp. pp. 418–31 • J. Teixidor 1969, esp. pp. 347–49 • E. Y. Kutscher, J. Naveh, and S. Shaked 1969–70, esp. pp. 129–36 • F. Altheim and R. Stiehl 1970, esp. pp. 344–55 • H. Humbach 1971 • G. Itō 1977 • F. Rosenthal 1978, esp. pp. 194–96 • G. Itō 1979 • H. Humbach

1979, esp. pp. 194–96 • M. N. Bogolyubov 1979 • J. Naveh 1982, pl. 16A.

B.6.9   Asoka IV (Kandahar, Afghanistan, 3d c.)   Asok.4

Fragmentary limestone block (24 x 18.5 cm.)

```
1 [              ]        [שׁ שׂיתיהס שׁיש[
  [              ]        י[שׁינאכיהינאי אתנלט זי ף.[
           י[תיהס הנמתפונא ןאכו אננכ קרא יתיה[ס]
           אנכיתסתפל ןורתוהיו ןריתוה ףא ןכ[ל]
5        ןרימג אנכיתסתפל יתיה[ס]       [
           איתפיטפונא ןאכל [א]המויו       [
  [        ] ידבע ןריצׂ֗נׁ֗ל[       ]
```

Ed. Pr.   E. Benveniste and A. Dupont-Sommer 1966.

LITERATURE

D. Schlumberger 1964 • C. Caillat 1966, esp. pp. 194–96 • A. Dupont-Sommer 1966b • J. Teixidor 1969, esp. pp. 349–50 • S. Shaked 1969 • E. Y. Kutscher, J. Naveh, and S. Shaked 1969–70, esp. pp. 128–29 • G. D. Davary and H. Humbach 1974 • V. A. Livshitz and I. Sh. Shifman 1977.

B.6.10   Asoka V (Laghman, Afghanistan, 3d c.)   Asok.5

Inscription carved in a vertical slab set in a hillside. In situ.

```
1 אחר קדז אכלמ שׁרדירפ 16 תנשׁב
  ןתשׁק קיר דבע המ (ירוכ) ׂירוכ תוירב דצמ המׂ ןרירשׁ ןמ
  יתהס יתפרכ אחרא הנז המשׁ רמדת ארות הנז 200
  80 אלע 100 ארתא חרת 120 ארתא אתנג
  אניד ושׁאו םע
```

Ed. Pr.   A. Dupont-Sommer 1970.

LITERATURE

S. Shaked 1969 • J. Teixidor 1971, esp. pp. 479–80 • F. Altheim and R. Stiehl 1972 • J. de Menasce 1972 • F. Rosenthal 1978 • G. Itō 1979 • H. Humbach 1979, esp. pp. 192–93.

B.6.11   Asoka VI (Laghman, Afghanistan, 3d c.)   Asok.6

Inscription carved on rock. In situ.

```
1 תנשׁ האמ לולאב
  אכלמ שׁרדירפ 16
  קקשׁ ןרירשׁ ןמ אחר קדז
  [ת...]וירב ירוכ דצמ המ
5 [...] ןתשׁק קיר דבע המ
```

זנה תורא אהותי שמה
זנה ארחא כרפתי ס>ה<יתי
גנתא אתר 300 תרח אתרה [....]
עמ ואשו שמה דינא [...]
10 וחשופרתבג שכן זכא [...]

Ed. Pr.   G. D. Davary and H. Humbach 1974.

LITERATURE   A. Dupont-Sommer 1949a, esp. p. 91.

B.7 Seals and Coins

B.7.1 Seals

The following table contains information on seals or seal impressions with names, scripts, or words considered to be, or once considered to be, Aramaic. The seals are listed by text in order of the Semitic alphabet. The readings are intended to be up-to-date, but they are based on the literature and do not represent new, independent readings. Note the following abbreviations: S: stamp seal; C: cylinder seal; SI: stamp seal impression; CI: cylinder seal impression; B: bulla, P. Bordreuil 1986; G: K. Galling 1941; H: L. G. Herr 1978; V: F. Vattioni 1971a.

#	Text	Prov.	Date	Editio princeps
1S	אבגד	?	8th–7th	P. Bordreuil and A. Lemaire 1976, p. 54 (pl. V.25).
2S	אבגד	Syria	8th–7th	L. Y. Rahmani 1964a, pp. 180–81 (pl. 41E).
3S	אבגד / הוזח	?	late 8th	R. Hestrin et al. 1973 (no. 10).
4S	אבגדה / וזחסי	?	7th	P. Bordreuil and A. Lemaire 1976, p. 54 (pl. V.26).
5S	אבגדה / וזחסי	?	ca. 600	H. H. Spoer 1907, p. 359 (pl. opposite p. 355).
6S	אבגדה / וזחסי	?	7th	P. Bordreuil and A. Lemaire 1982, pp. 109–11 (pl. 1).
7S	אבגדהו / זחסיך	?	early 6th	P. Bordreuil 1986.
8S	אבגדה / יוזחך	?	late 6th	P. Bordreuil 1986.
9S	אבה	Palestine	?	P. Schröder 1914, pp. 176–77 (no. 3; fig. 10).
10S	אבח	?	ca. 550	P. Bordreuil 1986.
11S	אלא ננא י	?	5th?	S. Shaked and J. Naveh 1986, pp. 23–24 (pl. 2–3).
12B	אדנלות	Hama	8th	B. Otzen 1990, pp. 276–77.
13C	אדנרי	?	ca. 700	L. Delaporte 1920–23 (A1146).
14S	אדנשע	Syria	late 8th	P. Berger 1894.
15C	אזאדשם זנומן	?	4th–3rd	W. H. Ward 1886, p. 155.
16CI	אחמלך	?	ca. 600	W. H. Ward 1920 (no. 271).
17S	אחז פקחי	Jericho	mid–8th	E. Sachau 1896, p. 1064.
18S	אחצר	Palestine	750–700	N. Avigad 1968, pp. 44–47.
19B	אלאן	Hama	8th	B. Otzen 1990, pp. 279 and 281.
20S	אלדלה	?	late 8th	R. D. Barnett 1940, p. 31.
21S	אלהעזר	?	early 8th	A. Lemaire 1990b, pp. 16–18 (pl. II.2).
22S	אלנורי	?	ca. 700	K. Galling 1941.
23B	אלעזר	Jerusalem	ca. 500	N. Avigad 1976, pp. 9–10 (no. 11).
24SI	אנאחאתן	?	?	C. C. Torrey, in M. Rostovtzeff 1932, pp. 18–19 (pl. III.4).
25S	ארבדי	?	Neo-Ass.	W. H. Ward 1920 (no. 284).

#	Collections	Literature
1S		A. Lemaire 1985d, p. 47; F. Israel 1987, p. 143; W. E. Aufrecht 1989, pp. 222–23 (no. 82).
2S	H 90	J. Naveh 1964–65, p. 185; J. Naveh 1966, p. 22; F. Vattioni 1981b (no. 79); A. Lemaire 1985d, p. 47; W. E. Aufrecht 1989, pp. 344–45 (no. 54a).
3S	H 18	R. Hestrin and M. Dayagi-Mendels 1979 (no. 129).
4S		A. Lemaire 1978, p. 227.
5S	ESE 3:68; RES 925	A. Lemaire 1978, p. 227; A. Lemaire 1985d, p. 47; F. Israel 1987, p. 142; W. E. Aufrecht 1989, pp. 53–54 (no. 22).
6S		W. E. Aufrecht 1989, p. 286 (no. 115).
7S	B 116	
8S	B 120	
9S	RES 1868; V 105	
10S	B 117	
11S		
12B		
13C	G 156; V 68; H 80; B 96	
14S	RES 1239; H 91; B 5	A. Reifenberg 1950 (no. 30); F. Israel 1986, p. 72; F. Israel 1987, p. 145; W. E. Aufrecht 1989, p. 148 (no. 17a).
15C	G 171; V 83	W. H. Ward 1910 (no. 1054); J. Boardman 1970a, pp. 320–21 and 350 (fig. 309); D. Collon 1987, pp. 92–93 (no. 431).
16CI	G 159; V 71 = 134	W. H. Ward 1910 (no. 1152); F. Rosenthal in E. Porada 1948 (no. 816).
17S	G 8; H 83	D. Diringer 1934, pp. 202–3 (no. 44); S. Moscati 1951 (pl. XV.8); F. Vattioni 1969b (no. 44); L. Jakob-Rost 1975 (no. 180); F. Israel 1986, p. 72.
18S	H 102	R. Hestrin and M. Dayagi-Mendels 1979 (no. 130); D. Parayre 1990 (no. 70).
19B		
20S		S. Moscati 1951, pp. 58–59 (pl. XII.8); D. Parayre 1990 (no. 122).
21S		
22S	G 12; V 2; H 46	L. Jakob-Rost 1975 (no. 178); F. Israel 1986, p. 72.
23B	H 42	
24SI	V 124	R. P. Dougherty, in M. Rostovtzeff 1932, pp. 94–97.
25S	G 127; V 54 = 133	F. Rosenthal, in E. Porada 1948 (no. 790); A. Lemaire 1985d, p. 42; F. Israel 1987, p. 143; W. E. Aufrecht 1989, pp. 59–60 (no. 24).

#	Text	Prov.	Date	Editio princeps
26C	ארפקדבן	?	8th	L. Speleers 1943 pp. 128–30 (no. 1499).
27S	ארתד	?	7th	L. Delaporte 1920-23 (A1145).
28S	ארתד	?	late 7th	L. Delaporte 1920-23 (A1142).
29CI	[....] ארתדר זי רב	Persepolis	Persian	R. A. Bowman, in G. G. Cameron 1948 (no. 4).
30SI	בא	Engedi	Persian	B. Mazar 1967, p. 227.
31C	בבן	?	4th	P. Bordreuil 1986.
32C	בגדת	?	Persian	A. R. Millard 1978, pp. 23–24 (pl. IV).
33C	בגדן	?	6th	P. Bordreuil and E. Gubel 1987, pp. 312–13.
34C	בגמרזדי	Egypt	?	N. Aimé-Giron 1939 (no. 117; pl. III).
35SI	ב]יב[נ	Nippur	464–404	L. Legrain 1925 (no. 829).
36C	בלאתן	Damascus	5th	H. C. Reichardt 1883.
37	בלטי	7th	Mesop.	M. Heltzer in O. W. Muscarella 1981 (no. 109).
38S	בעלנתן	Tello	7th	E. Ledrain 1882, p. 286.
39S	בעלנתן	?	8th	P. Schröder 1880, p. 683 (fig. 8).
40CI	ברהד	Balawat	686	B. Parker 1963, p. 97.
41C	ברכא בר גדל בר תבלט	?	ca. 700	L. Delaporte 1920-23 (A1138).
42S	בר עתר	?	ca. 800	P. Bordreuil 1986.
43C	גבואה	Assyria	?	W. H. Ward 1910 (no. 710).
44C	גחז	Babylon	?	E. J. Pilcher 1901.
45S	גנת	?	late 6th–5th	P. Bordreuil and A. Lemaire 1974, pp. 25–27 (pl. on p. 31).
46C	דדי	?	8th	A. Lemaire 1983, pp. 27–28 (pl. III.13).
47S	דדעלה	?	ca. 700	CIS
48S	דחד	Beirut?	ca. 500	C. J. M. de Vogüé 1868a (no. 28).
49S	דיכלא	?	late 8th	CIS
50C	דשתחו	?	about 450	W. H. Ward 1910 (no. 1138).
51C	הדתכל	Iraq?	ca. 700	H. C. Rawlinson 1865, p. 229 (pl. IV).
52C	הוזת	?	?	ESE
53SI	הרמי	Tello	4th	V. Scheil 1901.
54C	ויזך	?	Persian	D. J. Wiseman, n.d. (pl. 111)
55C	וחתרו	?	4th	L. Delaporte 1910 (no. 502).
56S	ורעחל	?	?	A. A. Zakharov 1931 (no. 33).
57C	זבדי	?	ca. 500	M.-L. Vollenweider et al., p. 157 (no. 44).
58S	זנה חתם זי ראכתוס	Syria	?	J. Teixidor 1990, pp. 505–6 (fig. 22A–C).
59C	זרתשתרש	?	late 4th	A. Parrot 1961 (fig. 260).
60S	חב	Amrit	ca. 700	C. J. M. de Vogüé 1868a (no. 12).
61S	חור	?	ca. 650	C. J. M. de Vogüé 1868a (no. 19).

#	Collections	Literature
26C	V 132	
27S	G 94; V 33; H 59; B 105	J. Naveh 1980, p. 75.
28S	G 96; V 34; H 60; B 106	P. Amiet 1973 (no. 547); J. Naveh 1980, p. 75; D. Parayre 1990 (no. 51).
29CI	V 135	E. F. Schmidt 1957 (no. 33); J. C. Greenfield 1962, p. 298.
30SI	V 163	E. Stern 1982, p. 209.
31C	B 138	
32C	V 169	
33C		
34C	V 126	J. C. Greenfield 1962, p. 298.
35SI	V 115	
36C	CIS 92; G 162; V 74	A. D. H. Bivar 1970, p. 48.
37		E. Borowski 1965, p. 66 (no. 11).
38S	ESE 1:138-40; RES 1822; V 20; H Moabite 8	J. Offord 1900, pp. 379–80; L. Delaporte 1920–23 (T242); H. Gressmann 1927 (fig. 584); R. Giveon 1961, pp. 41–42.
39S	RES 1823; G 54; V 21	D. Parayre 1990 (no. 15).
40CI	V 160	
41C	G 148; V 60; H 79; B 94	
42S	B 93	D. Parayre 1990 (no. 18).
43C	V 93	G. R. Driver 1957a, p. 46.
44C	ESE 1:275–76; RES 1831; V 104	
45S	H 85	
46C		
47S	CIS 107; V 46; H 18	A. Reifenberg 1950 (no. 41).
48S	CIS 96; G 83; V 27; H 105; B 119	M. A. Levy 1869, pp. 19–21; A. de Ridder 1911, pp. 489–90; D. Parayre 1990 (no. 71).
49S	CIS 106; G 89; V 31; H 20	A. Reifenberg 1950 (no. 37); G. R. Driver 1957a, p. 46; R. Hestrin and M. Dayagi-Mendels 1979 (no. 131).
50C	G 172; V 84; H 81; B 130	L. Delaporte 1920-23 (A779).
51C	CIS 89; G 155; V 67; H 70	M. A. Levy 1869, p. 15; W. H. Ward 1910 (no. 582 = no. 1149).
52C	ESE 2:400; RES 1825; G 168; V 80	O. Weber 1920 (no. 316); A. Moortgat 1940 (no. 764).
53SI	ESE 1:276; RES 244; V 98	A. Goetze 1944, pp. 100–1 (pl. XI.d).
54C		D. Collon 1987, pp. 156–57 (no. 698).
55C	G 167; B 135	F. Vattioni 1981b (no. 65).
56S	V 122	
57C		A. Lemaire 1985d, pp. 36–37 (fig. 4).
58S		
59C	B 136	
60S	G 104; H 101; B 9	M. A. Levy 1869, p. 27; A. de Ridder 1911, pp. 492–93; F. Vattioni 1981b (no. 18).
61S	G 39; B 104	M. A. Levy 1869, pp. 30–31; A. de Ridder 1911, pp. 491–92; F. Vattioni 1981b (no. 22).

#	Text	Prov.	Date	Editio princeps
62S	חמר זנה זי מתרצתר	?	early 5th	O. Blau 1864.
63S	חנכי	?	early 6th	F. Lajard 1847 (pl. 44.17).
64S	חר חבי	Egypt?	early 5th	C. Clermont-Ganneau 1887, p. 238.
65SI	חת[ם] אמדת בר [הדדת]	?	450	CIS
66CI	חתם [ארשם] בר ב[נ]יתא]	Egypt?	5th	P. Kahle 1948-49, p. 207.
67C	חתם אתו	5th–4th	Iran	E. Williams-Forte and M. Heltzer in O. W. Muscarella 1981 (no. 171).
68C	חתם בני בר זתו הי שן	Turkey	6th–4th	A. Parrot 1961 (fig. 256).
69C	חתם ברק עבד עתרשמן	Lebanon	late 9th	H. Seyrig 1955, p. 42.
70SI	חתם דתמ[תר]	Persepolis	?	E. F. Schmidt 1957 (no. 20).
71CI	חת[ם הומ]דת בר [בגדת]	?	450	C. Clermont-Ganneau 1883a (no. 33).
72C	חתם המתר	?	5th	S. Shaked and J. Naveh 1986, pp. 24–25, pl. 4.
73C	חתם וחוש	?	?	W. H. Ward 1910 (no. 1140).
74C	חתם יפעהד מפשר	?	ca. 800	O. Weber 1920 (no. 311).
75S	חתם מנגאנרת ברך למלכם	?	ca. 650	N. Avigad 1965, pp. 222–28 (pl. 40).
75a	חתם נגאנרת ברך למלכם	?	?	J. Naveh and H. Tadmor 1968, pp. 448–50.
75b	חתם לגאדת ברך למלכם	?	?	G. Garbini 1967.
76S	חתם מנן ברכבעל	Aleppo	7th–6th	C. J. M. de Vogüé 1868a (no. 21).
77C	חתם מתרש בר שעי	Jaffa	early 5th	P. Berger 1888.
78S	חתם נרגש בר שרש	?	5th	C. J. M. de Vogüé 1868a (no. 33).
79C	חתם סמסך	Iran	5th	M. Heltzer in O. W. Muscarella 1981 (no. 170).
80C	חתם עבדכדאה	?	?	D. Collon 1986, pp. 425–26 (no. III.3; fig. 10).
81CI	חתם פרנך בר ארשם	Persepolis	Persian	G. G. Cameron 1948, p. 53, n. 52.
82C	חתם פרשנדת בר ארתדת	Assyria	early 5th	F. Lajard 1847 (pl. 50.4).
83S	חתם שמש	Syria	8th–6th	ESE
84CI	חתם...הי	Persepolis	Persian	E. F. Schmidt 1957 (no. 39).
85S	טבשלם	Engedi	ca. 600	B. Mazar and I. Dunayevsky 1964, p. 123.
86SI	יאל בר ישׁעֹ / יהוד	Belmont Castle	5th	A. R. Millard 1989a, p. 61 (fig. 14).
87C	יבת	?	?	L. Speleers 1943 pp. 176–77(no. 1469).
88S	יהד	Jerusalem	ca. 500	N. Avigad 1976, p. 10 (no. 13; pl. 15).
89B	יהד	Jerusalem	ca. 500	N. Avigad 1976, pp. 3–4 (no. 1; pl. 3).

#	Collections	Literature
62S	CIS 102; G 42; V 14; H 7	M. A. Levy 1869, p. 17; J. Euting 1883 (no. 9); F. Imhoof-Blumer and O. Keller 1889 (pl. 19.51); J. Naveh 1980, p. 76; P. Bordreuil and E. Gubel 1985, pp. 173–74 (fig. 2).
63S	G 114a; V 45; B 113	
64S	CIS 140; V 91; H 6	
65SI	CIS 66; V 88	L. Delaporte 1920-23 (A797.G).
66CI	V 140	G. R. Driver 1957, p. 4, n. 1; J. C. Greenfield 1962, p. 299; A. F. Rainey 1966, p. 188; A. D. H. Bivar 1970, p. 52.
67C		
68C		M. Mellink and R. S. Young 1966, p. 196. D. Collon 1987 pp. 90–91 (no. 424).
69C	V 142; H 78; B 85	J. T. Milik 1958-59, p. 338; F. M. Cross 1983, p. 61; P. Bordreuil 1983a (no. 250).
70SI	V 143	J. C. Greenfield 1962, p. 299; R. A. Bowman 1970, pp. 6–7 (pl. 1.B).
71CI	CIS 66; V 88; B 125	S. Schiffer 1911, p. 182; L. Delaporte 1920-23 (A797).
72C		B. Zuckerman 1987, pp. 28–30.
73C	V 96	
74C	G 160; V 72	
75S	H Ammonite 9; B 76	H. Tadmor 1965; J. Naveh and H. Tadmor 1968, pp. 448–50; F. Vattioni 1969b (no. 225); F. Vattioni 1978a (no. 225); L. G. Herr 1980; J. Naveh 1980, p. 76; P. Bordreuil 1986b (no. 178); P. Bordreuil 1987, p. 285; W. E. Aufrecht 1989, pp. 141–44 (no. 55).
75a		F. Israel 1987, p. 143; W. E. Aufrecht 1989, pp. 166–67 (no. 61).
75b		J. Naveh and H. Tadmor 1968, pp. 448–51.
76S	G 47; V 17	M. A. Levy 1869, pp. 28–29.
77C	CIS 101; G 169; V 81; H 71; B 128	M. Ohnefalsch-Richter 1893 (pl. LXXVII.12).
78S	CIS 105; G 48; V 18	M. A. Levy 1869, pp. 18–19 (pl. I.17); E. Ledrain 1884d, pp. 66–67; A. F. Rainey 1966, p. 188.
79C		P. Bordreuil and E. Gubel 1987, p. 316 (fig. 6).
80C		D. Collon 1987, pp. 83 and 85 (no. 398).
81CI	V 136	
82C	CIS 100; G 163; V 75 = 76; H 72	A. H. Layard 1853, p. 517; M. A. Levy 1857, p. 40 (pl. 14); H. C. Rawlinson 1865, p. 233; M. A. Levy 1869, p. 18; M. Ohnefalsch-Richter 1893 (pl. LXXVII); W. H. Ward 1910 (no. 1125); A. R. Millard 1977, p. 484; A. R. Millard 1982, p. 151.
83S	ESE 3:186–87; G 40; V 12	
84CI	V 144	
85S	V 162	B. Mazar 1967, p. 226; J. Teixidor 1967, p. 180; F. M. Cross 1969, pp. 26–27.
86SI		
87C	V 131	
88S	H 44	
89B	H 32	

#	Text	Prov.	Date	Editio princeps
90B	יהד	Jerusalem	ca. 500	N. Avigad 1976, p. 2 (no. 2; pl. 4).
91SI	יהוד אוריו	Jericho	late 6th	P. C. Hammond 1957.
92B	יהוד חננה	Jerusalem	ca. 500	N. Avigad 1976, pp. 4–5 (no. 3; pl. 5).
93SI	יהוד חננה	Ramat Raḥel	Persian	Y. Aharoni 1956, p. 146 (pl. 26.4); Y. Aharoni 1964a, p. 46 (fig. 37.10; pl. 20.7).
94SI	יהוד יהועזר פחוא	Ramat Raḥel	Persian	Y. Aharoni 1962a, pp. 7–8 (fig. 9.1; pl. 9.2), 33 (fig. 22.8; pl. 30.10) and 1964a, pp. 21–22 (pl. 20.6) and 44–45 (pl. 20.9).
95B	יהוד.. .נ.	Jerusalem	ca. 500	N. Avigad 1976, p. 5 (no. 4; pl. 5).
96S	יחזק	?	early 8th	L. G. Herr 1978.
97S	יעדראל	Damascus	8th–6th	C. Clermont-Ganneau 1883a (no. 13).
98C	ירפאל בר הדעדר	Assyria	ca. 700	M. A. Levy 1857, pp. 28–30 (pl. 3).
99S	ישעא	Beirut	late 8th	ESE
100S	כנבו	?	ca. 700	L. Delaporte 1920–23 (A736).
101S	כני	?	ca. 650	A. Reifenberg 1950 (no. 38).
102C	כנתרֹ	Baghdad	Persian	W. H. Ward 1886, p. 155.
103C	כרדע	?	?	T. G. Pinches 1890 (no. 2).
104S	כרוזא	N. Syria	8th–6th	A. Bossier 1939, p. 63 (fig. 3).
105C	כרעדד	?	?	W. H. Ward 1910 (no. 1150).
106C	כרש	?	late 6th	G. A. Cooke 1922, pp. 270–71.
107C	כרתֹיר	?	?	W. H. Ward 1910 (no. 1053).
108S	לאבא	?	late 8th	C. Clermont-Ganneau 1883a (no. 14).
109S	לאבא ב...	Jerusalem	ca. 500	A. Reifenberg 1942-43, p. 111 (no. 6; pl. XIV.6).
110S	לאבגד	?	8th–7th	N. Avigad 1968b.
111S	לאבגד הוזֹח	?	late 7th	M. F. Martin 1964, p. 209 (pl. III.5).
112S	לאֹבחלל	?	late 8th	L. G. Herr 1978.
113S	לאדי בר חרי	?	early 5th	J. M. Unvala 1935, pp. 160–61.
114S	לאחאבי	?	early 7th	L. Delaporte 1920–23 (A1144).
115SI	לאחזי פחוא	Ramat Raḥel	Persian	Y. Aharoni 1962a, pp. 33–34 (fig. 22.10; pl. 30.12–13) and 1964a, pp. 22 and 45 (pl. 20.4–5).
116SI	לאחזי פחוא	T. en-Naṣbeh	Persian	F. M. Cross 1969, p. 26 (fig. 1.7–9).
117S	לאחימן	?	7th–6th	G. R. Driver 1938, p. 188 (pl. XIV.1).
118S	לאחלכן	Amrit	early 7th	C. J. M. de Vogüé 1868a (no. 29).
119S	לאאמה	?	ca. 700	C. J. M. de Vogüé 1868a (no. 9).

#	Collections	Literature
90B	H 33	
91SI	H 28	P. C. Hammond 1957a,b; W. F. Albright 1957a, pp. 28–30; N. Avigad 1957; Y. Yadin 1957; J. Naveh 1971c, p. 59; N. Avigad 1976, p. 22 (fig. 17.6).
92B	H 34	
93SI		J. Naveh 1971c, p. 59; N. Avigad 1976, p. 22.
94SI		F. M. Cross 1969, pp. 24–26; J. Naveh 1971c, pp. 60–61; N. Avigad, 1976, p. 22.
95B	H 35	
96S	H 63	
97S	G 50; V 19	
98C	CIS 77; G 152; V 64; H 73	M. A. Levy 1869, pp. 7–8 (no. 7; pl. I.2); C. J. M. de Vogüé 1868a (no. 25); G. A. Cooke 1903, p. 361 (no. 3); W. H. Ward 1910 (no. 1157); S. A. Cook 1930, p. 49, n. 5, and pl. IX.2.
99S	ESE 1:11 (no. 2); RES 61; G 72; H 21	C. Clermont-Ganneau 1901, p. 193 (no. 2); D. Diringer 1934, pp. 242–43 (no. 85); F. Vattioni 1969b (no. 85); J. Naveh 1980, p. 76; A. R. Millard 1988a (no. 295); W. E. Aufrecht 1989, no. 20; D. Parayre 1990 (no. 113).
100S	G 113; V 43; H 61; B 99	
101S	V 137; H 22; B 103	J. Boardman 1970 (no. 172); J. Teixidor 1971, p. 466.
102C	RES 1827; G 170; V 82	A. Furtwängler 1900 (fig. 82); A. Moortgat 1926, p. 20, n. 4.
103C	V 177	
104S	V 164	M.-L. Vollenweider 1967–83 (no. 145); J. Teixidor 1971, p. 465 (no. 65); A. Lemaire 1985d, pp. 32–33.
105C	V 97	G. R. Driver 1957a, p. 50.
106C	V 114	
107C	V 94 = 95	F. Rosenthal in E. Porada et al. 1948 (no. 833); G. R. Driver 1957a, p. 50; J. C. Greenfield 1962, p. 298.
108S	G 5; V 1; H 17	L. Jakob-Rost 1975 (no. 179).
109S	H 89	S. Moscati 1951, p. 65 (pl. XIV.6); R. Hestrin and M. Dayagi-Mendels 1979 (no. 135).
110S		A. Lemaire 1978, p. 226; R. Hestrin and M. Dayagi-Mendels 1979 (no. 127); A. Lemaire 1985d, p. 47; W. E. Aufrecht 1989, pp. 164–65 (no. 60).
111S		J. Naveh 1964–65, p. 183; J. Naveh 1966, pp. 22–23.
112S	H 108	
113S	B 127	J. Teixidor 1973, p. 412 (no. 72); P. Amiet 1977 (no. 2223).
114S	G 95; V 110; H 58; B 100	
115SI		F. M. Cross 1969, p. 26; J. Naveh 1971c, p. 60; N. Avigad 1976, p. 22; Y. Aharoni 1979, p. 414, n. 113.
116SI		
117S	G 118; V 49	
118S	CIS 93; G 121; V 51; H 5; B 97	M. A. Levy 1869, p. 16; J. Menant 1886, p. 224 (fig. 219); A. de Ridder 1911, pp. 487–88.
119S	G 18; V 4; H 92	S. A. Cook 1930, p. 60 and pl. IX.19; A. Lemaire 1990b, p. 13.

#	Text	Prov.	Date	Editio princeps
120S	לאחמם בר בחס	?	mid–5th	E. Ledrain 1892, p. 93.
121S	לאחנדב	Sidon?	ca. 700	E. Ledrain 1884e, p. 35.
122S	לאחת ברת נצרי	Jerusalem?	late 8th	N. Avigad 1958.
123S	ל[א]יעזר [ב]ר גבטי	?	late 7th–6th	P. Bordreuil and A. Lemaire 1979, pp. 76–78 (pl. IV.9).
124C	לאכדבן בר גנרד סרסא זי הקרב להדד	Assyria	early 7th	M. A. Levy 1857, pp. 24–27 (pl. 1).
125S	לאכמֿא	?	mid 6th	P. Bordreuil 1986.
126S	לאל	Syria	8th	E. Y. Rahmani 1964a, pp. 181–84 (pl. 41F).
127S	לאלבר[ך]	?	ca. 750	C. J. M. de Vogüé 1868a (no. 10).
128C	לאליהב	Syria	late 8th–7th	CIS
129S	לאלכֹני	?	5th	A. Lemaire 1982, pp. 111–12 (pl. 2).
130S	לאלנתן	Syria?	8th–7th	A. Reifenberg 1939, p. 196 (no. 2; pl. XXXIV.2).
131B	לאלנתן פחוא	Jerusalem	ca. 500	N. Avigad 1976, pp. 5–7 (no. 5; pl. 6).
132S	לאלסמכי	?	7th	A. Reifenberg 1938, p. 113 (no. 1; pl. VI.1).
133S	לאסראדנֹי	?	?	W. Wright 1883, p. 101 (pl. 4a).
134S	לאלרם	?	7th	C. C. Torrey 1921-22, p. 106 (no. 5).
135C	לארתים	Lycia?	ca. 400	A. D. H. Bivar 1961a.
136S	לאלש בֹֿר מֿל	?	ca. 400	A. Lemaire 1982, pp. 114–15 (pl. 4).
137S	לאשא	8th	?	P. Bordreuil and A. Lemaire 1974, pp. 27–30 (pl. on p. 31).
138S	לאשה	Syria	8th–7th	A. Lemaire 1982, pp. 109–11 (pl. 1).
139S	לאשל	Carchemish	?	L. Woolley and R. D. Barnett 1952, p. 183.
140S	לבידאל עבד גדעל	Lebanon?	ca. 700	C. Clermont-Ganneau 1883a (no. 10).
141S	לביתאל רעי	?	early 5th	P. Bordreuil 1986.
142S	לבכא	?	8th–7th	C. J. M. de Vogüé 1868a (no. 4).
143SI	לבלחי	Babylon	?	R. Koldewey 1900.
144S	לבסי	?	late 8th	N. Avigad 1969, pp. 5–6 (no. 13).
145C	לבעלרגם	Syria	late 8th	ESE
146S	לבקסת	?	?	F. Vattioni 1971a.
147S	לבקשאבא עבדירח	Mesop.	?	W. F. Prideaux 1877.
148S	לברכא / ל ב	Syria	ca. 700	S. H. Horn 1962.

#	Collections	Literature
120S	V 107; H 57; B 132	L. Delaporte 1920-23 (A1139).
121S	RES 898; G 35; V 109; H 84; B 79	E. Ledrain 1888, p. 168 (no. 414); L. Delaporte 1920–23 (A1141); G. Garbini 1977c, p. 482; P. Bordreuil and A. Lemaire 1979, p. 80; K. P. Jackson 1983a, pp. 75–76; F. Israel 1986, p. 72; P. Bordreuil 1986a (no. 181); F. Israel 1987, p. 143; W. E. Aufrecht 1989, pp. 38–39 (no. 16).
122S	V 145; H 15	D. Parayre 1990 (no. 40).
123S		
124C	CIS 75; G 151; V 63; H 68	H. C. Rawlinson 1865, p. 232; M. A. Levy 1869, p. 6; F. Hitzig 1871, pp. 252–53 (no. 2); E. Sachau 1891, pp. 432–36; G. A. Cooke 1903 p. 360 (no. 2); W. H. Ward 1910 (no. 1156); G. R. Driver 1948 pl. 61.1; J. C. Greenfield 1962, p. 297, n. 77; A. R. Millard 1962, pl. XXIIId; J. Naveh and H. Tadmor 1968, pp. 450–52 (pl. III.1).
125S	B 115	
126S		J. Naveh 1964–65, p. 184; J. Naveh 1966, p. 22 (no. 7.II); A. Lemaire 1990b, p. 14.
127S	G 23; V 8; H 103; B 88	M. A. Levy 1869, pp. 25–26; E. Ledrain 1888, p. 167 (no. 412); L. Delaporte 1920–23 (A1143); A. Lemaire 1985d, pp. 43–44; F. Israel 1987, p. 145; W. E. Aufrecht 1989, pp. 17–18 (no. 7).
128C	CIS 78; G 158; V 70; H 69	W. H. Ward 1910 (no. 1151).
129S		
130S	H 110	A. Reifenberg 1950 (no. 15); S. Moscati 1951, pp. 57–58 (pl. XII.6); R. Hestrin and M. Dayagi-Mendels 1979 (no. 133); A. Lemaire 1985d, pp. 45–46; W. E. Aufrecht 1989, pp. 77–78 (no. 32).
131B	H 36	
132S		R. Hestrin and M. Dayagi-Mendels 1979 (no. 132); F. Israel 1987, p. 144; W. E. Aufrecht 1989, p. 344 (no. 30a).
133S	G 112; V 42	C. Clermont-Ganneau 1883a (no. 45).
134S	V 113	A. Lemaire 1985d, pp. 41–42 (fig. 8); F. Israel 1987, p. 143; W. E. Aufrecht 1989, pp. 67–68 (no. 28).
135C	V 157	J. C. Greenfield 1962, p. 299.
136S		
137S		
138S		A. Lemaire 1990b, p. 14.
139S	V 90	
140S	CIS 76; G 30; V 9; H Amm. 3	W. E. Aufrecht 1989, pp. 30–33 (no. 13).
141S	B 126	
142S	G 131; V 56	
143SI	V 116	E. Unger 1931, p. 103.
144S	H 51	
145C	ESE 1:12; RES 66; G 150; V 62; H 67	B. Buchanan 1966 (no. 644).
146S	V 178	J. Boardman 1970 (no. 181).
147S	V 86	
148S	V 158; H 19	J. Naveh 1964-65, p. 184; J. Naveh 1966, p. 22 (no. 7.I).

#	Text	Prov.	Date	Editio princeps
149S	לברכי	?	ca. 700	E. Ledrain 1891, p. 143.
150SI	לברדכב בר פנמו	Zinjirli	?	F. von Luschan 1943, p. 73 (pl. 38b).
151SI	לג	Ur	?	L. Legrain 1951 (no. 823).
152C	לגבאל	Mesop.	6th	M. Heltzer in O. W. Muscarella 1981, p. 147 (no. 110).
153S	לגבׄרׄת מרחׄד	Iraq	?	P. Schröder 1914, pp. 177–79 (no. 4; fig. 11).
154S	לגדרם	Syria	8th–7th	C. Clermont-Ganneau 1885–1924, 3:193.
155C	לדלנת	?	3rd	P. Bordreuil 1986.
156S	להאמן בר פרקל	?	mid–8th	ESE
157S	להדדעזר	Saqqara	mid–8th	G. Maspero 1883, p. 396.
158S	להדדקיע בר הדבעד	?	early 8th	M. A. Levy 1857, pp. 30–31 (pl. 4).
159S	להודו ספרא	?	late 8th	U. F. Kopp 1817-29, 4:110.
160S	להוזי בר תד	?	ca. 500	P. Bordreuil and A. Lemaire 1979, pp. 78–79 (pl. IV.10).
161S	להושע בעלידגל	Egypt	?	E. Sachau 1911, p. 251 (no. 12; pl. 71.12)
162S	להמל דדה	T. el Mazar	early 5th	K. Yassine and P. Bordreuil 1982, pp. 192–93.
163SI	לזבדיו ט יהד	R. Raḥel	Persian	Y. Aharoni 1964a, pp. 46–47 (fig. 37.8; pl. 20.10-11).
164S	לחםמת	?	6th–5th	R. Hestrin and M. Dayagi-Mendels 1979, 134.
165S	לחכש	?	ca. 700	N. Avigad 1978, p. 68 (fig. 5).
166S	לחלליו ברת מתאי	Abu Gosh	?	W. R. Taylor 1930, p. 21 (pl. II.A).
167S	לחנא	Iraq?	8th	A. Reifenberg 1950 (no. 42).
168S	לחנן	?	8th–7th	ESE
169S	לחננדת דתננא	?	late 6th–5th	S. Shaked and J. Naveh 1986, pp. 21–23 (pl. 1).
170S	ליאש בר גדי	?	late 6th	P. Bordreuil 1986
171S	לידאׄח	?	early 6th	L. De Clercq 1903, pp. 19–20.
172S	ליכל עבד אברם	?	ca. 800	C. Clermont-Ganneau 1883a (no. 12).
173S	לילא	?	ca. 700	P. Bordreuil and A. Lemaire 1976, pp. 53–54.
174S	לכלוזרשמש	?	750–700	C. J. M. de Vogüé 1868a (no. 31).
175C	לכנתגם	?	?	M. A. Levy 1869, p. 53 (pl. I.4a).
176S	לכפר	Tyre	6th–5th	C. J. M. de Vogüé 1868a (no. 17).
177C	לכפר	?	8th	C. H. Gordon 1939 (no. 89).
178S	לכרזי	?	ca. 700	C. J. M. de Vogüé 1868a (no. 27).

#	Collections	Literature
149S	RES 959; G 105; V 37; H 56; B 95	L. Delaporte 1920-23 (A733).
150SI	V 129	Y. Yadin 1967a, p. 34.
151SI	V 146	
152C		P. Bordreuil and E. Gubel 1987, pp. 314–16 (fig. 4).
153S	RES 1829; G 88; V 30	
154S	G 19; V 5	A. Lemaire 1990b, p. 13.
155C	B 139	
156S	ESE 1:12 (no. 5); RES 64; H 14	D. Diringer 1934, p. 258 (no. 101; pl. 22.14); F. Vattioni 1969b (no. 101); A. R. Millard 1988a (no. 299).
157S	CIS 124; G 103; V 36; H 1	J. Euting 1885a (no. 45).
158S	CIS 74; G 129; V 55; H 12	O. Blau 1858, p. 726; H. C. Rawlinson 1865, p. 240; M. A. Levy 1869, p. 7; C. J. M. de Vogüé 1868a (no. 23); A. Lemaire 1978a.
159S	CIS 84; G 111; V 41; H 2	F. Lajard 1847 (pl. XXXVI.3); M. A. Levy 1857, pp. 37–38 (pl. 11); M. A. Levy 1869, p. 9; J. Euting 1883 (no. 10); S. A. Cook 1930, p. 57 and pl. IX.4.
160S		
161S	V 168	
162S		P. Bordreuil and E. Gubel 1983, p. 337; K. Yassine and P. Bordreuil, 1984, pp. 132–33 (fig. 9.4; 57.184); E. A. Knauf 1984, p. 24; A. Lemaire 1989a, p. 90.
163SI		F. M. Cross 1969, p. 26; J. Naveh 1971c, p. 60; P. Colella 1973, p. 551; N. Avigad 1976, p. 23.
164S		
165S	H 109; B 67	
166S	V 121	
167S	H 93	
168S	ESE 1:10 (no. 1) and 1:277; G 58; H 107	C. Clermont-Ganneau 1901, (no. 1); S. A. Cook 1930, p. IX.14; S. Ronzevalle 1932, p. 59 (pl. X.15); D. Diringer 1934, p. 246; (no. 91); F. Vattioni 1969b (no. 91); A. R. Millard 1988a (no. 294).
169S		
170S	B 118	
171S	CIS 104; G 114; V 44; B 114	
172S	H 82; B 90	A. de Ridder 1911, pp. 495–96; D. Diringer 1934, pp. 222–23 (no. 66); A. Bergman 1936, pp. 221–24; S. Moscati 1951, p. 70; J. Naveh 1980, p. 76; R. Zadok 1984a, pp. 211–12.
173S		
174S	CIS 97; G 120; V 50; H 86	M. A. Levy 1869, pp. 12–13; M. Ohnefalsch-Richter 1893 (pl. LXXVII.15).
175C	CIS 99; G 165; V 78	W. H. Ward 1910 (no. 1148).
176S	G 87; V 29; H Phoen. 18; B 24	M. A. Levy 1869, pp. 29–30; C. Clermont-Ganneau 1883a (no. 26); A. de Ridder 1911, pp. 493–94.
177C	V 69	S. M. Paley 1986, p. 218 (pl. 49.Ill.12).
178S	CIS 86; G 138; V 57; H 3; B 14	M. A. Levy 1869, pp. 10–12; L. Delaporte 1928, p. 53 (no. 42); J. Naveh 1971c, pp. 12–13.

#	Text	Prov.	Date	Editio princeps
179B	למיכה	Jerusalem	ca. 500	N. Avigad 1976, p. 10 (no. 12; pl. 14).
180S	למלך חרם	?	?	L. Delaporte 1920–23 (A1140).
181S	לממה	Babylon?	8th	F. Lajard 1847 (pl. XXXVI.1).
182S	למנן	?	6th	C. Clermont-Ganneau 1883a (no. 26).
183S	למנחם	?	7th	L. Delaporte 1920-23 (A737).
184S	לֹמֹנֹחֹם	?	?	P. Bordreuil and A. Lemaire 1976, p. 55 (pl. VI.27).
185S	לֹמֹנֹחֹם	Syria?	ca. 700	G. R. Driver 1955b, p. 183 (fig. 2).
186S	למראהד	?	ca. 700	W. Gesenius 1837 (pl. 31.LXVIII).
187S	למראישע	Syria?	early 7th	N. Aimé-Giron 1922, p. 63.
188C	למר ברך	?	early 7th	M. A. Levy 1857, pp. 27–28 (pl. 2).
189S	למרסמך	?	late 8th	C. Clermont-Ganneau 1883a (no. 21).
190S	למרעלי	?	end of 8th	P. Bordreuil 1986.
191S	למרתשמן	late 6th	Gibeon	J. B. Pritchard 1962, p. 116 (fig. 79).
192S	לנבושגב	?	end of 7th	P. Bordreuil 1986.
193C	לנבחתן	?	5th–4th	E. Williams-Forte and M. Heltzer in O. W. Muscarella 1981 (no. 111).
194S	לנברב	?	ca. 650	F. Lajard 1837, p. 146 (pl. III.8).
195S	לננו	?	end of 6th	P. Bordreuil 1986.
196S	לנרי	?	8th	D. Diringer 1950, pp. 65–67 (pl. I.1).
197S	לנרשא עבד עתרסמך	?	ca. 800	P. Bordreuil 1986.
198S	לנשכבר	?	late 7th	P. Bordreuil 1986.
199S	לנשכנאד	?	ca. 500	P. Bordreuil 1986.
200S	לסארה	Jerusalem?	late 8th	C. C. Torrey 1921–22, p. 106 (no. 4).
201S	לססראל	?	ca. 750	M. A. Levy 1857, pp. 32–33 (pl. 6).
202S	לסעלי	?	mid–8th	H. C. Rawlinson 1865, p. 239 (pl. XIII).
203C	לסרגד	?	late 8th	W. Gesenius 1837, pp. 221–22 (pl. 28.LXVII.bis).
204S	לסרי	Palestine	ca. 600	M. F. Martin 1964, pp. 208–9 (pl. II.4).
205S	לעבד	?	early 8th	P. Bordreuil 1986.
206S	לעבדהדד	Syria	850–750	C. Clermont-Ganneau 1885–1924 1:167.
207S	לעבדחורן	?	late 9th	C. Clermont-Ganneau 1883a (no. 17).
208S	לעזא	Dan	850–750	R. Giveon 1961, p. 42 (pl. III.B).
209S	לעזא	?	ca. 500	C. J. M. de Vogüé 1868a (no. 3).

#	Collections	Literature
179B	H 43	
180S	V 108	
181S	ESE 1:137–38; RES 1821; G 93; V 32	
182S	CIS 95; G 86; V 28	
183S	G 117; V 48; H 55; B 108	A. Lemaire 1985d, pp. 46–47; F. Israel 1987, p. 145; W. E. Aufrecht 1989, pp. 69–70 (no. 29).
184S		A. Lemaire 1985d, p. 46; F. Israel 1987, p. 146; W. E. Aufrecht 1989, p. 224 (no. 83).
185S	H 47	F. Vattioni 1969b (no. 182); M. Heltzer 1971, p. 188 (no. 182); M. Heltzer 1971, p. 188 (no. 16); A. R. Millard 1988a (no. 291); E. Gubel 1990.
186S	CIS 79; G 44; V 15; H 8	H. C. Rawlinson 1865, p. 242; C. J. M. de Vogüé 1868a (no. 15); M. A. Levy 1869, p. 13.
187S	G 61a; V 24; H 53	
188C	CIS 85; G 154; V 66; H 74	M. A. Levy 1869, p. 7; W. H. Ward 1910 (no. 1153); S. A. Cook 1930, pl. XIII.4; H. Frankfort 1939 (pl. XXXIIIe); D. Collon 1987, pp. 79–80 (no. 355).
189S	G 61; V 23; H 65	J. Euting 1883 (no. 5); S. A. Cook 1930, pp. 56–57 and pl. IX.29–30.
190S	B 92	
191S		E. Stern 1982, p. 201.
192S	B 112	
193C		P. Bordreuil and E. Gubel 1987, p. 316 (fig. 5).
194S	CIS 91; G 32; V 10; H 4; B 101	M. A. Levy 1857, pp. 36–37; M. A. Levy 1869, p. 30.
195S	B 122	D. Parayre 1990 (no. 124).
196S	H 94	S. Moscati 1951, p. 53 (pl. XI.3).
197S	B 86	A. R. Millard 1988b, p. 70.
198S	B 110	
199S	B 123	
200S	H 23	
201S	CIS 82; G 73; V 26; H 95; B 91	M. A. Levy 1869, p. 8; J. Menant 1886, p. 223 (fig. 217); Reifenberg 1950 (no. 39); G. R. Driver 1957a, p. 53; D. Parayre 1990 (no. 88).
202S	CIS 83; G 22; V 7; H 106	M. A. Levy 1869, p. 13; A. Lemaire 1990b, p. 13.
203C	CIS 81; G 149; V 61; H 75	H. C. Rawlinson 1865, p. 239; M. A. Levy 1869, p. 5; M. Ohnefalsch-Richter 1893 (pl. LXXVII.6); W. H. Ward 1910 (no. 1155); S. A. Cook 1930, p. 48 and pl. XIII.3; G. R. G. R. Driver 1948 (pl. 61.1); D. Collon 1987, pp. 84–85 (no. 395); D. Parayre 1990 (no. 111).
204S		J. Naveh 1964-65, p. 185; J. Naveh 1966, p. 23.
205S	B 87	
206S	G 57; V 22; H 97	
207S	G 141; H 16; B 2	F. Vattioni 1981b (no. 30).
208S	H 99	
209S	G 98; V 33; B 30	M. A. Levy 1869, p. 25. L. Delaporte 1928, pp. 52–53 (no. 40).

#	Text	Prov.	Date	Editio princeps
210S	לעין[...]	?	ca. 650	P. Bordreuil 1986.
211C	לעלנסחמלכי	?	Persian	V. Scheil 1895, p. 81 (no. XXI).
212S	לעפי	?	late 5th	E. Babelon 1899 (no. 89).
213S	לעתרעזר	Kuyunjik	ca. 700	A. H. Layard 1853, p. 131.
214S	לפטאס	Samaria	ca. 700	I. Ben-Dor 1946.
215C	לפלתחדן	Iraq	early 7th	A. H. Layard 1853, p. 517.
216SI	[ל]פנאסר[ל]מר סרס ז[י] סרגן	Khorsabad	ca. 710	M. Sprengling 1932.
217S	לפקד יהד	Mesop.	late 6th	P. Bordreuil 1986a, pp. 305–7 (fig. 9).
218S	לפרע	Syria?	ca. 700	A. Reifenberg 1939, p. 197 (no. 4).
219SI	לקחי	Babylon	7th	J. Hager 1801 (pl. IV).
220S	לקתרא	?	7th–6th	C. J. M. de Vogüé 1868a (no. 5).
221S	לרפא	Syria?	ca. 700	A. Reifenberg 1950 (no. 32).
222S	לשאל	Baghdad	8th–7th	W. H. Ward 1886, p. 155.
223S	לשגם	Til-Barsib	?	F. Thureau-Dangin and M. Dunand 1936, p. 77 (fig. 18).
224C	לשדה	?	late 8th–7th	D. Collon 1984, p. 102 (no. 136a).
225C	לשלם	Assyria	8th–7th	E. Borowski 1965, p. 64 (no. 4; pl. XVI.d).
226S	לשלמית אמת אל[נ]תן פ[חוא]	Jerusalem	ca. 500	N. Avigad 1976, pp. 11–13 (no. 14; pl. 15).
227S	לשמשעזר עבדשהר	Syria?	8th–7th	F. M. Cross 1983, p. 61.
228S	לשנחצר	?	ca. 700	N. Avigad 1978, pp. 68–69 (fig. 6).
229C	לשנחתן	?	Neo-Bab.?	R. A. Bowman in G. A. Eisen 1940 (no. 100).
230C	לשנחתן	?	7th	U. Moortgat-Correns 1955 (no. 41).
231S	לשעינב	Israel	8th	N. Avigad 1964, pp. 190–91 (pl. 44A).
232C	לשתח	?	ca. 800	W. H. Ward 1910 (no. 1154).
233S	לתמכאל בדמלכם	?	late 6th	F. Lajard 1847 (pl. XLIII.1).
234C	מידן	?	ca. 450	P. Bordreuil 1986.
235S	מנך	?	ca. 500	C. J. M. de Vogüé 1868a (no. 4).
236I	נב	Babylon	?	R. Koldewey 1902, p. 10.
237C	נבוכסר	Iran	650–500	E. Williams-Forte and M. Heltzer in O. W. Muscarella 1981 (no. 169).
238SI	נבושרי	Nippur	late 6th–5th	L. Legrain 1925 (no. 831).
239C	נבותר	Iran	5th	E. Borowski 1965, p. 66 (no. 7; pl. XVI.g).

#	Collections	Literature
210S	B 102	
211C	V 167	
212S	B 133	J. Boardman 1968 (no. 226).
213S	CIS 52; G 62; V 25	M. A. Levy 1857, pp. 38–39; M. A. Levy 1869, p. 9; A. R. Millard 1965, p. 14, n. 7.
214S	H 48	A. Reifenberg 1950 (no. 9); S. Moscati 1951, p. 55 (pl. XI.12).
215C	CIS 80; G 153; V 65; H 77	M. A. Levy 1857, p. 33 (pl. 7); C. H. Rawlinson 1865, p. 235; W. H. Ward 1910 (no. 684); S. A. Cook 1930, pl. XIII.5; D. Collon 1987, pp. 105–7 (no. 464).
216SI	V 123	J. C. Greenfield 1962, p. 297; S. A. Kaufman 1983, pp. 53–54; S. A. Kaufman 1984, p. 94.
217S		
218S	H 100	A. Reifenberg 1950 (no. 31); S. Moscati 1951, pp. 52–53 (pl. XI.2); W. E. Aufrecht 1989, pp. 81–82 (no. 34).
219SI	ESE 1:236–38; RES 1824; V 165	F. Delitzsch 1900.
220S	G 139; V 58	
221S	H 25	R. Hestrin and M. Dayagi-Mendels 1979 (no. 121); D. Parayre 1990 (no. 16).
222S	ESE 2:146–47; RES 1828; G 107; V 39 = 103	M. Ohnefalsch-Richter 1893 (pl. LXXVII.1).
223S	V 127	
224C		D. Collon 1986, p. 424 (no. III.2); D. Collon 1987, p. 79 (no. 358).
225C	H 66	R. Hestrin and M. Dayagi-Mendels 1979 (no. 136).
226S	H 45	
227S		N. Avigad 1986, pp. 52–53; P. Bordreuil and E. Gubel 1986, p. 429 (no. III.5; fig. 12).
228S	B 98	
229C	V 128	
230C	V 141	
231S		J. Naveh 1965–66a, pp. 74–75 (no. 14); J. Teixidor 1967, p. 168; F. Vattioni 1969b (no. 216); A. Lemaire 1990b, p. 13.
232C	G 161; V 73	
233S	CIS 94; G 45; V 16; H 10	M. A. Levy 1857, pp. 31–32; H. C. Rawlinson 1865, p. 236; M. A. Levy 1869, pp. 15–16; G. A. Cooke 1903, p. 361 (no. 4); S. A. Cook 1930, p. 58 and pl. IX.22; J. Boardman 1970 (no. 173); J. Teixidor 1971, p. 466; P. Bordreuil and A. Lemaire, 1976, p. 57; N. Avigad 1985, pp. 5–6; F. Israel 1987, p. 143; W. E. Aufrecht 1989, pp. 3–5 (no. 1).
234C	B 131	
235S	CIS 103; G 116; V 47; H 11; B 124	
236I	V 166	
237C		
238SI	H 50	
239C	V 171	E. Williams-Forte and M. Heltzer in O. Muscarella 1981 (no. 172).

#	Text	Prov.	Date	Editio princeps
240B	נדת לדק	?	?	C. C. Torrey in M. Rostovtzeff 1932, no. 44.
241S	נחם בר חלקיו	Mesop.	late 6th	N. Avigad 1965, pp. 230–31 (pl. 40F).
242C	נערני	?	375–350	A. Lemaire 1982, pp. 112–13 (pl. 3).
243S	נתו	?	?	F. Lajard 1847 (pl. 43.26).
244S	עבדא	?	?	M. L. Vollenweider 1967–83 (no. 150; pl. 61.7).
245S	עבדאים	?	ca. 700	C. Clermont-Ganneau 1884-1924, 6:116.
246S	לעבדבעל	Khorsabad	ca. 700	A. de Longpérier 1855, p. 422.
247S	עבדחנם	?	5th–4th	A. Lemaire 1982, pp. 115–16 (pl. 5).
248S	עבדכחבן	?	ca. 700	C. Clermont-Ganneau 1883a (no. 20).
249S	עבכא	?	8th	C. Clermont-Ganneau 1883a (no. 28).
250C	עדרי	?	5th	L. Delaporte 1910 (no. 501).
251S	עזי	?	ca. 400	P. Bordreuil 1986.
252S	עזריו שחז	?	5th–4th	A. Lemaire 1986b, pp. 324–25 (no. 16).
253S	עלה	?	early 8th	A. Lemaire 1979.
254C	פגזו	?	7th	F. Lajard 1847 (pl. XXV.4).
255S	פגל	?	5th	A. Lemaire 1986b, pp. 323–24 (no. 15).
256S	פדה	?	early 8th	N. Avigad 1969, p. 2 (no. 2).
257S	פהשף	Oxus valley	5th–4th	G. A. Cooke in O. M. Dalton 1964 (no. 105).
258S	פמן	Jerusalem?	6th	N. Avigad 1954, p. 238 (pl. 21.3).
259S	פת	?	5th–4th	P. Bordreuil 1986.
260S	צדקרמן	?	late 8th	C. J. M. de Vogüé 1886, p. 191.
261SI	צר ידד	?	8th–7th	G. Garbini 1978.
262C	רבבת	Oxus valley	6th	G. A. Cooke in O. M. Dalton 1964 (no. 115).
263S	רפתי	Khorsabad	ca. 750	C. J. M. de Vogüé 1868a (no. 26).
264S	שלמאל בר עמשא	Ashdod?	late 6th	A. Reifenberg 1938, pp. 115–16 (no. 10).
265S	סמאב	Egypt?	ca. 700	A. Reifenberg 1939, p. 198 (no. 5; pl. XXXIV.5).
266S	שמשעדרי	?	7th	M. A. Levy 1857, pp. 39–40 (no. 14; pl. 13).
267S	שנסרצר	Babylon	late 7th	E. Ledrain 1883, p. 73.
268SI	שסחמר	Tello	4th	V. Scheil 1901, p. 568.
269C	שציא	?	ca. 700	E. Borowski 1952, pp. 178–79 (no. 11).
270S	תנגי	?	late 7th	P. Bordreuil 1986.
271S	תסמר	Aleppo	late 6th	ESE
272S	תרתן	?	early 5th	A. D. Mordtmann 1860, p. 556.
273S	ת..	Egypt	?	W. M. Müller 1907.

#	Collections	Literature
240B	V 125	R. P. Dougherty in M. Rostovtzeff 1932, pp. 94–97.
241S	V 161; H 29	J. Boardman 1970 (no. 182); J. Naveh 1971, p. 31.
242C		
243S	G 181; V 85	M. Ohnefalsch-Richter 1893 (pl. 32.7, 77.13 142.4);J. Boardman 1970 (no. 158); J. Teixidor 1971, p. 466.
244S		J. Teixidor 1971, p. 465 (no. 66).
245S	ESE 2:147–48; RES 616; G 52; H 96; B 16	D. Diringer 1934, pp. 243–44 (no. 87); A. Reifenberg 1950 (no. 17); S. Moscati 1951, p. 71; F. Vattioni 1969b (no. 87); W. E. Aufrecht 1989, pp. 148–49 (no. 21a).
246S	G 55; H 104; B 8	M. A. Levy 1869, p. 6; J. Menant 1886, p. 234 (fig. 231); E. Ledrain 1888, pp. 165–66 (no. 409); L. Delaporte 1920–23 (K13); F. Vattioni 1981b (no. 56); D. Parayre 1990 (no. 21).
247S		
248S	G 124; V 53; H 24	S. A. Cook 1930, p. 64, n. 4, and pl. IX.3.
249S	G 109; V 40; H 98; B 29	A. Reifenberg 1950 (no. 34).
250C	G 164; V 77; B 129	
251S	B 134	
252S		
253S		A. Lemaire 1990b, p. 14.
254C	CIS 98; G 166; V 79; H 76	M. A. Levy 1869, p. 16; G. Perrot and C. Chipiez 1884, II (fig. 156); W. H. Ward 1910 (no. 1082).
255S		
256S	H 52	J. Naveh 1980, p. 76.
257S	V 119	
258S	H 49	
259S	B 137	
260S	CIS 73; G 16; V 3; H 87	
261SI		
262C	V 120	
263S	CIS 51; G 20; V 6; H 88; B 89	M. A. Levy 1869, pp. 8–9; L. Ledrain 1888, pp. 166–67 (no. 411); L. Delaporte 1920–23 (K12); A. Lemaire 1990b, p. 13.
264S	H 26	S. Moscati 1951, p. 60 (pl. XIII.1).
265S	H 62	A. Reifenberg 1950 (no. 2); S. Moscati 1951, pp. 53–54 (pl. XI.4); J. Naveh 1980, p. 76; W. E. Aufrecht 1989, pp. 83–84 (no. 35).
266S	CIS 87; G 106; V 38; H 54; B 111	M. A. Levy 1869, p. 17; L. Delaporte 1920-23 (A734).
267S	CIS 88; G 123; V 52; H 9; B 109	C. Clermont-Ganneau 1883a (no. 32); L. Delaporte 1920-23 (A732).
268SI	ESE 1:276; RES 245; V 99	A. Goetze 1944, pp. 98–99 (pl. XIa); A. D. H. Bivar 1970, p. 56.
269C	V 139	
270S	B 107	
271S	ESE 3:298; G 147; V 59; B 121	S. Ronzevalle 1914–21, pp. 185–86 (no. 2); G. Fussman 1972 (pl. II.15).
272S		P. Bordreuil and E. Gubel 1988, p. 445.
273S	V 92	

B.7.2   Coins   Coins

M. A. Levy 1862, esp. pp. 147–53 • F. W. Madden 1864, esp. pp. 249–320 • F. W. Madden 1881, esp. pp. 5, 7, 24–41 • E. Drouin 1889 • E. Babelon 1893 • W. Wroth 1899, esp. pp. 29, 138, pl. vi, n. 1; pl. xvii, n. 7 • G. F. Hill 1900 • E. Babelon 1901, esp. pp. 2:344–79; 2:379–478, 3 pls. 105–115. • W. Wroth 1903 • B. V. Head 1911 • E. Rogers 1914, esp. p. 9 • G. F. Hill 1914 • A. de la Fuye 1919 • G. F. Hill 1922 • E. T. Newell 1926 • O. R. Sellers 1933 • E. L. Sukenik 1934, esp. pp. 178–82, pls. 1–3 • W. F. Albright 1934a • E. S. G. Robinson 1936, esp. pp. 196–97, 199–200 • M. Narkiss 1936–38 • E. S. G. Robinson 1958 • B. Simonetta 1961 • A. D. H. Bivar 1961a • C. M. Kraay 1962 • D. G. Sellwood 1962 • O. Mørkholm 1962 • B. Simonetta 1964 • L. Y. Rahmani 1964 • O. Mørkholm 1964 • D. G. Sellwood 1965 • D. W. MacDowall 1965 • G. le Rider 1965 • J. Naveh 1964–65, esp. p. 194 • A. M. Simonetta 1966 • B. Simonetta 1967 • D. G. Sellwood 1967 • B. Simonetta 1967a • J. Naveh 1968 • A. D. H. Bivar 1970, esp. pp. 56–57; pl. II • M. T. Abgarians and D. G. Sellwood 1971 • J. Naveh 1972a • L. Mildenberg 1979 • E. Lipiński 1982 • D. Barag 1984 • M. A. Rizack 1984 • A. Lemaire 1985d, esp. pp. 37–38 • J. W. Betlyon 1986 • Y. Meshorer 1989, esp. p. 288.

C. BIBLICAL ARAMAIC

C.1 General

(See also s.vv. Grammars, Grammatical Studies, and Lexicography.)

C. R. Brown 1884 • E. Kautzsch 1884 • R. Duval 1884 • M. Lambert 1893 • K. Marti 1896 • H. H. Powell 1907 • G. Bergsträsser 1912, esp. pp. 515–17 • H. L. Strack 1921 • W. F. Albright 1921, esp. p. 117 • C. C. Torrey 1923 • H. S. Gehman 1924 • W. B. Stevenson 1924 • W. Baumgartner 1927 • P. Leander 1927 • H. H. Rowley 1929 • S. R. Driver 1929, esp. p. 508 • E. Littmann 1930 • P. Leander 1930 • J. Cantineau 1931a • J. A. Montgomery 1931 • J. Cantineau 1932 • H. J. Polotsky 1932 • W. Baumgartner 1947 • E. Y. Kutscher 1951 • F. R. Blake 1951 • E. Y. Kutscher 1954a • S. Segert 1956, esp. pp. 384–91 • S. Segert 1956b, esp. pp. 12–17, 20–21, 237–302 • J. A. Fitzmyer 1957 • P. Nober 1957 • W. Baumgartner 1957 • S. Segert 1958 • H. L. Ginsberg 1959, esp. pp. 143–45 • N. H. Tur-Sinai (Torczyner) 1960 • R. Murray 1960–61 • P. Nober 1961a • K. Beyer 1962 • M. Ellenbogen 1962 • W. F. Stinespring 1962 • A. F. Johns 1963 • S. Morag 1964 • J. Carmignac 1964–66 • N. H. Richardson 1965 • T. Muraoka 1966 • E. Jenni 1968, esp. pp. 112–19 • M. Sokoloff 1969–70 • S. Rin 1972 • R. Degen 1975 • D. Boyarin 1975–76 • D. R. Cohen 1975–76 • Y. Avishur 1975–76 • Z. Beşar 1976–77 • P. Coxon 1977 • P. Coxon 1977–78 • I. Jerusalmi 1978 • P. Coxon 1978 • G. H. Wilson 1979 • P. Coxon 1979 • R. I. Vasholz 1979–81 • R. I. Vasholz 1979–81a • D. C. Snell 1980 • F. Rundgren 1982–83 • G. McEwan 1983, esp. pp. 172–73 • J. Teixidor 1984 • M. Görg 1984 • J. P. Asmussen 1988 • S. E. Fassberg 1989 • W. R. Garr 1990 • J. A. Naudé 1990.

C.2 Ezra

C. C. Torrey 1908 • C. C. Torrey 1910, esp. pp. 140–207 • L. W. Batten 1913 • A. B. Ehrlich 1914, esp. pp. 156–82 • J. A. Bewer 1922 • T. Nöldeke 1924 • M. Haller 1925 • P. Joüon 1927 • H. H. Schaeder 1930a • R. de Vaux 1937 • A. Gelin 1953 • J. Harmatta 1954 • K. Galling 1954 • R. A. Bowman and C. W. Gilkey 1954 • S. B. Sperry 1955 • F. Rundgren 1957a (7:26) • F. Rundgren 1958 (6:6) • C. G. Tuland 1958a • P. Nober 1958a (7:23) • Z. W. Falk 1959 (7:26) • H. L. Ginsberg 1960 (1:4) • P. Nober 1960a • P. Nober 1961 • A. Spitaler 1962, esp. pp. 112–14 (5:10) • F. Altheim and R. Stiehl 1963, esp. pp. 109–81 • J. M. Myers 1965 • R. A. Bowman 1965 (5:8) • S. Mowinckel 1965 • A. F. Rainey 1969 • S. A. Kaufman 1974, esp. p. 55 • B. Porten 1978–79a • F. Parente 1979 (6:11) • F. Rundgren 1981 • A. H. J. Gunneweg 1982 • H. Williamson 1983, esp. pp. 15–23 (4:6–6:22) • P.-E. Dion 1983 • G. Garbini 1985 (7:12) • W. S. Morrow and E. G. Clarke 1986 • A. Dodi 1989, esp. pp. 64–67 • J. A. Naudé 1990.

C.3 Daniel

General
A. Barnes 1853 • E. O. A. Merx 1865 • S. Baer 1882 • C. F. Keil 1884 • J. E. H. Thomson 1893 • A. A. Bevan 1892, esp. pp. 33–40, 69–127 • A. Kamphausen 1896 • S. R. Driver 1900 • H. Preiswerk 1902 • C. C. Torrey 1909 • R. D. Wilson 1912 • A. B. Ehrlich 1914, esp. pp. 126–55 • R. D. Wilson 1917–38 • M. Haller 1920–21 • W. St. C. Tisdall 1921 • W. St. C. Tisdall 1921a • W. Baumgartner 1926 • G. R. Driver 1926a • A. F. von Gall 1926, esp. pp. 266–69; 412–13 • W. Baumgartner 1927a • P. Joüon 1927 • J. A. Montgomery 1927 • R. H. Charles 1929 • C. Boutflower 1931 • B. D. Eerdmans 1932 • O. Eissfeldt 1932 • H. H. Rowley 1932 • H. H. Rowley 1933 • G. Messina 1934 • J. Linder 1935 • F. Zimmermann 1938 • W. Baumgartner 1939 • F. Zimmermann 1939 • P. Joüon 1941 • H. L. Ginsberg 1948 • J. H. Hospers 1948 • J.-P. Audet 1950 • C. C. Torrey 1952 • R. Augé 1954 • E. Vogt 1954, esp. pp. 266–67 • J. J. Rabinowitz 1955 • G. G. Cameron 1958, esp. p. 162 • G. Geiss 1961, esp. p. 11 • H. B. Rosen 1961 • F. Zimmermann 1961 • F. Zimmermann 1964–65 • K. A. Kitchen 1965 • O. Plöger 1965 • J. G. Landels 1966 • H. H. Rowley 1966 • M. Delcor 1971 • A. Mertens 1971 • S. Morag 1973 • S. A. Kaufman 1974, esp. pp. 80, 102 • S. Morag 1974 • A. Lacocque 1976 • B. K. Waltke 1976 • F. F. Bruce 1977 • P. Coxon 1977b • A. R. Millard 1977 • L. F. Hartman and A. A. Di Lella 1978 • R. I. Vasholz 1978 • H. H. P. Dressler 1979 • J. Day 1980 • B. Margalit 1980 • E. M. Yamauchi 1980 • G. F. Hasel 1981 • G. F. Hasel 1981a • A. A. Di Lella 1982 • J. Schaberg 1982 • A. J. Ferch 1983 • W. H. Shea 1983 • P.-M. Bogaert 1984 • W. H. Shea 1985a • J. C. Trever 1985 • G. H. Wilson 1985 • E. M. Cook 1986 • P. Coxon 1986 • W. S. Morrow and E. G. Clarke 1986 • A. S. van der Woude 1986 • G. Boccaccini 1987 • Z. Stefanovic 1987 • W. H. Shea 1988 • J. W. Wesselius 1988.

Chapter 2
W. Baumgartner 1926a (2:48) • H. H. Rowley 1928 (2:5) • W. B. Stevenson 1934–35 • J. W. Swain 1940 (2:37) • W. Baumgartner 1945 (2:37) • M. J. Gruenthaner 1946 (2:37) • J. T. Nelis 1954 (2:37) • E. F. Siegman 1956 (2:34) • J. V. K. Wilson 1957 (2:10) • J. Vergote 1957–58, esp. p. 93 (2:10) • H. Wehr 1964 (2:49) • B. Z. Bergman 1968 (2:25) • H. P. Rüger 1969 (2:49) • B. A. Mastin 1973 (2:46) • F. Rundgren 1976–77 (2:5) • W. S. LaSor 1980, esp. pp. 113–14 (2:20–23).

Chapter 3
C. Kuhl 1930 • H. Nyberg 1931 (3:21) • A. T. Olmstead 1944 (3:5) • J. B. Alexander 1950 (3:6) • S. Grill 1953 • G. N. Knauer 1954 (3:27) • B. G. Sanders 1955 (3:6) • S. Gevirtz 1957 (3:18) • F. Vattioni 1958 (3:8, 6:25) • E. M. Yamauchi 1970 (3:5) • P. Coxon 1976 (3:17) • P. Grelot 1979 (3:5, 7, 10, 15) • W. H. Shea 1982 • S. Paul 1983 (3.29) • E. Haag 1987 • E. M. Cook 1989 (3:1).

Chapter 4
I. Eitan 1941, esp. pp. 16–17 (4:33) • B. Segall 1955 • D. N. Freedman 1957 (4:24) • H. L. Ginsberg 1959 (4:9, 18) esp. p. 145 • P. Nober 1960 (4:33) • P. Grelot 1974 • A. A. Di Lella 1981 (4:7–14) • W. H. Shea 1985.

Chapter 5

J. M. Fuller 1885 (5:1) • R. P. Dougherty 1929, esp. p. 15 (5:1) • C. Clermont-Ganneau 1886 (5:25) • T. Nöldeke 1886 (5:25) • J. D. Prince 1893 (5:25) • J. P. Peters 1896, esp. pp. 114–17 (5:25) • E. König 1901 (5:25) • C. Boutflower 1916 • H. H. Rowley 1924 (5:1) • W. F. Albright 1925 • H. Bauer 1925 (5:25) • B. Alfrink 1928 (5:1) • H. H. Rowley 1930–31 • W. von Soden 1935 • J. Melkman 1939 • E. G. Kraeling 1944 (5:25) • C. Torres 1944 (5:30) • H. F. D. Sparks 1946 (5:31) • M. J. Gruenthaner 1949 (5:1) • A. de Guglielmo 1949 (5:25) • O. Eissfeldt 1951 (5:1) • P. P. Saydon 1951 (5:30–31) • A. Alt 1954 (5:25) • B. Couroyer 1955 (5:2, 23) • H. L. Ginsberg 1959, esp. p. 145 (5:17) • H. Kruse 1959 (5:25) • J. A. Emerton 1960 (5:12) • M. A. Beek 1966 (5:25) • R. Schmitt 1967 • P. Grelot 1974a • P. Coxon 1977a (5:3–5) • W. H. Shea 1982b (5:31) • P. Grelot 1985 • A. R. Millard 1985, esp. p. 77 • A. R. Millard 1987 (5:5) • L. L. Grabbe 1988a.

Chapter 6

B. Alfrink 1928a (6:1) • H. H. Rowley 1935 (6:1) • L. Waterman 1946 (6:1) • A. Bentzen 1950 • E. Cassin 1951 • K. Galling 1954a (6:1) • S. Cavalletti 1957, esp. pp. 126–28 (6:8) • W. von Soden 1963 (6:18) • B. Z. Bergman 1968 (6:19) • W. H. Shea 1982a, esp. pp. 138–39 • S. Paul 1984 (6:8) • L. L. Grabbe 1988 (6:1), esp. p. 205.

Chapter 7

H. Gunkel 1895, pp. 323–35 • G. H. Dix 1925, esp. pp. 248–50 (7:13) • O. Procksch 1927 (7:13) • E. G. Kraeling 1933 • W. B. Stevenson 1934–35 • P. Parker 1941 (7:13) • C. C. Torrey 1946 (7:5) • L. Waterman 1946 (7:5) • E. Sjöberg 1948 (7:13) • T. W. Manson 1949–50 (7:13) • E. Sjöberg 1950 (7:13) • E. Sjöberg 1950–51 (7:13) • S. Morenz 1951 (7:7) • A. Feuillet 1953 (7:13) • A. Caquot 1955 (7:3) • J. Coppens 1955 (7:13) • M. Noth 1955 (7:18) • W. F. Albright 1957, esp. pp. 262, 378–80 (7:9–12) • J. A. Emerton 1958 (7:13) • L. Rost 1958 (7:13) • E. J. Young 1958 (7:13) • W. Eichrodt 1959 (7:13) • R. M. Frank 1959 (7:5) • J. Muilenburg 1960 • J. Coppens and L. Dequeker 1961 • C. Brekelmans 1965 (7:25) • A. Caquot 1967 • R. Hanhart 1967 • D. Flusser 1972 • M. Müller 1972 (7:13) • G. F. Hasel 1975 • V. S. Poythress 1976 • R. Roca-Puig 1976 (7:25–28) • M. Sokoloff 1976 (7:9) • J. Teixidor 1976, esp. p. 309 (7:18) • A. A. Di Lella 1977 (7:13) • J. Coppens 1978 • P. Grelot 1978 (7:9–10) • J. Lust 1978 (7:13) • T. Wittstruck 1978 • M. Casey 1979 • A. J. Ferch 1980 • H. S. Kvanvig 1981 • M. Müller 1984 (7:13) • P. R. Raabe 1985 • P. G. Mosca 1986 • C. C. Caragounis 1987 • J. Goldingay 1988.

PART TWO

REFERENCES

Aartun, K. 1959. Zur Frage des bestimmten Artikels im Aramäischen. *AcOr* 24:5–14.

———. 1973. Die hervorhebende Endung -w(V) an nordwestsemitischen Adverbien und Negationen. *UF* 5:1–5.

'Abada, K. 1974. Objects Acquired by The Iraq Museum -4- [Arabic]. *Sumer* 30:329–34 + 9 pls.

Abgarians, M. T., and D. G. Sellwood. 1971. A Hoard of Early Parthian Drachms. *NC* 7/11:103–19.

Abou Assaf, A. 1981. Die Statue des HDYS'Y, König von Guzana. *MDOG* 113:3–22.

———. 1982. Dumyat al-malik had-yis'î malik ğawzan [The statue of king HDYS'Y, king of Gozan]. *AASyr* 32:35–58.

Abou Assaf, A., P. Bordreuil, and A. Millard. 1982. *La statue de Tell Fekherye et son inscription bilingue assyro-araméenne.* Etudes assyriologiques 7. Paris: Editions Recherche sur les Civilisations ADPF.

Reviews: B. F. Batto 1985; G. Bunnens 1989: *Revue belge de philologie et d'histoire* 67:229–31; H. Cazelles 1984: *VT* 34:114–16; L. Diez Merino 1983: *AO* 1:117–19; J. A. Fitzmyer 1984; J. J. Glassner 1987: *Syria* 64:156; M. J. Geller 1983: *BSOAS* 46:545–46; J. Huehnergard 1986; F. Israel 1989: *RSO* 63:171; E. Jacob 1984: *Revue d'histoire et de philosophie religieuses* 64:168; S. A. Kaufman 1984; R. Lebrun 1989: *Langues orientales anciennes philologie et linguistique* 2:273–5; E. Lipiński 1984; J. Peirkovà 1984: *ArOr* 52:100–02; D. Pardee and R. D. Biggs 1984; E. Puech 1983; J. M. Sasson 1983; S. Segert 1985; W. von Soden 1982; E. Ullendorff 1983: *SOTS Book List*: 25; J. W. Wesselius 1983a.

Abramson, S. 1976–77. על קציעי (קציעין) צואריא, גזיר קדל, תביר קדל, ראש קטיעה. *Leš* 41:191–95.

Academia Inscriptionum et Litterarum Humaniorum. 1888, 1893. *Corpus Inscriptionum Semiticarum, pars 2: Inscriptiones aramaicae.* ed. C. J. de Vogüé. 2 vols. Paris: Imprimerie Nationale [Librairie C. Klincksieck].

Aggoula, B. 1985. Studia aramaica II. *Syria* 62:61–76.

Aharoni, Y. 1953. The land of 'Amqi. *IEJ* 3:153–61.

———. 1956. Excavations at Ramath Raḥel, 1954, Preliminary Report. *IEJ* 6:137–57.

———. 1960. Ramat Raḥel. *RB* 67:398–400.

———. 1962. Ramat Raḥel. *RB* 69:401–4.

———. 1962a. *Excavations at Ramat Raḥel Seasons 1959 and 1960.* Rome: Università di Roma, Centro di Studi Semitica.

———. 1963. Ramat Raḥel. *RB* 70:572–74.

———. 1963a. Ḥorvat Dorban (Khirbet esh-Sheikh Ibrahim). *IEJ* 13:337.

———. 1963b. Tel Arad. *IEJ* 13:334–37.

———. 1964. Tel Arad. *IEJ* 14:280–83.

————. 1964a. *Excavations at Ramat Raḥel Seasons 1961 and 1962*. Rome: Università di Roma, Centro di Studi Semitica.

————. 1965. Tel Arad. *IEJ* 15:249–51.

————. 1967. חותמות של פקידים ממלכתיים מערד. *EI (Sukenik Volume)* 8:101–3, pl. יג.

————. 1967a. Excavations at Tel Arad: Preliminary Report on the Second Season, 1963. *IEJ* 17:233–49.

————. 1968. Trial Excavation in the "Solar Shrine" at Lachish: Preliminary Report. *IEJ* 18:157–69.

————. 1968a. Arad: Its Inscriptions and Temple. *BA* 31:2–32.

————. 1969. The Israelite Sanctuary at Arad. In *New Directions in Biblical Archaeology*, ed. David Noel Freedman and Jonas C. Greenfield, 25–39. Garden City, N. Y.: Doubleday.

————. 1970–71. מזבח הלבונה מלכיש. *Leš* 35:3–6, pl. 1.

————. 1974. Excavations at Tel Beer-Sheba: Preliminary Report of the Fourth Season, 1972. *Tel Aviv* 1:34–42.

————. 1979. *The Land of the Bible, A Historical Geography*. Revised and Enlarged Edition. Transl. A. F. Rainey. Philadelphia: Westminster.

Aharoni, Y., and R. Amiran. 1962. Tel Arad. *IEJ* 12:144–45.

————. 1963. עונת החפירות הראשונה בתל ערד. *Yediot* 27:217–34 + 8 pls.

————. 1964. Excavations at Tel Arad: Preliminary Report on the First Season, 1962. *IEJ* 14:131–47.

Aimé-Giron, N. 1921. Fragments de papyrus araméens provenant de Memphis. *JA* 18:56–64.

————. 1922. Notes epigraphiques. *JA* 11/20:63–65.

————. 1923. Note sur une tombe découverte près de Cheikh-Fadl par Monsieur Flinders Petrie et contenant des inscriptions araméennes. In *Ancient Egyptians* 2.38–43. London: Williams & Norgate.

————. 1926. Trois ostraca araméens d'Éléphantine. *ASAE* 26:23–31.

————. 1931. *Textes araméens d'Egypte*. Service des antiquités de l'Egypte. Cairo: Imprimerie de l'Institut Français.

————. 1939. Adversaria semitica. *BIFAO* 38:1–63.

————. 1939a. Adversaria semitica. *ASAE* 39:339–63.

————. 1940. Adversaria semitica (III). *ASAE* 40:433–66.

Akurgal, E. 1956. Les fouilles de Daskyleion. *Anatolia* 1:20–24, pl. XII.

————. 1966. Griechisch-persische Reliefs aus Daskyleion. *Iranica antiqua* 6:147–56 + 6 pls.

————. 1981. Aramaean and Phoenician Stylistic and Iconographic Elements in Neo-Hittite Art. In *Temples and High Places in Biblical Times: Proceedings of the Colloquium in Honor of the Centennial of Hebrew Union College—Jewish Institute of Religion*, ed. A. Biran and I. Pommerantz, 131–41. Jerusalem: Hebrew Union College.

Albright, W. F. 1911. Recent Discoveries at Elephantine. *Upper Iowa Academician*: 18–20.

————. 1921. The Date and Personality of the Chronicler. *JBL* 40:104–24.

————. 1925. The Conquests of Nabonidus in Arabia. *JRAS*: 293–95.

————. 1926. Notes on Early Hebrew and Aramaic Epigraphy. *JPOS* 6:75–102.

————. 1927. The Names "Israel" and "Judah" with an Excursus on the Etymology of Tôdâh and Tôrâh. *JBL* 46:151–85.

————. 1932. *The Archaeology of Palestine and the Bible*. New York: Revell.

————. 1934. *The Vocalization of the Egyptian Syllabic Orthography*. AOS 5. New Haven, Conn.: American Oriental Society.

————. 1934a. Light on the Jewish State in Persian Times. *BASOR* 53:20–22.

————. 1941. Ostracon No. 6043 from Ezion-geber. *BASOR* 82:11–15.

————. 1942. A Votive Stele Erected by Ben-Hadad I of Damascus to the God Melcarth. *BASOR* 87:23–29 + 1 pl.

————. 1943. Books Received by the Editor: I. Near Eastern Archaeology and Related Subjects. *BASOR* 90:39–41.

————. 1945. The Chronology of the Divided Monarchy of Israel. *BASOR* 100:16–22.

————. 1949. The Biblical Period. In *The Jews: Their History, Culture, and Religion*, ed. L. Finkelstein. Philadelphia: Jewish Publication Society of America.

————. 1950. Baal-Zephon. In *Festschrift Alfred Bertholet zum 80. Geburtstag gewidmet von Kollegen und Freunden*, ed. W. Baumgartner, O. Eissfeldt, K. Elliger and L. Rost, 1–14. Tübingen: J. C. B. Mohr.

————. 1950a. Cilicia and Babylonia under the Chaldaean Kings. *BASOR* 120:22–25.

————. 1953. *Archaeology and the Religion of Israel*. Ayer Lectures of the Colgate-Rochester Divinity School. Baltimore: Johns Hopkins Univ. Press.

————. 1953a. Some Recent Publications. *BASOR* 132:46–47.

————. 1955. Recent Books on Archaeology and Ancient History. *BASOR* 139:19.

————. 1956. Northeast-Mediterranean Dark Ages and the Early Iron Age Art of Syria. In *The Aegean and the Near East: Studies Presented to Hetty Goldman*, ed. S. S. Weinberg, 144–64. Locust Valley, N.Y.: J. J. Augustin.

————. 1956a. The Date of the Kapara Period at Gozan (Tell Halaf). *Anatolian Studies* 6:75–85.

————. 1957. *From the Stone Age to Christianity: Monotheism and the Historical Process*. 2d ed. Baltimore: Johns Hopkins Univ. Press.

————. 1957a. The Seal Impression from Jericho and the Treasurers of the Second Temple. *BASOR* 148:28–30.

————. 1958. An Ostracon from Calah and the North-Israelite Diaspora. *BASOR* 149:33–36.

————. See also: G. Levi della Vida.

Alexander, J. B. 1950. New Light on the Fiery Furnace. *JBL* 69:375–76.

Alexander, P. S. 1978. Remarks on Aramaic Epistolography in the Persian Period. *JSS* 23:155–70.

Alfrink, B. 1928.   Der letzte König von Babylon. *Bib* 9:187–205.

———. 1928a.   Darius Medus. *Bib* 9:316–40.

Allchin, F. R. 1982.   How Old is the City of Taxila? *Antiquity* 56:8–14.

Alt, A. 1910.   Psammetich II. in Palästina und in Elephantine. *ZAW* 30:288–97.

———. 1934.   Die syrische Staatenwelt vor dem Einbruch der Assyrer. *ZDMG* 88:233–58. Reprinted in *Kleine Schriften* 3 (1959): 214–32.

———. 1954.   Zur Menetekel-Inschrift. *VT* 4:303–5.

Altheim, F. 1947.   Eine neue Aśoka-Inschrift. In *Festschrift Otto Eissfeldt zum 60. Geburtstage 1. September 1947*, ed. J. Fück, 29–46. Halle (Saale): Niemeyer.

———. 1947a.   *Weltgeschichte Asiens in griechischer Zeit.* Halle (Saale): Niemeyer.

———. 1947–48.   Eine neue Aśoka-Inschrift. In *Weltgeschichte Asiens im griechischen Zeitalter* 1:25–43 + 1 pl. Halle (Saale): Niemeyer.

———. 1948–50.   *Literatur und Gesellschaft im ausgehenden Altertum.* 2 vols. Halle (Saale): Niemeyer.

———. 1949.   *Awestische Textgeschichte.* Hallische Monographien 9. Halle (Saale): Niemeyer.

Altheim, F., and R. Stiehl. 1953.   Pahlawīk und Pārsīk. *ParPass* 8:307–17 + 3 pls.

———. 1957.   *Supplementum Aramaicum: Aramäisches aus Iran.* Baden-Baden: Grimm.

———. 1958.   The Aramaic Version of the Kandahar Bilingual Inscription of Aśoka. *EAW* 9:192–98.

———. 1959.   Zwei neue Inschriften: Die aramäische Fassung der Aśoka-Bilinguis von Kandahar. *ACA* 7:107–26 + 1 pl.

———. 1959a.   The Greek-Aramaic Bilingual Inscription of Kandahār and its Philological Importance. *EAW* 10:243–60.

———. 1959–62.   Die aramäische Fassung der Aśoka-Bilinguis von Kandahār. In *Geschichte der Hunnen.* 5 vols. 1:397–415, 431. Berlin: De Gruyter.

———. 1963.   *Die aramäische Sprache unter den Achaimeniden, I.* Frankfurt am Main: V. Klostermann.

———. 1964–69.   *Die Araber in der alten Welt.* 5 vols. Berlin: De Gruyter.

———. 1968.   Maṣḥafa falāsfā ṭabībān. In *In Memoriam Paul Kahle*, ed. M. Black and G. Fohrer, 3–9. BZAW 103. Berlin: Töpelmann.

———. 1969.   *Zur Bilinguis von Kandahar: Der Hellenismus in Mittelasien.* Darmstadt: Wissenschaftliche Buchgesellschaft.

———. 1970.   *Geschichte Mittelasiens im Altertum.* Berlin: De Gruyter.

———. 1971.   *Christentum am Roten Meer.* 2 vols. Berlin: De Gruyter.

———. 1972.   Die Handelsstrasse von Lagmān nach Tadmor (Die neue aramäische Inschrift Aśokas aus Lagmān). *Klio* 54:61–66.

Altheim, F., R. Stiehl, D. Metzler, and E. Schwertheim. 1983.   Eine neue gräko-persische Grabstelle aus Sultaniye Köy und ihre Bedeutung für die Geschichte und Topographie von Daskyleion. *Epigraphica anatolica* 1:1–23, pls. 1–2.

Altheim, F., R. Stiehl, and M. Cremer. 1985. Eine gräko-persische Türstele mit aramäischer Inschrift aus Daskyleion. *Epigraphica anatolica* 6:1–15.

Amadasi Guzzo, M. G. 1979. Review of *La langue de Ya'udi*, by P.-E. Dion. *RSO* 53:200–3.

———. 1985. Le scritture della Siria antica. In *Da Ebla a Damasco: Diecimila anni di archeologia in Siria*, ed. G. Garroni and E. Parcu, 62–67. Milan: Electa.

Amandry, P. 1958. A propos d'un récent catalogue des ivoires de Nimrud. *RA* 52:226–32.

Amiet, P. 1973. *Bas-reliefs imaginaires du Proche-Orient ancien*. Paris: Hôtel de la Monnaire.

———. 1977. *Glyptique susienne*, vol. I. Mémoires de la D. A. I.

Amiran, R. See: Y. Aharoni.

Ammassari, A. 1976. La redazione del Codice dell'Alleanza (Es 20,22 e 24,3–8) e lo stile degli atti giuridici de Elefantina. In *La religione dei Patriarchi*, 137–48. Rome: Città Nuova.

Andersen, F. I., and A. D. Forbes. 1986. *Spelling in the Hebrew Bible*. BibOr 41. Rome: Pontifical Biblical Institute.

Andersen, F. I., and D. N. Freedman. 1988. The Orthography of the Aramaic Portion of the Tell Fekherye Bilingual. In *Text and Context: Old Testament and Semitic Studies for F. C. Fensham*, ed. W. Claassen, 9–49. *JSOT* Supplement Series 48. Sheffield: JSOT.

———. 1989. Aleph as a Vowel Letter in Old Aramaic. In *To Touch the Text: Biblical and Related Studies in Honor of Joseph A. Fitzmyer, S.J.*, ed. M. P. Horgan and P. J. Kobelski, 3–14. New York: Crossroad.

Andersen, F. I. See also: D. N. Freedman.

Andersen, H. G. 1975. Book of Ahikar. In *The Zonde·van Pictorial Encyclopedia of the Bible, vol. 1*, ed. M. C. Tenney, 87. Grand Rapids, Mich.: Zondervan.

Andreas, F. C. 1932. Erklärung der aramäischen Inschrift von Taxila. *Nachrichten der göttingischen Gesellschaft der Wissenschaften, phil.-hist. Kl.* 1:6–17.

Angerstorfer, A. 1984. Gedanken zur Analyse der Inscriften der Beterstatue vom Tel Fecherije in *BN* 22 (1983) 91–106. *BN* 24:7–11.

———. 1984a. Hebräisch *dmwt* und aramäisch *dmw(t)*: Ein Sprachproblem der Imago-Dei-Lehre. *BN* 24:30–43.

Anneler, H. 1912. *Zur Geschichte der Juden von Elephantine*. Bern: M. Drechsel. Reviews: A. Grimme 1914.

Anon. 1907. Review of *Aramaic Papyri Discovered at Assuan*, by A. H. Sayce and A. E. Cowley. *GGA* 169:181–99.

———. 1929. Zeitschriftenschau. *ZAW* 47:150–51.

———. 1934. Notes of the Quarter: Recent Discoveries at Persepolis. *JRAS*: 226–32.

———. 1960. Inscriptions au pays de Moab. *RB* 67:243–44.

———. 1982. Syrian Inscriptions Published in Biblical Archaeologist Assist in Understanding Hebrew Bible. *BARev* 8/6:6–10.

———. 1985. Bible's Psalm 20 Adapted for Pagan Use. *BARev* 11/1:20–23.

Aristar, A. M. R. 1979. The IIwy Verbs and the Vowel System of Proto-West Semitic. *AAL* 6:209–17.

———. 1987. The Semitic Jussive and the Implications for Aramaic. *Maarav* 4:157–89.

Arnold, W. R. 1912. The Passover Papyrus from Elephantine. *JBL* 31:1–33.

Artzi, P. 1968. Some Unrecognized Syrian Amarna Letters (EA 260, 317, 318). *JNES* 27:163–69.

Asmussen, J. P. 1968. Iranica. *AcOr* 31:9–20.

———. 1988. Remarks on Judeo-Persian Translations of Some Aramaic Passages in the Hebrew Bible. *ArOr* 56:341–45.

Astour, M. C. 1979. The Arena of Tiglath-Pileser III's Campaign against Sarduri II (743 B.C.) *Assur* 2:69–91.

Attardo, E. 1984. La paleografia aramaica dagli inizi al 612 a.C. Ph.D. diss., Univ. of Padua.

———. 1987. Paleografia della statue di Tell Fekherye: Alcune considerazioni. In *Atti della 4a Giornata di Studi Camito-Semitici e Indo-europei*, ed. G. Bernini, 33–39. Milan: Unicopli.

Audet, J.-P. 1950. A Hebrew-Aramaic List of Books of the Old Testament in Greek Transcription. *JTS* n. s. 1:135–54.

Aufrecht, W. E. 1985. A Bibliography of the Deir 'Alla Plaster Texts. *NTCS Supplement* 2:1–7.

———. 1989. *A Corpus of Ammonite Inscriptions*. Ancient Near Eastern Texts and Studies 4. Lewiston, New York: Edwin Mellen Press.

Aufrecht, W. E., and G. J. Hamilton. 1988. The Tell Fakhariyah Inscription: A Bibliography. *NTCS Supplement* 4:1–7.

Aufrecht, W. E., and J. C. Hurd. 1975. *A Synoptic Concordance of Aramaic Inscriptions (According to H. Donner and W. Roellig)*. International Concordance Library 1. Missoula, Mont: Scholars Press.

Augé, R. 1954. *Daniel*. La Biblia de Montserrat 15/2. Montserrat: Monastery of Montserrat.

Augapfel, J. 1917. *Babylonische Rechtsurkunden aus der Regierungszeit Artaxerxes I. und Darius II*. Denkschriften der kaiserlichen Akademie der Wissenschaften in Wien, phil.-hist. Kl. 59/3. Wien: A. Hölder.

Aurès, A. 1884. Lettre à M. Ledrain sur la distinction à établir entre la mine du roi et la mine du pays. *RA* 1:11–16.

Avanzini, A. 1987. Alcune osservazioni in margine all'iscrizione di Zakir. *EVO* 10:113–19.

Avigad, N. 1954. Three Ornamented Hebrew Seals. *IEJ* 4:236–38.

———. 1957. A New Class of *Yehud* Stamps. *IEJ* 7:146–53.

———. 1958. An Early Aramaic Seal. *IEJ* 8:228–30.

———. 1958a. New Light on the MṢH Seal Impressions. *IEJ* 8:113–19.

———. 1960. *Yehûd* or *Ha'îr*? *BASOR* 158:23–27.

———. 1964. Seals and Sealings. *IEJ* 14:190–94 + 1 pl.

———. 1965. Seals of Exiles. *IEJ* 15:222–32 + 1 pl.

———. 1966. כתובת ארמית על קערה מתל דן. *Yediot* 30:209–12.

———. 1968. Notes on Some Inscribed Syro-Phoenician Seals. *BASOR* 189:44–49.

———. 1968a. An Inscribed Bowl from Dan. *PEQ* 100:42–44, pl. XVIII.

———. 1968b. The Seal of Abigad. *IEJ*:52–53; pl. 4C.

———. 1969. קבוצת חותמות עבריים. *EI (Albright Volume)* 9:1–9 + 2 pls.

———. 1974. More Evidence on the Judean Post-Exilic Stamps. *IEJ* 24:52–58 + 1 pl.

———. 1976. *Bullae and Seals from a Post-Exilic Judean Archive.* Qedem 4. Jerusalem: The Institute of Archaeology, The Hebrew University of Jerusalem.

———. 1978. Gleanings from Unpublished Ancient Seals. *BASOR* 230:67–69.

———. 1985. Some Decorated West Semitic Seals. *IEJ*:1–7; pl. 1.

———. 1986. Three Ancient Seals. *BA* 49:51–53.

Avishur, Y. 1975–76. זוגות מלים מקבילות המצומדים בארמית היהודית בסמיכות בארמית בארמית המקראית ובתרגומים הארמים. *BM* 21:247–62.

———. 1984. *Stylistic Studies of Word-Pairs in Biblical and Ancient Semitic Literatures.* AOAT 210. Neukirchen-Vluyn: Neukirchener.

Ayad, B. A. 1967. *The Topography of Elephantine according to the Aramaic Papyri.* Cairo: Institute of Coptic Studies.

———. 1972. The Topography of Elephantine according to the Aramaic Papyri. In *Medieval and Middle Eastern Studies in Honor of Aziz Suryal Atiya,* ed. S. A. Hanna, 23–37. (Revised version of Ayad, 1967.) Leiden: Brill.

———. 1975. *The Jewish-Aramean Communities in Ancient Egypt.* Cairo: Institute of Coptic Studies.

Babelon, E. 1893. *Les Perses achéménides, les satrapes et les dynastes tributaires de leur empire, Chypre et Phénicie.* Catalogue des monnaies grecques de la Bibliotheque Nationale. Paris: C. Rollin and Feuardent.

———. 1899. *Collection pauvert de la Chapelle: Intailles et camées donnés au département des médailles et antiques de la Bibliothéque Nationale.* Paris: E. Leroux.

———. 1901. *Traité des monnaies grecques et romaines.* 2 vols. Paris: E. Leroux., pls. CV–CXV.

Bacher, W. 1906–7. The Origin of the Jewish Colony of Syene (Assuan). *JQR* 19:441–44.

Badian, E. 1978. A Document of Artaxerxes IV? In *Greece and the Eastern Mediterranean in Ancient History and Prehistory: Studies Presented to F. Schachermeyr on the Occasion of his 80th Birthday,* ed. K. Kinzl, 40–50. Berlin: De Gruyter.

Baer, S. 1882. *Libri Danielis, Ezrae et Nehemiae.* Leipzig: Tauchnitz.

Bahnam, G. P. 1976. *Aḥīqār al-Ḥakīm.* Baghdad: Syriac Academy Publications.

Bahnassi, 'A. 1982. Maṣdar ism sūriyah wal-asmā' al-uḫrā al-qadīmah [The origin of the name Syria and the other ancient names]. *AASyr* 32:105–11 + 4 pls.

Balensi, J. 1985. [Section VI: Discussion]. *BAT,* 368.

Balkan, K. 1959. Inscribed Bullae from Daskyleion-Ergili. *Anatolia* 4:123–28, figs. 1–3, nos. 26–34; pl. 34a–d.

Baneth, D. H. 1914. Bemerkungen zu den Achikarpapyri. *OLZ* 17:248–52; 295–99; 348–53.

———. 1919. Zu dem aramäischen Brief aus der Zeit Assurbanipals. *OLZ* 22:55–58.

————. 1932–33. Review of *Laut- und Formenlehre des Aegyptisch-Aramäischen*, by P. Leander. *Kiryat Sepher* 9:89–91.

Bange, L. A. 1971. *A Study of the Use of Vowel-Letters in Alphabetic Consonantal Writing.* Munich: Verlag UNI-Druck.
Reviews: K. Petráček 1975: *ArOr* 43:92–93.

Barag, D. 1984. A Silver Coin of Yohanan, the High Priest. *Qadmoniot* 17:59–61.

Bar-Asher, M. 1978. *M.A. and Doctoral Theses on Hebrew and Aramaic Submitted in Israeli Universities (1938–1977).* Jerusalem: Ha-Moatsah le-Hanhalat Ha-Lašon.

Bardtke, H. 1960. Elephantine und die jüdische Gemeinde der Perserzeit. *Das Altertum* 6:13–31.

————. 1971. Review of *Archives from Elephantine*, by B. Porten. *TLZ* 96:96–98.

Bargès, J. 1856. Nouvelle interprétation de l'inscription phénicienne découverte par M. Mariette. *Revue de l'Orient* n.s. 3:190–206.

————. 1862. *Papyrus égypto-araméen appartenant au musée égyptien du Louvre.* Paris: B. Duprat.

Barnes, A. 1853. *Notes, critical, illustrative and practical, on the Book of Daniel with an introductory dissertation.* New York: Leavitt and Allen.

Barnett, L. D. 1915. An Aramaic Inscription from Taxila. *JRAS*: 340–42 + 1 pl.

Barnett, R. D. 1935. The Nimrud Ivories and the Art of the Phoenicians. *Iraq* 2:179–210.

————. 1939. Phoenician and Syrian Ivory Carving. *PEQ*:4–19, pls. I-XI.

————. 1940. Hebrew, Palmyrene and Hittite Antiquities. *British Museum Quarterly* 14:31.

————. 1957. *A Catalogue of the Nimrud Ivories.* London: British Museum.

————. 1963. Shell Fragments from Hamath and the Provenance of the Nimrud Ivories. *Iraq* 25:81–84.

————. 1964. The Gods of Zinjirli. In *Compte rendu de l'onzième rencontre assyriologique internationale organisée à Leyde du 23 au 29 Juin 1962*, 59–87. Leiden: Nederlands Instituut voor het Nabije Oosten.

————. 1967. Layard's Nimrud Bronzes and Their Inscriptions. *EI (Sukenik Volume)* 8:1–7, figs. I–VIII.

————. See also: L. Woolley.

Barré, M. L. 1983. *The God-List in the Treaty between Hannibal and Philip V of Macedonia: A Study in Light of the Ancient Near Eastern Treaty Tradition.* Baltimore: Johns Hopkins Univ. Press.

————. 1985. The First Pair of Deities in the Sefire I God-List. *JNES* 44:205–10.

Barrois, A. See: F. Thureau-Dangin.

Barth, J. 1901. Erklärung zu E. König's "The Emphatic State in Aramaic." *AJSL* 18:52.

————. 1907. Zu den neuen Papyrusfunden in Elephantine. *JJLG* 5:323–34.

————. 1907a. Bemerkungen zu den aramäischen Papyri von Assuan. *RevSém* 15:522–24.

————. 1908. Zu den Papyrusurkunden von Elephantine. *ZA* 21:188–94.

————. 1908a. Zur Bauinschrift des Bar-Rkhb. *RevSém* 16:241–242.

————. 1909. Zur altaramäischen Inschrift des Königs Zkr. *OLZ* 12:10–12.

————. 1912. Zu den Papyri von Elephantine (ed. Sachau). *OLZ* 15:10–11.

Barthélemy, M. l'abbé. 1768. Explication d'un bas-relief égyptien, et de l'inscription phénicienne qui l'accompagne. *Mémoires de literature tiréz des regîtres de l'Académie royale des inscriptions et belles lettres* 32:725–38.

Barton, G. A. 1926. The Problem of the Origin and Early History of the Deity NIN-IB (Ninurta, Nin-urash). *JAOS* 46:231–36.

Batten, L. W. 1913. *A Critical and Exegetical Commentary on the Books of Ezra and Nehemiah.* ICC 24–25. New York: Scribner.

Batto, B. F. 1985. Review of *La statue de Tell Fekherye*, by A. Abou Assaf et al. *CBQ* 47:501–3.

Bauer, H. 1914. Semitische Sprachprobleme: 2. Die Herkunft der Objektspartikel *yāt*, את usw. *ZDMG* 68:369–71.

————. 1925. Menetekel. In *Vierter deutscher Münzforschertag zu Halle (Salle): Festgabe den Teilnehmern gewidmet,* 27–30.

————. 1926. Überreste der kananäischen Unterschicht in den aramäischen Sprachen. *OLZ* 29:801–3.

————. 1932–33. Ein aramäischer Staatsvertrag aus dem 8. Jahrhundert v. Chr: Die Inschrift der Stele von Sudschīn. *AfO* 8:1–16.

Bauer, H., and B. Meissner. 1936. Ein aramäischer Pachtvertrag aus dem 7. Jahre Darius I. *SPAW* 72:414–24, taf. 1, 2.

Bauer, H., and P. Leander. 1927. *Grammatik des Biblisch-Aramäischen.* Halle (Saale): Niemeyer.
Reviews: E. Bräunlich 1928: *Dts. Ltztg.* 1753–56; E. Bräunlich 1931: *Dts. Ltztg.* 1063–64; W. Eichrodt 1929: *Th. d. Gegenwart* 23:303; J. Horovitz 1928: *MGWJ* 72:628; E. Littmann 1930: *OLZ* 33:449–51; J. A. Montgomery 1931; R. Savignac 1928: *RB* 37:310–11.

————. 1929. *Kurzgefasste biblisch-aramäische Grammatik mit Texten und Glossar.* Halle (Salle): Niemeyer.
Reviews: K. Holzhey 1929: *Theologische Revue* 28:348–49; E. Littmann 1930; J. A. Montgomery 1931.

Bauer, H. See also: J. Hempel.

Baumgartner, W. 1924. Zur Form der assyrischen Königsinschriften. *OLZ* 27:313–17.

————. 1926. *Das Buch Daniel.* Giessen: Töpelmann.

————. 1926a. Neues keilschriftliches Material zum Buche Daniel? *ZAW* 44:38–56.

————. 1927. Aramäisches in der Bibel. *RGG*[2] 1:468–70.

————. 1927a. Das Aramäische im Buche Daniel. *ZAW* 4:81–133. Reprinted in *Zum Alten Testament und seiner Umwelt: Ausgewählte Aufsätze* (Leiden: Brill,1959), 68–123.

————. 1939. Ein Vierteljahrhundert Danielforschung. *TRu* 11:59–83, 125–44, 201–28.

————. 1945. Zu den vier Reichen von Daniel 2. *TZ* 1:17–22.

————. 1947. Vom neuen biblisch-aramäischen Wörterbuch. In *Festschrift Otto Eissfeldt zum 60. Geburtstag 1. September 1947*, ed. J. Fück, 47–55. Halle (Saale): Niemeyer.

————. 1953. A Dictionary of the Aramaic Parts of the Old Testament in English and German. In *Lexicon in Veteris Testamenti libros*, ed. L. Koehler and W. Baumgartner, 1045–1138. Second ed., with supplement, 1958. Leiden: Brill.

————. 1957. Aramäisches — im AT. *RGG*[3] 1:532–34.

Bausani, A. 1980. La scrittura pahlavica frutto di bilinguismo aramaico-iranico. *VO* 3:269–76.

Bawden, G. et al. 1980. Typological and Analytical Studies: a. Preliminary Archaeological Investigations at Taymā. *Atlal* 4:69–106, pl. 69.

Bea, A. 1946. Papyri aramaicae nuper detectae. *Bib* 27:295.

————. 1948. De papyris aramaicis nuper inventis. *Bib* 29:307–8.

————. 1949. Epistula aramaica saec. VII exeunte ad Pharaonem scripta. *Bib* 30:514–16.

Becking, B. 1988. Kann das Ostrakon ND 6231 von Nimrud für ammonitisch gehalten werden? *ZDPV* 104:59–67.

Beek, M. A. 1966. Zeit, Zeiten und eine halbe Zeit. In *Studia biblica et semitica Theodoro Christiano Vriezen qui munere professoris theologiae per XXV annos functus est, ab amicis, collegis, discipulis dedicata*, 19–24. Wageningen: H. Veenman en Zonen.

Beer, E. F. F. 1833. *Inscriptiones et papyri veteres semitici quotquot in Aegypto reperti sunt*. Bk. 1. 2–21. Leipzig: Typographia Fridericinies.

Belger, C. 1893. Sendschirli II. *Berliner philologische Wochenschrift* 13:355–56, 385–88.

Belléli, L. 1909. *Interprétations erronées et faux monuments: Remarques sur quelques inscriptions récemment éditées suivies d'un sommaire analytique de l'ouvrage "An Independent Examination of the Assuan and Elephantine Aramaic Papyri."* Casal Montferrat: Rossi et Lavagno.

————. 1909a. *An Independent Examination of the Assuan and Elephantine Aramaic Papyri*. London: Luzac.

Ben-David, I. 1980–81. בוני. *Leš* 45:151–52.

Ben-Dor, I. 1946. A Hebrew Seal from Samaria. *Quarterly of the Department of Antiquities in Palestine* 12:78–83; pl. 25a.

Ben-Ḥayyim, Z. 1951. הנסתרות בארמית הקדמונית. *EI (Schwabe Volume)* 1:135–39.

————. 1970–71. עם העיון בכתובות ספירה. *Leš* 35:243–53.

————. 1980–81. ערכי מלים, ג'. *Tarbiz* 50:192–208.

Ben-Ḥayyim, Z., and S. E. Loewenstamm. 1958. יב. *EM* 3:425–44 + 1 pl.

Bennett, S. F. 1984. Objective Pronominal Suffixes in Aramaic. Ph.D. diss., Yale Univ.

————. 1987. Note on the Saqqâra Aramaic Texts. *Or* 56:87–88.

Bentzen, A. 1950. Daniel 6. Ein Versuch zur Vorgeschichte einer Märtyrerlegende. In *Festschrift A. Bertholet zum 80. Geburtstag gewidmet von Kollegen und Freunden*, 58–64. Tübingen: J. C. B. Mohr.

Benveniste, E. 1934. Termes et noms achéménides en araméen. *JA* 225:177–93.

————. 1954. Éléments perses en araméen d'Égypte. *JA* 242:297–310.

————. 1958. Notes sur les tablettes Elamites de Persépolis. *JA* 246:49–65.

————. 1958a. Review of *Persepolis*, by E. F. Schmidt. *JA* 246:203–4.

————. 1964. Édits d'Asoka en traduction grecque. *JA* 252:137–57.

Benveniste, E., and A. Dupont-Sommer. 1966. Une inscription indo-araméenne d'Asoka pro-venant de Kandahar (Afghanistan). *JA* 254:437–65 + 3 pls. and 3 figs.

Beṣar, Z. 1976–77. על מערכת הזמנים במגילה החיצונית לבראשית. *Leš* 41:196–204.

Benveniste, E. See also: D. Schlumberger.

Berger, P. 1884. [Communication about CIS II 47, 48, 46, 49; I 164]. *PSBA* 6:119–23.

————. 1885. *L'Arabie avant Mahomet, d'après les inscriptions.* Paris: Maisonneuve.

————. 1888. Cylindre perse avec légende araméenne. *Gazette archéologique* 13:143–44.

————. 1891. *Histoire de l'écriture dans l'antiquité.* Paris: Imprimerie Nationale.

————. 1894. [no title]. *CRAIBL*:356–57.

Berger, P.-R. 1975. Der Kyros-Zylinder mit dem Zusatzfragment BIN II Nr. 32 und die akka-dischen Personennamen im Danielbuch. *ZA* 64:192–234.

Bergman, A. 1936. Two Hebrew Seals of the 'Ebed Class. *JBL* 55:221–26.

Bergman, B. Z. 1968. *Han'el* in Daniel 2:25 and 6:19. *JNES* 27:69–70.

Bergsträsser, G. 1912. Review of *Hebräische Grammatik mit Übungsbuch*, by H. Strack; *Grammatik des Biblisch-Aramäischen mit den nach Handschriften berichtigten Texten und einem Wörterbuch*, by H. Strack; *Kurzgefasste Grammatik der biblisch-aramäischen Sprache*, by K. Marti. *ZDMG* 66:513–17.

Bernard, P. 1969. Les bas-reliefs gréco-perses de Dascylion à la lumière de nouvelles découvertes. *RArch* n.s. 1:17–28.

Betlyon, J. W. 1986. The Provincial Government of Persian Period Judea and the Yehud Coins. *JBL* 105:633–42.

Bevan, A. A. 1892. *A Short Commentary on the Book of Daniel.* Cambridge: Cambridge Univ. Press.

Bevan, W. L. 1896. Weights and Measures. In *A Dictionary of the Bible*, ed. W. Smith, 3:1727–42. London: J. Murray.

Bewer, J. A. 1922. *Der Text des Buches Ezra.* Göttingen: Vandenhoeck & Ruprecht.

Beyer, K. 1962. *Semitische Syntax im Neuen Testament.* Band I: Satzlehre Teil 1. Göttingen: Vandenhoeck & Ruprecht. 2. verbesserte Auflage, 1968.

————. 1970. Review of *Die lexikalischen und grammatikalischen Aramaismen im alttes-tamentlichem Hebräisch*, by M. Wagner. *ZDMG* 120:195–98.

————. 1970a. Review of *Altaramäische Grammatik der Inschriften des 10.-8. Jh. v. Chr.*, by R. Degen. *ZDMG* 120:198–204.

————. 1977. Der Ausfall der drucklosen kurzen Vokale in offener Silbe und die Trennung silbenanlautender Doppelkonsonanz. In *XIX. Deutscher Orientalistentag vom 28. Sep-tember bis 4. Oktober 1975 in Freiburg im Breisgau*, ed. W. Voigt, 649–53. ZDMGSupp III/1. Wiesbaden: Steiner.

————. 1979. Review of *Lexicon linguae aramaicae Veteris Testamenti documentis antiquis illustratum*, by E. Vogt. *ZDMG* 129:375–77.

————. 1984. *Die aramäischen Texte vom Toten Meer samt den Inschriften aus Palästina, dem* Testament Levis aus der Kairoer Genisa, der Fastenrolle und den alten talmudischen Zitaten. Göttingen: Vandenhoeck & Ruprecht.

———. 1986. *The Aramaic Language: Its Distribution and Subdivisions.* Tr. J. F. Healey. Göttingen: Vandenhoeck & Ruprecht.

———. 1988. Akkadisches *līmu* und aramäisches לאם "Eponymat." *Or* 57:82–83.

Beyer, K., and A. Livingstone. 1987. Die neuesten aramäischen Inschriften aus Taima. *ZDMG* 137:285–96.

———. 1990. Eine neue reichsaramäische Inschrift aus Taima. *ZDMG* 140:1–2.

Biggs, R. D. See: D. Pardee.

Bilabel, F. 1921. Beiträge zu lydischen Inschriften. *ZA* 33:148–56.

Biran, A. 1976. Tel Dan, 1976. *IEJ* 26:202–6 + 1 pl.

———. 1977. Tel Dan. *RB* 84:256–63, pl. VIIa.

———. 1980. Tell Dan Five Years Later. *BA* 43:168–83.

———. 1981. "To the God Who is in Dan." In *Temples and High Places in Biblical Times: Proceedings of the Colloquium in Honor of the Centennial of Hebrew Union College—Jewish Institute of Religion,* ed. A. Biran and I. Pommerantz, 142–51. Jerusalem: Hebrew Union College.

Biran, A., and R. Cohen. 1979. Tell 'Ira. *IEJ* 29:124–25.

Biran, A., and V. Tzaferis. 1977–78. כתובת-הקדשה דו-לשונית מתל דן. *Qadmoniot* 10:114–15.

Biran, A. See also: B. Mazar.

Birkeland, H. 1934. Drei Bemerkungen zu der Elephantine-Papyri 1–3 (ed. Sachau). *AcOr* 12:81–90.

———. 1938. Eine aramäische Inschrift aus Afghanistan. *Acta orientalia [Batava]* 16:222–33.

Birnbaum, S. A. 1954–57, 1971. *The Hebrew Scripts.* 2 vols. London: Palaeographia.

———. 1957. Inscriptions. In *The Objects from Samaria,* ed. J. W. Crowfoot, G. M. Crowfoot and K. M. Kenyon, 9–42. Samaria-Sebaste 3. London: Palestine Exploration Fund.

Bivar, A. D. H. 1961. A Rosette *phialē* Inscribed in Aramaic. *BSOAS* 24:189–99.

———. 1961a. A "Satrap" of Cyrus the Younger. *NC* 7th s., 1:119–27.

———. 1970. A Persian Monument at Athens, and Its Connections with the Achaemenid State Seals. In *W. B. Henning Memorial Volume,* ed. M. Boyce and I. Gershevitch, 43–61. London: Lund Humphries.

Blake, F. R. 1951. Hebrew Influence on Biblical Aramaic. In *A Resurvey of Hebrew Tenses,* 81–96. Scripta Pontificii Instituti Biblici 103. Rome: Pontifical Biblical Institute.

Blau, J. 1970. *On Pseudo-Corrections in Some Semitic Languages.* Jerusalem: Israel Academy of Sciences and Humanities.
Reviews: R. Degen 1977.

———. 1972. Marginalia Semitica II. *IOS* 2:57–82.

———. 1980. The Parallel Development of the Feminine Ending *-at* in the Semitic Languages. *HUCA* 51:17–28.

————. 1983. The Influence of Living Aramaic on Ancient South Palestinian Christian Arabic. In *Arameans, Aramaic and the Aramaic Literary Tradition*, ed. M. Sokoloff, 141–43. Ramat-Gan: Bar-Ilan Univ. Press.

————. 1984–85. Review of *Aramaic Texts from North Saqqâra*, by J. B. Segal. *Leš* 48–49:216–17.

————. 1985–86. On Some Arabic Dialectal Features Paralleled by Hebrew and Aramaic. *JQR* 76:5–12.

————. 1987. Minutiae Aramaicae. In *Perspectives on Language and Text: Essays and Poems in Honor of Francis I. Andersen's Sixtieth Birthday, July 28, 1985*, ed. E. W. Conrad and E. G. Newing, 3–10. Winona Lake, Ind.: Eisenbrauns.

Blau, L. 1907–08. Az assuani aram papyrusok talmudi világításban. *Magyar-Zsidó Szemle* 24:222–38; 25:236–61.

————. 1911–12. *Die jüdische Ehescheidung und der jüdische Scheidebrief: Eine historische Untersuchung.* 2 vols. Strassburg: Trübner.

————. 1912. Az elephantinei zsidó katonai telep ujabb aram papyrusai. *Magyar-Zsidó Szemle* 29:41–61.

————. 1913. *Papyri und Talmud in gegenseitiger Beleuchtung.* Schriften herausgegeben von der Gesellschaft zur Förderung der Wissenschaft des Judentums. Leipzig: Gustav Fock .

————. 1919. Die Strafklauseln der griechischen Papyrusurkunden beleuchtet durch die aramäischen Papyri und durch den Talmud. *MGWJ* 63:138–55.

Blau, O. 1858. Review of *Phönizischen Studien*, by M. A. Levy. *ZDMG* 12:723–28.

————. 1864. Über einen aramäisch-persischen Siegelstein. *ZDMG* 18: 299–300.

Bloch, J. 1950. *Les inscriptions d'Asoka.* Collection Émile Senart 8. Paris: Société d'édition "Les Belles lettres."

Block, D. I. 1984. The Role of Language in Ancient Israelite Perceptions of National Identity. *JBL* 103:321–40.

Blois, F. de. 1985. "Freemen" and "Nobles" in Iranian and Semitic Languages. *JRAS*: 5–15.

Blomqvist, J. 1982. Translation Greek in the Trilingual Inscription of Xanthus. *Opuscula atheniensia* 14:11–20.

Boardman, J. 1968. *Archaic Greek Gems.* London: Thames and Hudson.

————. 1970. Pyramidal Stamp Seals in the Persian Empire. *Iran* 8:19–45.

————. 1970a. *Greek Gems and Finger Rings, Early Bronze Age to Late Classical.* London: Thames and Hudson.

Boccaccini, G. 1987. E Daniele un testo apocalittico? Una (ri)definizione del pensiero del libro di Daniele in rapporto al Libro dei Sogni e all' apocalittica. *Henoch* 9:267–302.

Bogaert, M. 1964. Les suffixes verbaux non accusatifs dans le sémitique nord-occidental et particulièrement en hébreu. *Bib* 45:220–47.

Bogaert, P.-M. 1984. Relecture et refonte historicisantes du livre de Daniel attestées par la première version grecque (Papyrus 967). In *Études sur le judaïsme hellénistique: Congrès de Strasbourg*, ed. R. Kuntzmann and J. Schlosser, 197–224. Lectio divina, vol. 119. Paris: Cerf.

Bogolyubov, M. N. 1966.   Arameyskaya stroitelynaya nadpisy iz Asuana. *PalSb* 15 (= 78):41–46.

———. 1969.   To the Reading of the Strasburg [sic] Aramaic Papyrus (in Russian). *PalSb* 19 (82):69–75.

———. 1971.   O neskol'kich terminach v rasporjazenii Aršama o remonte korablja [Einige Termini in (aramäischen) Anordnungen Aršamas zur Schiffsreparatur]. *Voprosy filologii stran Azii i Afriki* 1:15–19.

———. 1973.   Arameyskie nadpisi na ritya predmetach iz Persepolyi (Inscriptions aramaicae de sacris ritibus e Persepoli). In *Izvestiya Ak. Nauk SSSR* 172–77. Seriya literatury i Jazyka 32/2. Moscow: Academy of Sciences.

———. 1974.   La version araméenne du texte bilingue lydien-araméen. *Voprosy Iazykoznaniya* 23:106–12.

———. 1976.   An Aramaic Inscription from Taxila. *Voprosy Iazykoznaniya* 25/6:64–69.

———. 1977.   Dating of Aramaic Inscriptions of the Ašoki Epoch. *Voprosy Iazykoznaniya* 26/5:72–77.

———. 1979.   Example of Perfect with Prothetic Vowel in Imperial Aramaic. *Uenyje zapiski Leningradskogo universiteta Serija vostokovedeskin nauk, Vypusk 6* 401:14–17.

Böhl, E. 1860.   *De Aramaismis Libri Koheleth*. Erlangen: T. Blaesing.

Böhl, F. M. T. de Liagre. 1937.   *Der babylonische Fürstenspiegel*. MAOG 11/3.

———. 1946.   Een schuldvordering uit de Regeering van Darius I met een arameesch bijschrift (492 v. Chr.) In *Symbolae ad ius et historiam antiquitatis pertinentes Julio Christiano van Oven dedicatae*, ed. M. D. B. A. van Groningen and E. M. Meijers, 63–70. Leiden: Brill.

Bondi, J. H. 1918.   Zu Sachau APO 4, 10. *OLZ* 21:17.

Bonfante, G. 1980.   L'origine della formazione perifrastica it. *sta insegnando*, ingl. He Is Teaching. In *The Bible World: Essays in Honor of Cyrus H. Gordon*, ed. G. Rendsburg et al., 9–11. New York: Ktav.

Bongard-Levin, G. M. 1956.   Taxila Inscription. *Sovietskoye Vostokovedenie*.

Borchardt, L. 1932.   Das Elephantine-Mondjahr. *MGWJ* 76:299–310.

———. 1933.   Nachricht von einem weiteren Funde aramäischer Urkunden. In *Allerhand Kleinigkeiten seinen Wissensch. Freunden und Bekannten ... uberreicht*, 47–49. Leipzig.

Bork, F. 1918.   Zum Jahresrätsel der Achiqargeschichte. *OLZ* 21:226–27.

Bornstein, H. 1908.   פליטה מני קדם או שרידי קביעת שנים מדור עזרא ונחמיה. In *Festschrift zu Ehren des Dr. A. Harkavy ... gewidmet*, ed. D. Günzburg and I. Markon, Hebräische Abteilung, 63–104. St. Petersburg [Berlin]: H. Itzkowski.

Bordreuil, P. 1973.   Une tablette araméenne inédite de 635 av. J.-C. *Sem* 23:95–102, pls. I–V.

———. 1979.   Les noms propres transjordaniens de l'ostracon de Nimroud. *Revue d'histoire et de philosophie religieuses* 59:313–17.

———. 1986.   *Catalogue des sceaux ouest-sémitiques inscrits de la Bibliothèque Nationale, du Musée du Louvre et du Musée biblique de Bible et Terre Sainte*. Paris: Bibliothèque Nationale.

Reviews: M. G. Amadasi Guzzo 1989: *Rivista di studi fenici* 17:147–48; P. Amiet 1988: *RA* 82:117–18; F. Bron 1987: *Museum Helveticum* 44:265; G. Bunnens 1989: *Abr Nahrain* 27:174–76; A. Caquot 1987: *CRAIBL*:163–64; A. Caquot 1987: *Syria* 64:352–53; P.-E. Dion 1989; F. Israel 1988: *Or* 57:93–96; A. R. Millard 1988: *SOTS Book List*: 29; J. Naveh 1988: *JSS* 33:115–16; E. Puech 1989: *RB* 96:588–92; W. Röllig 1988: *WO* 19:194–97; S. Segert 1988: *ZAW* 100:311; J. Teixidor forthcoming: *AO*.

———. 1986a. Charges et fonctions en Syrie-Palestine d'après quelques sceaux ouest-sémitiques du second et du premier millénaire. *CRAIBL*: 290–308, esp. 305–7.

———. 1986b. Sceaux transjordaniens inscrits. In *La voie royal; 9000 ans d'art au royaume de Jordanie*. Paris: Association Française d'Action Artistique.

———. 1987. Perspectives nouvelles de l'épigraphie sigillaire ammonite et moabite. In *Studies in the History and Archaeology of Jordan*, vol. 3, ed. A. Hadidi, 283–86. Amman: Department of Antiquities.

Bordreuil, P., and E. Gubel, eds. 1983. Bulletin d'antiquités archéologiques du Levant inédites ou méconnues I. *Syria* 60:335–41.

———. 1985. Bulletin d'antiquités archéologiques du Levant inédites ou méconnues II. *Syria* 62:171–86.

———. 1986. Bulletin d'antiquités archéologiques du Levant inédites ou méconnues III. *Syria* 63:417–35.

———. 1987. Bulletin d'antiquités archéologiques du Levant inédites ou méconnues IV. *Syria* 64:309–21.

———. 1988. Bulletins d'antiquités archéologiques du Levant inédites ou méconnues V. *Syria* 65:437–56.

———. 1990. Bulletins d'antiquités archéologiques du Levant inédites ou méconnues VI. *Syria* 67:483–520.

Bordreuil, P., and A. Lemaire. 1974. Trois sceaux nord-ouest sémitiques inédits. *Sem* 24:25–34.

———. 1976. Nouveaux sceaux hébreux, araméens et ammonites. *Sem* 26:45–63 + 3 pls.

———. 1979. Nouveau groupe de sceaux hébreux, araméens et ammonites. *Sem* 29:71–84.

———. 1982. Nouveaux sceaux hébreux et araméens. *Sem* 32:21–34.

Bordreuil, P., and J. Teixidor. 1983. Nouvel examen de l'inscription de Bar-Hadad. *AO* 1:271–76.

Bordreuil, P. See also: A. Abou Assaf, A. R. Millard, K. Yassine.

Borger, R. 1957. Anath-Bethel. *VT* 7:102–4.

———. 1982. Die Chronologie des Darius-Denkmals am Behistun-Felsen. *Nachrichten der Akademie der Wissenschaften in Göttingen, phil.-hist. Kl.* 3:103–32.

Borowski, E. 1952. Siegel der Sammlung Layard. *Or* 21:168–83 + 5 pls.

———. 1965. Inscriptions (Borowski Collection). In *The Bible in Archaeology. Catalogue 6*, ed. P. P. Kahane, 64–67. Jerusalem: The Israel Museum.

Bossert, H. T. 1951. *Altsyrien: Kunst und Handwerk in Cypern, Syrien, Palästina, Transjordanien und Arabien von den Anfängen bis zum völligen Aufgehen in der griechisch-römischen Kultur.* Die ältesten Kulturen des Mittelmeerkreises 3. Tübingen: E. Wasmuth.

———. 1958. Neues von Zincirli und Maraş. *Or* 27:399–406.

Bossier, A. 1939. Melanges d'archéologie orientale. *RA* 36:61–67.

Bostrup, P. O. 1927. Aramäische Ritualtexte in Keilschrift. *AcOr* 5:257–301.

Bouriant, U. 1889. Notes de voyage. *Recueil de travaux relatifs à la philologie et à l'archéologie égyptiennes et assyriennes* 11:131–59.

Bousquet, J. 1986. Une nouvelle inscription trilingue à Xanthos? *RArch* n.s. 1:101–6.

Boutflower, C. 1916. The Historical Value of Daniel V and VI. *JTS* 17:43–60.

———. 1923. *In and Around the Book of Daniel.* London: SPCK.

———. 1931. *Dadda-'Idri; or, The Aramaic of the Book of Daniel.* London: SPCK.

Bovier-Lapierre, P. See: A. Strazzulli.

Bowman, R. A. 1936. An Interpretation of the Asshur Ostracon. In *Royal Correspondence of the Assyrian Empire.* Vol. 4, ed. L. Waterman, 273–82. University of Michigan Studies, Humanistic Series 20. Ann Arbor: Univ. of Michigan Press.

———. 1939. Anu-uballiṭ—Kefalon. *AJSL* 56:231–43.

———. 1941. The Old Aramaic Alphabet at Tell Halaf: The Date of the "Altar" Inscription. *AJSL* 58:359–67 + 1 fig.

———. 1941a. An Aramaic Journal Page. *AJSL* 58:302–13 + 2 pls.

———. 1944. An Aramaic Religious Text in Demotic Script. *JNES* 3:219–31.

———. 1948. Arameans, Aramaic, and the Bible. *JNES* 7:65–90.

———. 1965. 'Eben gelal — aban galâlu (Ezra 5:8; 6:4). In *Doron: Hebrew Studies in Honor of Professor Abraham I. Katsh* 64–74. New York: Nat. Assoc. of Prof. of Hebrew in American Institutions of Higher Learning.

———. 1970. *Aramaic Ritual Texts from Persepolis.* OIP 91. Chicago: Univ. of Chicago Press.
Reviews: H. J. W. Drijvers 1971; P. Gignoux 1972: *RHR* 181:86–87; P. Grelot 1973a; B. A. Levine 1972a; J. Oelsner 1975: J. Z. Smith 1971.

———. 1970a. Review of *Archives from Elephantine*, by B. Porten. *Or* 39:454–59.

Bowman, R. A., and C. W. Gilkey. 1954. The Book of Ezra and the Book of Nehemiah. *Interpreter's Bible* 3:549–819.

Boyarin, D. 1972–73. סידרוס סדר השם ולואו בארמית ובעברית. *Leš* 37:113–16.

———. 1975–76. עיונים בארמית בבלית. *Leš* 40:172–77.

———. 1981. An Inquiry into the Formation of the Middle Aramaic Dialects. In *Bono Homini Donum: Essays in Historical Linguistics, in Memory of J. Alexander Kerns.* 2 vols., ed. Y. L. Arbeitman and A. R. Bomhard, 2:613–49. Current Issues in Linguistic Theory 16. Amsterdam: John Benjamins.

Boyd, J. L., III. 1982. The Development of the West Semitic Qal Perfect of the Double-'Ayin Verb with Particular Reference to Its Transmission into Syriac. *JNSL* 10:11–23.

Boylan, P. 1912. The New Aramaic Papyri from Elephantine. *ITQ* 7:40–50.

Branden, A. van den. 1956. *Les textes thamoudéens de Philby.* 2 vols. Inscriptions du Nord. Bibliothèque du Muséon 41. Louvain: Publications Universitaires.

Brandenstein, W. 1929. Die lydische Sprache I. *WZKM* 36:263–304.

———. 1931–32. Die Nominalformen des Lydischen. *Caucasica* 9:25–40; 10:67–94.

———. 1932. Die lydische Sprache II. *WZKM* 38:1–67.

Brandis, J. 1866. *Das Münz-, Mass-, und Gewichtswesen in Vorderasien bis auf Alexander den Grossen.* Berlin: W. Hertz.

Brauner, R. 1974. A Comparative Lexicon of Old Aramaic. Ph.D. diss., Dropsie Univ.

———. 1975. The Old Aramaic *Zakir A* Inscription and Comparative Semitic Lexicography. *Gratz College Annual of Jewish Studies* 4:9–27.

———. 1977. Aramaic and Comparative Semitic Lexicography. *Gratz College Annual of Jewish Studies* 6:25–33.

Bravmann, M. M. 1977. The Aramaic Nomen Agentis *qāṭōl* and Some Similar Phenomena of Arabic. In *Studies in Semitic Philology*, 171–80. Studies in Semitic Languages and Linguistics, vol. 6. Leiden: Brill.

———. 1977a. Aramaic *m^{e}sar*, Neo-hebraic *māsar* 'to surrender (someone)'. In *Studies in Semitic Philology*, 513–16. Leiden: Brill.

———. 1977b. The Origin of Aramaic *d^{e}mā* 'to be like, to resemble'. In *Studies in Semitic Philology* 556–58. Leiden: Brill.

Brekelmans, C. 1963. Sefire I A 29–30. *VT* 13:225–28.

———. 1965. The Saints of the Most High and Their Kingdom. *OTS* 14:305–29.

Brentjes, B. 1981. Archäologie Afghanistans. *Das Altertum* 27:133–46.

Bresciani, E. 1958. Nuovi documenti aramaici dall'Egitto. *ASAE* 55:273–83.

———. 1958a. Alcuni nuovi monumenti di epoca persiana. *ASAE* 55:267–72, pl. Ib, facs. p 269.

———. 1958b. La satrapia d'Egitto. *Studi classici e orientali* 7:132–88.

———. 1959. Un papiro aramaico da El Hibeh del Museo Archeologico di Firenze. *Aeg* 39:3–8 + 1 pl.

———. 1960. Papiri aramaici egiziani di epoca persiana presso il Museo Civico di Padova. *RSO* 35:11–24 + 5 pls.

———. 1960a. Postilla a RSO, XXXV, 11–24. *RSO* 35:211.

———. 1962. Un papiro aramaico di età tolemaica. *AANL Rendiconti* 17, 5/6:258–64 + 1 pl.

———. 1967. Nouveaux papyrus araméens d'époque perse provenant d'Hermopolis. *CRAIBL*: 301–4.

———. 1971. Frammenti di un testo aramaico da Saqqara del V sec. a. Cr. In *Studi in onore di Edoardo Volterra*. Vol. 6, 529–32 + 1 pl. Milan: Giuffrè.

———. 1971a. Una statuina fittile con iscrizione aramaica dall'Egitto. *HomAD-S*, 5–8.

———. 1975. Review of *Documents araméens d'Égypte*, by P. Grelot. *OrAnt* 14:174–75.

———. 1980. L'attività archeologica dell'Università di Pisa in Egitto: 1977–80. *EGO* 3:1–36, pl. XVIb.

———. 1985. I semiti nell'egitto di età saitica e persiana. In *Egitto e società antica: Atti del convegno, Torino 8/9 VI–23/24 XI 1984*, 93–104. Milan: Vita e Pensiero.

Bresciani, E., and M. Kamil. 1966. Le lettere aramaiche di Hermopoli. *AANL Memorie* 8-9:357–428.

Bright, J. 1949. A New Letter in Aramaic Written to a Pharaoh of Egypt. *BA* 12:46–52.

Brinkman, J. A. 1977. Notes on the Aramaeans and Chaldeans in Southern Babylonia in the Early Seventh Century B.C. *Or* 46:304–25.

Brock, S. P. 1968. Review of *The Aramaic Inscriptions of Sefîre*, by J. A. Fitzmyer. *JTS* 19:713–14.

———. 1977. Review of *Textbook of Syrian Semitic Inscriptions II*, by J. C. L. Gibson. *JTS* 28:184–85.

———. 1984. Review of *The Bisitun Inscription of Darius the Great: Aramaic Version*, by J. C. Greenfield and B. Porten. *JRAS*:138–39.

———. 1985. Review of *Aramaic Texts from North Saqqâra*, by J. B. Segal. *JJS* 36:109–10.

———. 1989. Three Thousand Years of Aramaic Literature. *Aram* 1:11–23.

Brockelmann, C. 1939. Eine vermeintliche aramäische Präposition. *OLZ* 42:666–69.

———. 1940. Neuere Theorien zur Geschichte des Akzents und des Vokalismus im Hebräischen und Aramäischen. *ZDMG* 94:332–71.

———. 1954. Das Aramäische, einschliesslich des Syrischen. In *Semitistik*, Handbuch der Orientalistik 1/3, 135–62. Leiden: Brill.

Bron, F., and A. Lemaire. 1979–84. Notes de lexicographie ouest-sémitique. *Comptes rendus du GLECS* 24-28:7–30.

———. 1983. Poids inscrits phénico-araméens du VIIIème siècle av. J.-C. In *Atti del I Congresso Internazionale di Studi Fenici e Punici Roma, 5-10 Novembre 1979, volume terzo*, 763–70. Rome: Consiglio Nazionale delle Ricerche.

———. 1983a. Inscriptions d'Al-Mina. In *Atti del I Congresso Internazionale di Studi Fenici e Punici Roma, 5-10 Novembre 1979, volume terzo*, 677–86. Rome: Consiglio Nazionale delle Ricerche.

———. 1989. Les inscriptions araméennes de Hazaël. *RA* 83:35–44.

Brown, C. R. 1884. *An Aramaic Method: A classbook for the study of the elements of Aramaic from Bible and Targums*. Chicago: American Publication Soc. of Hebrew.

Brown, F., S. R. Driver, and C. A. Briggs. 1907. *A Hebrew and English Lexicon of the Old Testament With An Appendix Containing the Biblical Aramaic*. Oxford: Clarendon.

Brown, M. L. 1987. "Is It Not?" or "Indeed!": *HL* in Northwest Semitic. *Maarav* 4:201–19.

Bruce, F. F. 1977. The Oldest Greek Version of Daniel. *OTS (Instruction and Interpretation: Studies in Hebrew Language, Palestinian Archaeology and Biblical Exegesis)* 20:22–40.

Brugnatelli, V. forthcoming. *5th International Hamito-Semitic Congress, Vienna 27.9–2.10.1987*.

Bruston, C. 1908. Les papyrus judéo-araméens d'Éléphantine. *RTP* 41:97–113.

Buccellati, G. 1962. Review of *Il semitico di nord-ovest*, by G. Garbini. *RSO* 37:135–36.

———. 1964. The Enthronement of the King and the Capital City in Texts from Ancient Mesopotamia and Syria. In *Studies Presented to A. Leo Oppenheim: June 7, 1964*, ed. R. D. Biggs and J. A. Brinkman, 54–61. Chicago: Oriental Institute of the University of

Chicago.

———. 1967. *Cities and Nations of Ancient Syria*. Studi Semitici 26. Rome: Università degli studi "La Sapienza."

Buchanan, B. 1966–88. *Catalogue of Ancient Near Eastern Seals in the Ashmolean Museum*. 3 vols. Oxford: Clarendon.

Buckler, W. 1924. *Lydian Inscriptions*. Leiden: Brill.

Büchler, A. 1912. Zu Sachaus aramäischen Papyrus aus Elephantine. *OLZ* 15:126–27.

Budde, K. 1918. Die Inschrift von 'Arāḳ el-emīr. *ZDMG* 72:186–88.

Buhl, F. 1908. Remarques sur les papyrus juifs d'Éléphantine. *Oversigt over det Kongelige Danske Videnskabernes Selskabs forhandlinger*: 37–64.

Burchardt, M. 1911. Datierte Denkmäler der berliner Sammlung aus dem Achämenidenzeit. *ZÄS* 49:69–80, pls. VIII/2, X/6.

Burney, C. F. 1912. New Aramaic Papyri and Old Testament History. *Church Quarterly Review* 74:392–409.

———. 1912a. The Priestly Code and the New Aramaic Papyri from Elephantinê. *Expositor* 8/3:97–108.

Buth, R. 1987. Word Order in Aramaic from the Perspectives of Functional Grammar and Discourse Analysis. Ph.D. diss., UCLA.

Cagni, L. 1990. Considérations sur les textes babyloniens de Neirab près d'Alep. *Transeuphratène* 2:169–85.

Caillat, C. 1966. La séquence *shyty* dans les inscriptions indo-araméennes d'Asoka. *JA* 254:467–70.

Cameron, G. G. 1948. *Persepolis Treasury Tablets*. OIP 65. Chicago: Univ. of Chicago Press.
Reviews: A. Falkenstein 1952: *WO* 1:503–6; I. Gershevitch 1952: *Asia Major* 2:132–44.

———. 1958. Persepolis Treasury Tablets Old and New. *JNES* 17:161–76.

———. 1960. The Elamite Version of the Bisitun Inscriptions. *JCS* 14:59–68.

———. 1965. New Tablets from the Persepolis Treasury. *JNES* 24:167–92.

Campbell Thompson, R., and R. W. Hamilton. 1932. An Aramaic Inscription on a Piece of Black painted Ware from Nineveh. *JRAS*: 29–31.

Cannuyer, C. 1985. A propos de l'origine du nom de la Syrie. *JNES* 44:133–37.

Canova, R. 1954. *Iscrizioni e monumenti protocristiani del paese di Moab*. Sussidi allo studio delle antichità cristiane 4. Vatican City: Pontificio Istituto di Archeologia Cristiana.

Cantera, F. 1961. Review of *Il semitico di nord-ovest*, by G. Garbini. *Sef* 21:377–78.

Cantineau, J. 1931. Remarques sur la stèle araméenne de Sefiré-Soudjin. *RA* 28:167–178.

———. 1931a. De la place de l'accent de mot en hébreu et en araméen biblique. *Bulletin d'études orientales de l'Institut Français de Damas* 1:81–98.

———. 1932. Elimination des syllabes brèves en hébreu et en araméen biblique. *Bulletin d'études orientales de l'Institut Français de Damas* 2:125–44.

Caquot, A. 1951–52. La déesse Šegal. *Sem* 4:55–58.

———. 1955. Sur les quatre bêtes de *Daniel* VII. *Sem* 5:5–13.

———. 1962. L'alliance avec Abram (Genèse 15). *Sem* 12:51–66.

———. 1967. Les quatre bêtes et le 'Fils d'homme' (Daniel 7). *Sem* 17:37–71.

———. 1971. Une inscription araméenne d'époque assyrienne. *HomAD-S*, 9–16.

———. 1977. Review of *La langue de Ya'udi*, by P.-E. Dion. *Syria* 54:134–36.

———. 1978. Un nouveau témoignage sur le prophète Balaam. *RHR* 193:143–44.

———. 1984. Hébreu et araméen. In *Annuaire du collège de France 1983-84*, 603–22. Paris: Collège de France.

Caquot, A., and A. Lemaire. 1977. Les textes araméens de Deir 'Alla. *Syria* 54:189–208.

Caragounis, C. C. 1987. The Interpretation of the Ten Horns of Daniel 7. *ETL* 63:106–13.

Cardascia, G. 1951. *Les archives des Murašû: une famille d'hommes d'affaires babyloniens à l'époque perse (455–403 av. J.-C.).* Paris: Imprimerie Nationale.
Reviews: W. Eilers 1955: *ZA* 51:270–73; W. von Soden 1954: *BO* 11:205–7.

———. 1958. Review of *Neubabylonisches Pfandrecht*, by H. Petschow. *BO* 15:31–36.

Carmignac, J. 1964–66. Un aramaïsme biblique et qumrânien: L'infinitif placé après son complément d'objet. *RevQ* 5:503–20.

Carruba, O. 1977. Commentario alla trilingue licio-greco-aramaica di Xanthos. *Studi micenei ed egeo-anatolici* 18:273–318.

Carruba, O. et al. 1978. Sull'interpretazione delle righe 20-21 della trilingue di Xanthos. *Incontri linguistici* 4:89–98.

Casey, M. 1979. *Son of Man: The Interpretation and Influence of Daniel 7.* London: SPCK.

Cassin, E. 1951. Daniel dans la 'fosse' aux lions. *RHR* 139:129–61.

Cassuto, M. D. 1942. אלוהיהם של יהודי יב. *Kedem* 1:47–52.

Catastini, A. 1987. Observations on Aramaic Epigraphy. *JSS* 32:273–77.

Cavalletti, S. 1957. Ebraico biblico ed ebraico mishnico. *Sef* 17:122–29.

Caylus, A. C. P., Comte de. 1752. *Recueil d'antiquités égyptiennes, etrusques, grecques et romaines.* 8 vols. Paris: Desaint et Saillant.

Cazelles, H. 1954. Documents araméens d'Égypte nouvellement publiés. *CRAIBL*: 505–11.

———. 1955. Nouveaux documents araméens d'Égypte. *Syria* 32:75–100 + 2 pls.

———. 1962. Connexions et structure de *Gen.* XV. *RB* 69:321–49.

———. 1971. Tal'ayim, Tala et Muṣur. *HomAD-S*, 17–26.

———. 1982. La rupture de la Berît selon les Prophètes. *JJS* 33:133–44.

Chabot, J.-B. 1909. Les papyri araméens d'Éléphantine sont-ils faux? *JA* 10/14:515–22.

———. 1910. *Les langues et les littératures araméennes.* Paris: Geuthner.

———. 1944. Les fouilles de Clermont-Ganneau à Éléphantine. *Journal des savants*: 87–92, 136–42.

Charbel, A. 1970. 'Shelamim' nei documenti di Elefantina. *BeO* 12:91–94.

Charbonnet, A. 1986. Le dieu aux lions d'Erétrie. *AION–Archeologia e storia antica* 8:117–56.

Charles, R. H. 1929. *A Critical and Exegetical Commentary on the Book of Daniel.* Oxford: Clarendon.

Charlesworth, J. H. 1981. *The Pseudepigrapha and Modern Research with a Supplement.* SBL Septuagint and Cognate Studies, vol. 7. Chico, Cal: Scholars Press.

Chaumont, M.-L. 1963. A propos de quelques personnages feminins figurant dans l'inscription trilingue de Šāhpuhr Ier à la Ka'ba de Zoroastre. *JNES* 22:194–99.

———. 1965. Le culte de la déesse Anāhitá (Anahit) dans la religion des monarques d'Iran et d'Arménie au Ier siècle de notre ère. *JA* 253:167–81.

Childs, W. A. P. 1981. Lycian Relations with Persians and Greeks in the Fifth and Fourth Centuries Re-examined. *Anatolian Studies* 31:55–80.

Choudhary, R. 1958. Asóka and the Taxila Inscription. *Annals of the Bhandarkar Oriental Research Institute* 39:127–32.

Clarke, E. G. 1977. Review of *Altaramäische Grammatik*, by S. Segert. *JBL* 96:573–75.

———. See also: W. S. Morrow.

Clay, A. T. 1904. *Business Documents of Murashû Sons of Nippur: Dated in the Reign of Darius II 424–404 B. C.* The Babylonian Expedition of the University of Pennsylvania, series A: Cuneiform Texts 10. Philadelphia: Univ. of Pennsylvania Press.

———. 1906–7. Ellil, the God of Nippur. *AJSL* 23:269–79.

———. 1907. The Origin and Real Name of NIN-IB. *JAOS* 28:135–44.

———. 1908. Aramaic Indorsements on the Documents of the Murašu Sons. In *Old Testament and Semitic Studies in Memory of William Rainey Harper*, ed. R. F. Harper et al., 285–322. Chicago: Univ. of Chicago Press.

———. 1912. *Business Documents of Murashu Sons of Nippur Dated in the Reign of Darius II.* The University Museum, Publications of the Babylonian Section II/1. Philadelphia: Univ. of Pennsylvania Museum.

———. 1912a. *Babylonian Records in the Library of J. Pierpont Morgan. Part I: Babylonian Business Transactions of the first Millennium B. C.* New York: privately published.

———. See also: H. V. Hilprecht.

Clermont-Ganneau, C. 1878. Origine perse des monuments araméens d'Egypte. *RArch* 36:93–107.

———. 1879. Origine perse des monuments araméens d'Egypte (Notes d'archéologie orientale). Deuxième article. *RArch* 37:21–39.

———. 1880–97. *Études d'archéologie orientale.* 2 vols. Bibliothèque de l'École des Hautes Études, Sciences historiques et philologiques, vol. 113. Paris: F. Viewig.

———. 1883. Notes d'archéologie orientale. *Revue critique d'histoire et de littérature* n. s. 15:413–18.

———. 1883a. Sceaux et cachets israélites, phéniciens et syriens. *JA* 8/1:123–59; 8/2:304–5.

———. 1884. Notes d'archéologie orientale. *Revue critique d'histoire et de littérature* 18:265–66 [no. XV], 442–44 [no. XVII].

———. 1885–1924. *Recueil d'archéologie orientale.* 8 vols. Paris: E. Leroux.

———. 1886. Maná Thécel Pharès et le festin de Balthasar. *JA* 8/1:36–67.

———. 1896. Mitteilung über die Inschriften von Nêrab. *CRAIBL* 4/24:118–19.

———. 1897. *Album d'antiquités orientales: Recueil de monuments inédits ou peu connus.* Paris: E. Leroux.

———. 1898. Inscription araméenne de Cappadocie. *CRAIBL* 4/26:630–40, 808–10.

———. 1903. Traduction et interprétation du Papyrus d'Euting (Notes). *CRAIBL*: 364.

———. 1904. [No title]. *CRAIBL*: 212.

———. 1909. Stèle araméenne inédite de la nécropole de Memphis. In *Annuaire du Collège de France*: 64.

Cody, A. 1979. The Phoenician Ecstatic in Wenamūn: A Professional Oracular Medium. *JEA* 65:99–106.

Cogan, M. 1974. *Imperialism and Religion.* SBL Monograph Series, vol. 19. Missoula, Mont: Scholars Press.

Cohen, C. 1982. Some Overlooked Akkadian Evidence Concerning the Etymology and Meaning of the Biblical Term *mšl* [in Hebrew]. In *Te'uda II: Bible Studies: Y. M. Grintz in Memoriam*, ed. B. Uffenheimer, 315–24. Tel Aviv: Tel Aviv Univ.

Cohen, D. R. 1975–76. Subject and Object in Biblical Aramaic: A Functional Approach Based on Form-Content Analysis. *AAL* 2:1–23.

Cohen, N. G. 1966–67. שמותיהם של יהודי יֵב כמקור לידיעות היסטוריות. *Leš* 31:97–106, 199–210.

Cohen, R. 1986. Horvat Rogem. *Excavations and Surveys in Israel* 5:91–92.

Colella, P. 1973. Les abréviations ט et ᴘ✕ (XP). *RB* 80:547–58.

Collon, D. 1984. Phoenicia and the Punic World. In *The Cambridge Ancient History*, plates to Volume 3: *The Middle East, the Greek World and the Balkans to the Sixth Century B.C.* New edition. Ed. J. Boardman, 93–111. Cambridge: Cambridge University Press.

———. 1986. In BAALIM [P. Bordreuil and E. Gubel 1986]. *Syria* 63:424–26.

———. 1987. *First Impressions, Cylinder Seals in the Ancient Near East.* Chicago: Univ. of Chicago Press.

Colombo, D. 1953–58. Elefantina. In *Dizionario Ecclesiastico*, ed. A. M. Bozzone, 952–53. Turin: Editrice Torinese.

Commission du *CIS*. 1900–5, 1907–14. *Répertoire d'épigraphie sémitique.* 8 vols. Ed. C. J. de Vogüé. Paris: Imprimerie Nationale [Librairie C. Klincksieck].

Conder, C. R. 1896. The Syrian Language. *PEFQS* 28:60–78.

Contini, R. 1979. Problemi dell'aramaico antico. *EGO* 2:197–213.

———. 1981. Review of *Fouilles de Xanthos, Tome VI: La stèle trilingue de Létôon*, ed. H. Metzger. *OrAnt* 20:231–35.

———. 1982. *Tipologia della frase nominale nel semitico nordoccidentale del I millennio a. C.* Studi e ricerche 1. Pisa: Giardini.

———. 1986. I documenti aramaici dell'Egitto persiano e tolemaico. *RivB* 34:73–109.

Conybeare, F. C., J. R. Harris, and A. S. Lewis. 1898. *The Story of Ahikar from the Syriac, Arabic, Armenian, Ethiopic, Greek and Slavonic Versions.* London: C. J. Clay and Sons. 2nd, enlarged and corrected ed. Cambridge: Cambridge Univ. Press, 1913.

Conybeare, F. C. See also: J. R. Harris.

Coogan, M. D. 1975. The Use of Second Person Singular Verbal Forms in Northwest Semitic Personal Names. *Or* 44:194–97.

Cook, E. M. 1986. Word Order in the Aramaic of Daniel. *AAL* 9/3:1–16.

———. 1989. "In the Plain of the Wall" (Dan 3:1). *JBL* 108:115–16.

———. 1990. The Orthography of Final Unstressed Long Vowels in Old and Imperial Aramaic. In *Sopher Mahir: Northwest Semitic Studies Presented to Stanislav Segert*, ed. E. M. Cook (= *Maarav* 5–6), 53–67. Winona Lake, Ind.: Eisenbrauns.

Cook, S. A. 1898. *A Glossary of the Aramaic Inscriptions*. Cambridge: Cambridge Univ. Press. Reprint. Hildesheim: Olms, 1974.

———. 1904. Notes on Semitic Inscriptions. *PSBA* 26:32–35.

———. 1907. The Jewish Temple of Yahu, God of Heavens, at Syene. *Expositor* 7/4:497–505.

———. 1908. Supplementary Notes on the New Aramaic Papyri. *Expositor* 7/5:87–96.

———. 1912. The Elephantinê Papyri and the Old Testament. *Expositor* 8/3:193–207.

———. 1915. The Significance of the Elephantine Papyri for the History of Hebrew Religion. *AJT* 19:346–82.

———. 1917. A Lydian-Aramaic Bilingual. *JHS* 37:77–87, 219–31 + 1 pl.

———. 1930. *The Religion of Ancient Palestine in the Light of Archaeology*. London: British Academy.

Cooke, G. A. 1903. *A Text-Book of North-Semitic Inscriptions: Moabite, Hebrew, Phoenician, Aramaic, Nabataean, Palmyrene, Jewish*. Oxford: Clarendon.

———. 1907. The Assuan Papyri. *JTS* 8:615–24.

———. 1922. Epigraphical Notes. *JRAS* 54:270–73.

Coppens, J. 1955. Le messianisme sapiential et les origines littéraires du Fils de l'Homme daniélique. In *Wisdom in Israel and in the Ancient Near East: Presented to Professor Harold Henry Rowley*, ed. M. Noth and D. Winton Thomas, 33–41. VTSup 3. Leiden: Brill.

———. 1968. Review of *The Aramaic Inscriptions of Sefîre*, by J. A. Fitzmyer. *ETL* 44:244.

———. 1978. Le chapitre VII de Daniel: Lecture et commentaire. *ETL* 54:301–22.

Coppens, J., and L. Dequeker. 1961. Le Fils de l'homme et les saints du Très-Haut en Daniel, VII, dans les apocryphes et dans le Nouveau Testament. *Analecta Lovaniensia Biblica et Orientalia* series 3, 23:108.

Couroyer, B. 1952. L'origine égyptienne du mot 'Pâque'. *RB* 62:481–96.

———. 1954. Termes égyptiens dans les papyri araméens du Musée de Brooklyn. *RB* 61:554–59.

———. 1954a. Review of *The Brooklyn Museum Aramaic Papyri*, by E. G. Kraeling. *RB* 61:251–53, 592–95.

———. 1955. *Lḥn*: chantre? *VT* 5:83–88.

———. 1968. Le temple de Yaho et l'orientation dans les papyrus araméens d'Éléphantine. *RB* 75:80–85.

——. 1970. A propos de la stèle de Carpentras. *Sem* 20:17–21.

——. 1970a. Eléphantine. *RB* 77:463–65.

——. 1970b. Review of *Archives from Elephantine*, by B. Porten. *BO* 27:249–51.

——. 1973. Sapin vrai et sapin nouveau. *Or* 42:339–56.

——. 1973a. Review of *Documents araméens d'Egypte*, by P. Grelot. *RB* 80:465–69.

——. 1980. Nm'ty: Osiris ou "justifiés." *RB* 87:594–96.

——. 1988. *'Édut*: Stipulation de traité ou enseignement? *RB* 95:321–31.

Cowley, A. 1909. [no title]. In *The Palace of Apries (Memphis II)*, by W. M. F. Petrie and J. H. Walker, 12–13, pls. 13a, 14.(unseen). London.

——. 1915. The First Aramaic Inscription from India. *JRAS*: 342–47.

——. 1915a. Notes on the Two Ostraka Referred to Above. *PSBA* 37:221–23.

——. 1915b. Another Aramaic Papyrus of the Ptolemaic Age. *PSBA* 37:217–21.

——. 1919. *Jewish Documents of the Time of Ezra: Translated from the Aramaic*. London: Society for Promoting Christian Knowledge.

——. 1921. L'inscription bilingue araméo-lydienne de Sardes. *CRAIBL*: 7–14.

——. 1923. *Aramaic Papyri of the Fifth Century B. C: Edited with Translations and Notes*. Oxford: Clarendon. Reprint. Osnabrück: Zeller, 1967.
Reviews: E. L. Sukenik 1924: *JPOS* 4:211–14.

——. 1929. Two Aramaic Ostraka. *JRAS*: 107–12.

——. 1932. [Quoted report]. In *Beth Pelet II: Prehistoric Fara*, by E. MacDonald, J. L. Starkey and L. Harding, Publications of the British School of Archaeology in Egypt, vol. 52. London: British School of Archaeology in Egypt.

Cowley, A., and G. Buchanan Gray. 1903. Some Egyptian Aramaic Documents. *PSBA* 25:202–8, 259–66, 311–14 + pls.

Cowley, A. See also: A. H. Sayce.

Coxon, P. 1976. Daniel iii 17: A Linguistic and Theological Problem. *VT* 26:400–409.

——. 1977. The Problem of Nasalization in Biblical Aramaic in the Light of 1QGA. *RevQ* 9:253–58.

——. 1977a. A Philological Note on אשתיו Dan 5 3f. *ZAW* 89:275–76.

——. 1977b. The Syntax of the Aramaic of Daniel: A Dialectical Study. *HUCA* 48:107–22.

——. 1977–78. The Distribution of Synonyms in Biblical Aramaic in the Light of Official Aramaic and the Aramaic of Qumran. *RevQ* 9:497–512.

——. 1978. A Morphological Study of the *h*-Prefix in Biblical Aramaic. *JAOS* 98:416–19.

——. 1979. The Problem of Consonantal Mutations in Biblical Aramaic. *ZDMG* 129:8–22.

——. 1986. The "List" Genre and Narrative Style in the Court Tales of Daniel. *JSOT* 35:95–121.

Craig, J. A. 1893. The Panammu Inscription of the Zinjirli Collection. *The Academy* 43:351–52, 441.

Cremer, M. See: F. Altheim.

Cross, F. M. 1955. Geshem the Arabian, Enemy of Nehemiah. *BA* 18:46–47.

———. 1963. La découverte des papyrus de Samarie. *Nouvelles chrétiennes d'Israël* 14:27–37 + 5 figs.

———. 1963a. The Discovery of the Samaria Papyri. *BA* 26:110–21.

———. 1964. An Ostracon from Nebī Yūnis. *IEJ* 14:185–86, pl. 41/H.

———. 1966. An Aramaic Inscription from Daskyleion. *BASOR* 184:7–10.

———. 1966a. Aspects of Samaritan and Jewish History in Late Persian and Hellenistic Times. *HTR* 59:201–11.

———. 1968. Jar Inscriptions from Shiqmona. *IEJ* 18:226–33, pl. 25.

———. 1969. Judean Stamps. *EI (Albright Volume)* 9:20–27, pls. V/1–2.

———. 1969a. Papyri of the Fourth Century B.C. from Dâliyeh: A Preliminary Report on Their Discovery and Significance. In *New Directions in Biblical Archaeology*, ed. D. N. Freedman and J. C. Greenfield, 41–62. Garden City, N. Y.: Doubleday.

———. 1969b. Epigraphic Notes on the Ammān Citadel Inscription. *BASOR* 193:13–19.

———. 1969c. Two Notes on Palestinian Inscriptions of the Persian Age. *BASOR* 193:19–24.

———. 1972. The Stele Dedicated to Melcarth by Ben-Hadad of Damascus. *BASOR* 205:36–42 + 1 pl.

———. 1974. The Papyri and Their Historical Implications. In *Discoveries in the Wâdī ed-Dâliyeh*, ed. P. W. Lapp and N. L. Lapp, 17–29, 59–63. Annual of the American Schools of Oriental Resarch 41. Cambridge, Mass.: American Schools of Oriental Research.

———. 1978. The Historical Importance of the Samaria Papyri. *BARev* 4/1:25–27.

———. 1981. An Aramaic Ostracon of the Third Century B. C. E. from Excavations in Jerusalem. *EI (Aharoni Volume)* 15:67*–69* + 1 pl.

———. 1983. The Seal of Miqnêyaw. In *Ancient Seals and the Bible*, ed. L. Gorelick and E. Williams-Forte, 55–63. Malibu: Undena.

———. 1985. [Section VI: Discussion]. *BAT*, 367, 369.

———. 1985a. Samaria Payrus 1: An Aramaic Slave Conveyance of 335 B.C.E. Found in the Wâdi ed-Dâliyeh. *EI (Avigad Volume)* 18:7*–17*, pl. II.

———. 1986. A New Aramaic Stele from Taymā. *CBQ* 48:387–94.

———. 1988. A Report on the Samaria Papyri. In *Congress Volume, Jerusalem 1986*, ed. J. A. Emerton, 17–26, photo, p. 24. VTSup 40. Leiden: Brill.

Cross, F. M., and D. N. Freedman. 1952. *Early Hebrew Orthography: A Study of the Epigraphic Evidence*. AOS 36. New Haven, Conn.: American Oriental Society.

Cumont, F. 1905. Une inscription gréco-araméenne d'Asie Mineure. *CRAIBL*: 93–104.

Cunchillos, J. L. 1983. Une formule inédite de salutation en ugaritique: *b'l yš'ul šlmk* 'que Ba'al s'occupe de ton bien-être!' RS. 17.117. Ses parallèles akkadien, hébreu et araméen. *AO* 1:61–66.

Cunningham, A. 1961. *Inscriptions of Asoka*. Corpus Inscriptionum Indicarum 1. Varanasi, India: Indological Book House.

Cuny, A. 1920–21. L'inscription lydo-araméenne de Sardes. *Revue des études anciennes* 22:259–72; 23:1–27.

———. 1923. Étrusque et Lydien. *Revue des études anciennes* 25:97–112.

Cussini, E. 1986. Epigrafi aramaiche su tavolette dei secoli vi-v a.C.: Le collezioni europee. Bacalaureate thesis, dept. of Oriental Languages and Literature, Univ. of Venice.

Dahood, M. 1960. La regina del cielo in Geremia. *RivB* 8:166–68.

———. 1960a. Ugaritic *ṭat* and Isaia 5,18. *CBQ* 22:73–75.

———. 1960b. Textual Problems in Isaia. *CBQ* 22:400–409.

———. 1975. Isaiah 51,19 and Sefîre III 22. *Bib* 56:94–95.

———. 1976. Review of *La langue de Ya'udi*, by P.-E. Dion. *Or* 45:381–83.

Daiches, S. 1907. ‏כתבות ארמיות מימי עזרא‎. *Ha-Shiloah* 17:8–20, 504–22.

———. 1909. Zu den Elephantine-Papyri. *ZA* 22:197–99.

———. 1912. The Aramaic Ostracon from Elephantinê and the Festival of Passover. *PSBA* 34:17–23.

———. 1910. *The Jews in Babylonia in the Time of Ezra and Nehemiah according to Babylonian Inscriptions.* Jews' College London Publication no. 2. London: Jews' College.

———. 1929. Some Notes on Ostrakon A. *JRAS*: 584–85.

Dalley, S. 1979. [d]NIN.LÍL = Mul(l)is(s)u, the Treaty of Barga'yah and Herodotus' Mylitta. *RA* 73:177–78.

Dalman, G. 1920. Die Tobia-Inschrift von ʿarāk el-emīr und Daniel 11,14. *PJB* 16:33–35 + 1 pl.

Dalton, O. M. 1964. *The Treasure of the Oxus with Other Examples of Early Metal-Work.* 3rd ed. London: British Museum.

Dandamaev, M., and V. G. Lukonin. 1989. *The Culture and Social Institutions of Ancient Iran.* Trans. Philip L. Kohl with the assistance of D. J. Dadson on the basis of a revised version of Russian edition, 1980: *Kultura i ekonomika drevnego Irana.* Cambridge: Cambridge Univ. Press.

Daniels, P. T. 1981. Frustulum aramaicum. *Or* 50:193.

———. 1984. A Calligraphic Approach to Aramaic Paleography. *JNES* 43:55–68.

Danielsson, O. A. 1917. Zu den lydischen Inschriften. *Skrifter utgifna af Kungl. Humanistiska Vetenskaps-Samfundet i Uppsala* 20/2:3–43.
Reviews: G. Herbig 1921.

Dankwarth, G., and C. Müller. 1988. Zur altaramäischen "Altar"-Inschrift vom Tell Ḥalaf. *AfO* 35:73–78.

Darmesteter, J. 1888. L'inscription araméenne de Limyra. *JA* 8/12:508–10.

Davary, G. D. 1981. Epigraphische Forschungen in Afghanistan. *Studia iranica* 10:53–59.

Davary, G. D., and H. Humbach. 1974. *Eine weitere aramäoiranische Inschrift der Periode des Aśoka aus Afghanistan.* Abh. d. Wissenschaften und d. Literatur, Mainz 1. Mainz: Akademie der Wissenschaften und der Literatur; Wiesbaden: Steiner. Also published separately under the same title (Kabul, 1974).

Reviews: J. Oelsner 1977.

Davidson, B. 1848. *The Analytical Hebrew and Chaldee Lexicon*. London: Bagster.

Davies, G. I. 1986. Review of *The Balaam Text from Deir 'Alla*, by J. A. Hackett. *VT* 36:507–08.

———. 1991. Response to J. Greenfield and J. Hoftijzer. In *BTDAR*, 143–48.

Day, J. 1980. The Daniel of Ugarit and Ezekiel and the Hero of the Book of Daniel. *VT* 30:174–84.

Dayagi-Mendels, M. See: R. Hestrin.

De Clercq, L. 1903. *Collection De Clerq: Catalogue méthodique et raisonné. Tome II: Cachets, briques, bronzes, bas-reliefs*. Paris: E. Leroux.

De Geus, C. H. J. 1979–80. Idumaea. *JEOL* 26:53–74.

Dearman, J. A., and J. M. Miller. 1983. The Melqart Stele and the Ben Hadads of Damascus: Two Studies. *PEQ* 115:95–101.

Deblauwe, F. 1987. The Sculpture in the Round of the Principality of Guzana: A Bibliography of the Sculptures from the 1st mill. B.C., found at Tell Halaf, Tell Fekherye and Tell Herbe. *AION* 47:333–59.

Degen, R. 1967. Zur Schreibung des Kaška-Namens in ägyptischen, ugaritischen und altaramäischen Quellen: Kritische Anmerkungen zu einer Monographie über die Kaškäer. [Review article: E. von Schuler, *Die Kaškäer. Ein Beitrag zur Ethnographie des alten Kleinasien*.] *WO* 4:48–60.

———. 1967–68. עדדן. *Leš* 32:409–11.

———. 1968–69. Review of *Die lexikalischen und grammatikalischen Aramaismen im alttestamentlichen Hebräisch*, by M. Wagner. *Oriens* 21–22:386–91.

———. 1969. *Altaramäische Grammatik der Inschriften des 10.–8. Jh. v. Chr.* Abh. f. d. Kunde d. Morgenlandes 38/3. Wiesbaden: F. Steiner.
Reviews: K. Beyer 1970a; H. Donner 1970; J. A. Fitzmyer 1970; G. Garbini 1970; E. Puech 1975.

———. 1969a. Die Präfixkonjugationen des Altaramäischen. In *XVII. deutscher Orientalistentag . . . Vorträge, Teil 2*, ed. W. Voigt, 701–6. *ZDMG* Supplement 1. Wiesbaden: Steiner.

———. 1969–70. הכתובת הארמית מטקסילה. *Leš* 34:314–17.

———. 1970. Aramäischer Einfluss bei der Bildung der altpersischen Relativ Pronomina? *Zeitschrift für vergleichende Sprachforschung* 84:202–6.

———. 1972. Der Räucheraltar aus Lachisch. *NESE* 1:39–48, pl. III.

———. 1972a. Zum Ostrakon CIS II 138. *NESE* 1:23–37.

———. 1972b. Ein neuer aramäischer Papyrus aus Elephantine: P. Berol. 23 000. *NESE* 1:9–22.

———. 1972c. Die aramäischen Tontafeln von Tell Halaf. *NESE* 1:49–57.

———. 1974. Ein Fragment des bisher ältesten aramäischen Papyrus. *NESE* 2:65–70 + 1 pl.

———. 1974a. Die aramäischen Inschriften aus Ṭaimā' und Umgebung. *NESE* 2:79–98.

———. 1974b. Neue Fragmente aramäischer Papyri aus Elephantine I. *NESE* 2:71–78.

————. 1974c. Review of *Aramaic Ritual Texts from Persepolis*, by R. Bowman. *BO* 31:124–27.

————. 1975. Eine neues Wörterbuch für das Biblisch-Aramäische. *Or* 44:116–25.

————. 1977. Review of *On Pseudo-Corrections in Some Semitic Languages*, by J. Blau. *OLZ* 72:384–86.

————. 1978. Die Zahlwörter in CIS II 2 und 3. *NESE* 3:11–14.

————. 1978a. Ein aramäisches Alphabet vom Tell Halaf. *NESE* 3:1–9 + drawing.

————. 1978b. Die aramäischen Ostraka in der Papyrus-Sammlung der österreichischen Nationalbibliothek. *NESE* 3:33–57.

————. 1978c. Neue Fragmente aramäischer Papyri aus Elephantine II. *NESE* 3:15–31.

————. 1978d. Zu den aramäischen Texten aus Edfu. *NESE* 3:59–66.

————. 1979. Review of *Altaramäische Grammatik*, by S. Segert. *GGA* 231:8–51.

Degen, R., W. W. Müller, and W. Röllig, eds. 1972, 1974, 1978. *Neue Ephemeris für semitische Epigraphik*. 3 vols. Wiesbaden: Harrassowitz.

Deist, F. E. 1970. "Van die duisternis tot sy merkwaardige lig" (1 Petr. 2:9) in die lig van Elephantine ["Out of the darkness into His marvelous light" in the light of Elephantine]. *Nederduitse gereformeerde teologiese Tydskrif* 11:44–48.

————. 1971. The Punishment of the Disobedient Zedekiah. *JNSL* 1:71–72.

Delaporte, L. 1910. *Catalogue des cylindres orientaux et des cachets assyro-babyloniens, perses et syro-cappadociens de la Bibliothèque Nationale*. Paris: E. Leroux.

————. 1912. *Épigraphes araméens: Étude des textes araméens gravés ou écrits sur des tablettes cunéiformes*. Paris: Geuthner.
Reviews: T. H. Pinches 1914: *JRAS*: 207; S. Schiffer 1914.

————. 1920–23. *Catalogue des cylindres, cachets et pierres gravées de style oriental*. 2 vols. Paris: Hachette.

————. 1928. Cachets orientaux de la collection de Luynes. *Aréthuse* 5:41–65; pls. VI–X.

Delaunay, J. A. 1974. A propos des "Aramaic Ritual Texts from Persepolis" de R. A. Bowman. In *Commémoration Cyrus: Actes du Congrès de Shiraz 1971 et autres études rédigées à l'occasion du 2500e anniversaire de la fondation de l'empire perse, Hommage universel, II*, 193–217. Acta Iranica 1/2. Leiden: Brill.

————. 1974a. L'araméen d'empire et les débuts de l'écriture en Asie centrale. In *Commémoration Cyrus: Actes du Congrès de Shiraz 1971 et autres études rédigées à l'occasion du 2500e anniversaire de la fondation de l'empire perse, Hommage universel, II*, 219–36, pls. iv–xv. Acta Iranica 1/2. Leiden: Brill.

————. 1976. Remarques sur quelques noms de personne des archives élamites de Persepolis. *Studia iranica* 5:9–31.

Delavault, B. See: A. Lemaire.

Delcor, M. 1966. Les attaches littéraires, l'origine et la signification de l'expression biblique "Prendre à témoin le ciel et la terre." *VT* 16:8–25.

————. 1967. Une inscription funéraire araméenne trouvée à Daskyleion en Turquie. *Le Muséon* 80:301–14 + 2 pls.

———. 1968. Review of *The Aramaic Inscriptions of Sefîre*, by J. A. Fitzmyer. *BO* 25:379–80.

———. 1971. *Le livre de Daniel*. SB. Paris: Gabalda.

———. 1981. Le texte de Deir 'Alla et les oracles bibliques de Bala'am. In *Congress Volume: Vienna 1980*, ed. J. A. Emerton, 52–73. VTSup 32. Leiden: Brill.

———. 1982. Bala'am pâtôrâh, "interprète de songes" au pays d'Ammon, d'après Num 22,5: Les témoignages épigraphiques parallèles. *Sem* 32:89–91.

Delitzsch, F. 1900. Eine aramäische Inschrift aus Babylon. MDOG 6:3.

Deller, K. 1965. Aramäische Personennamen aus Sultantepe. *Or* 34:473–76.

Delsman, W. C. 1983. Aramäische Dokumente. In *Rechts- und Wirtschaftsurkunden: Historisch-chronologische Texte*, ed. O. Kaiser, 253–63. TUAT 1. Gütersloh: G. Mohn.

———. 1985. Aramäische historische Inschriften. In *Rechts- und Wirtschaftsurkunden: Historisch-chronologische Texte*, ed. O. Kaiser, 625–37. TUAT 1. Gütersloh: G. Mohn.

———. 1988. Eine aramäische Beschwörung. In *Religiöse Texte*, ed. O. Kaiser, 432–34. TUAT 2. Gütersloh: G. Mohn.

———. 1988. Aramäische Grab- und Votivinschriften. In *Religiöse Texte*, ed. O. Kaiser, 573–81. TUAT 2. Gütersloh: G. Mohn.

Denis, A.-M. 1969–70. L'étude des pseudépigraphes: État actuel des instruments de travail. *NTS* 16:348–53.

———. 1970. Les fragments grecs de l'histoire et des maximes d'Aḥiqar. In *Introduction aux pseudépigraphes grecs d'Ancien Testament*, 201–14. Studia in Veteris Testamenti pseudepigrapha, vol. 1. Leiden: Brill.

Dequeker, L. See: J. Coppens.

Derenbourg, H. 1893. Pînamou, fils de Karîl. *REJ* 26:135–38.

Derenbourg, J. 1867. Sur l'inscription de l''Araq-el-émir: Lettre à M. de Saulcy. *JA* 6/10:188–93.

———. 1868. Notes épigraphiques. V. L'inscription dite de Carpentras. *JA* 6/11:277–87.

Desnoyers, L. 1907. Papyrus juifs araméens du Ve siècle avant Jésus Christ. *BLE* 3/9:138–48, 176–85.

———. 1908. Les nouveaux papyrus araméens d'Éléphantine. *BLE* 3/10:235–46.

Dhorme, P. 1908. Les pays bibliques au temps d'El-Amarna. *RB* 5:500–519.

———. 1911. 'Melanges': II. Le dieu de Zakir. *RA* 8:97–98.

———. 1928. Les tablettes babyloniennes de Nerab. *JPOS* 8:122–24.

———. 1928a. Les tablettes babyloniennes de Neirab. *RA* 25:53–82.

Di Lella, A. A. 1977. The One in Human Likeness and the Holy Ones of the Most High in Daniel 7. *CBQ* 39:1–19.

———. 1981. Daniel 4: 7–14: Poetic Analysis and Biblical Background. In *Mélanges bibliques et orientaux en l'honneur de M. Henri Cazelles*, ed. A. Caquot and M. Delcor, 247–58. AOAT 212.

———. 1982. Strophic Structure and Poetic Analysis of Daniel 2: 20–23; 3: 31–33 and 6: 26b–28. In *Studia hierosolymitana III: Nell' ottavo centenario francescano (1182–1982)*, ed. G. C. Bottini, 91–96. Studii biblici franciscani coll. maior, vol. 30. Jerusalem: Franciscan.

———. See also: L. F. Hartman.

Díaz Esteban, F. 1962. Una fórmula de cortesía epistolar de Ugarit, repetida en una carta judeo-aramea del siglo V. a. C. *Sef* 22:101–2.

Diem, W. 1982. Die Entwicklung des Derivationsmorphems der t-Stämme im Semitischen. *ZDMG* 132:29–84.

———. 1986. Alienable und Inalienable Possession im Semitischen. *ZDMG* 136:227–91.

Dietrich, M. 1963–65. Historia de Āḥīqār . *EncBib*, 264–66.

———. 1970. *Die Aramäer Südbabyloniens in der Sargonidenzeit (700–648).* AOAT 7.

Díez Macho, A. 1965. Persia, Inscripciones arameas de. *EncBib* 5:1057–61.

Díez Merino, L. 1982. Il vocabolario relativo alla "ricerca de Dio" nell'Antico Testamento. *BeO* 24:129–45.

———. 1982a. Il vocabolario relativo alla ricerca di Dio nell'Antico Testamento: La radice *šʾl. BeO* 24:207–18.

———. 1983. Il vocabolario relativo alla "ricerca di Dio" nell'Antico Testamento: La radice *šḥr. BeO* 25:35–38.

———. 1984. El sintagma *nš ʿynym* en la tradición aramaea. *AO* 2:23–41.

———. 1988. Diacronía de la partícula aramea *yât. RevQ (Mémorial Jean Carmignac)* 13:497–512.

Dijkema, F. 1931. De Tempel te Elefantine en de zoogenaamde Centralisatie van den Eeredienst te Jeruzalem. *Nieuw theologisch tijdschrift* 20:321–33.

Dijkstra, M. 1991. Response to E. Puech and Dr. G. van der Kooij. In *BTDAR*, 263–70.

Dion, P.-E. 1974. *La langue de Ya'udi: Description et classement de l'ancien parler de Zencirli dans le cadre des langues sémitiques du nord-ouest.* Editions SR 1. Waterloo: Corporation for the Publication of Academic Studies in Religion in Canada.
Reviews: M. G. Amadasi Guzzo 1979; A. Caquot 1977; M. Dahood 1976; J. A. Fitzmyer 1976; G. Fohrer 1975; G. Garbini 1976; O. Klíma 1979; E. Lipinski 1976; J. Oelsner 1980; E. Puech 1977, 1977a; W. Röllig 1977; F. Rosenthal 1976; D. Snell 1976; P. Swiggers 1981.

———. 1974a. Une inscription araméenne en style *awilum ša* et quelques textes bibliques datant de l'exil. *Bib* 55:399–403.

———. 1977. A Tentative Classification of Aramaic Letter Types. *SBL Seminar Papers* 11:415–41.

———. 1978. The Language Spoken in Ancient Samal. *JNES* 37:115–18.

———. 1979. Les types épistolaires hébréo-araméens jusqu'au temps de Bar Kokhbah. *RB* 86:544–79.

———. 1982. The Aramaic "Family Letter" and Related Epistolary Forms in Other Oriental Languages and in Hellenistic Greek. In *Studies in Ancient Letter Writing*, ed. J. L. White, 59–76. Semeia 22. Chico, Cal.: Scholars Press.

———. 1982a. Aramaic Words for "Letter." In *Studies in Ancient Letter Writing*, ed. J. L. White, 77–88. Semeia 22. Chico, Cal.: Scholars Press.

———. 1982b. La lettre araméenne passe-partout et ses sous-espèces. *RB* 89:528–75.

———. 1982c.   Image et ressemblance en araméen ancien (Tell Fakhariyah). *Science et esprit* 34:151–53.

———. 1983.   סס נורי and ששבצר. *ZAW* 95:111–12.

———. 1983a.   Review of *The Aramaic Proverbs of Ahiqar,* by J. M. Lindenberger. *SR* 12:342–44.

———. 1984.   Un nouvel éclairage sur le contexte culturel des malheurs de Job. *VT* 34:213–15.

———. 1985.   La bilingue de Tell Fekherye: Le roi de Gozan et son dieu: la phraséologie. In *Mélanges bibliques et orientaux en l'honneur de M. Mathias Delcor*, ed. A. Caquot et al., 139–47. AOAT 215.

———. 1986.   Review of *Les inscriptions araméenes de Sfiré et l'Assyrie de Shamshi-ilu,* by A. Lemaire and J.-M. Durand. *JBL* 105:510–12.

———. 1987.   Formulaic Language in the Book of Job: International Background and Ironical Distortion. *Studies in Religion / Sciences religieuses* 16:187–93.

———. 1988.   Review of *Ancient Damascus,* by W. T. Pitard. *BASOR* 270:97–100.

———. 1989.   Review of *Catalogue des sceaux ouest-sémitiques inscrits,* by P. Bordreuil. *BASOR* 275:74–77.

———. 1989a.   Medical Personnel in the Ancient Near East. *asû* and *āšipu* in Aramaic Garb. *ARAM* 1:206–16.

Dion, P.-E., and D. Fraikin. 1985.   Ressemblance et image de Dieu. In *Dictionnaire de la Bible: Supplément*, ed. L. Pirot, 10.365–414. Paris: Letouzey et Ané.

Diringer, D. 1934.   *Le iscrizioni antico-ebraiche palestinesi.* Florence: Felice le Monnier.

———. 1937.   *L'alfabeto nella storia della civiltà.* Florence: G. Barbèra.

———. 1950.   Three Early Hebrew Seals. *ArOr* 18/3:65–69; pl. 1.

———. 1955.   Review of *Aramaic Documents of the Fifth Century B.C.,* by G. R. Driver. *PEQ*:95–96.

Diringer, D., with the assistance of R. Regensburger. 1968.   *The Alphabet: A Key to the History of Mankind.* 2 vols. 3rd rev. edition. New York: Funk & Wagnalls.

Dix, G. H. 1925.   The Influence of Babylonian Ideas on Jewish Messianism. *JTS* 26:241–56.

Dodi, A. 1989.   Pausal Forms in Aramaic. In *Studies in the Hebrew Language and the Talmudic Literature, Dedicated to the Memory of Dr. Menahem Moreshet,* ed. M. Z. Kaddari and S. Sharvit, 63–74. Ramat Gan: Bar-Ilan Univ. Press.

Dohmen, C. 1983.   Die Statue von Tell Fechrīje und die Gottesebenbildlichkeit des Menschen: Ein Beitrag zur Bilderterminologie. *BN* 22:91–106.

Döller, J. 1907.   Der Papyrusfund von Assuan. *TQ* 89:497–507.

———. 1908.   Drei neue aramäische Papyri. *TQ* 90:376–84.

Dolunay, N. 1967.   Reliefs Discovered at Dascyleion (Ergili). *Annual of the Archaeological Museums of Istanbul* 13–14:97–111.

Dombrowski, B. W. W. 1984.   *Der Name* Europa *auf seinem griechischen und altsyrischen Hintergrund: Ein Beitrag zur ostmediterranen Kultur- und Religionsgeschichte in frühgriechischen Zeit.* Amsterdam: Hakkert.

Donner, H. 1955. Ein Orthostatenfragment des Königs Barrakab von Sam'al. MIO 3:73–98.

———. 1957. Neue Quellen zur Geschichte des Staates Moab in der zweiten Hälfte des 8. Jahrh. v. Chr. MIO 5:155–84.

———. 1957–58. Zur Inschrift von Südschīn Aa 9. *AfO* 18:390–92.

———. 1962. Zu Gen 28,22. *ZAW* 74:68–70.

———. 1963. Review of *A Grammar of Biblical Aramaic*, by F. Rosenthal. *OLZ* 58:358–62.

———. 1968. Elemente ägyptischen Totenglaubens bei den Aramäern Ägyptens. In *Religions en Egypte hellénistique et romaine. Colloque de Strasbourg—1967*, ed. P. Derchain, 35–44. Paris: Presses Universitaires de France.

———. 1968a. Review of *An Aramaic Handbook I-II*, ed. F. Rosenthal. *BO* 25:377–78.

———. 1970. Review of *Altaramäische Grammatik der Inschriften des 10.–8. Jh. v. Chr.*, by R. Degen. *BO* 27:246–49.

———. 1970a. Adadnirari III. und die Vasallen des Westens. In *Archäologie und Altes Testament: Festschrift für Kurt Galling zum 8. Januar 1970*, ed. A. Kuschke and E. Kutsch, 49–59. Tübingen: J. C. B. Mohr.

———. 1971. Bemerkungen zum Verständnis zweier aramäischer Briefe aus Hermopolis. In *Near Eastern Studies in Honor of William Foxwell Albright*, ed. H. Goedicke, 75–85. Baltimore: Johns Hopkins Univ. Press.

———. 1973. Aramäische Lexikographie. In *Studies on Semitic Lexicography*, ed. P. Fronzaroli, 127–43. Quaderni di Semitistica 2. Florence: Istituto di linguistica e di lingue orientali.

Donner, H., and W. Röllig. 1962, 1964. *Kanaanäische und aramäische Inschriften (Mit einem Beitrag von O. Rössler): Band I, Texte; Band II, Kommentar; Band III, Glossar und Indizes*. Wiesbaden: Harassowitz. 3rd rev. ed., 1971–73.
Reviews: J. Körner 1977; S. Segert: *ArOr* 41:223–25.

Dossin, G. 1930. Une inscription cunéiforme de Haute Syrie. *RA* 27:85–92.

———. 1932. Sur un proverbe araméen de la Sagesse d'Aḥiqar. *RA* 29:123–29.

———. 1944. BRG'YH, roi de KTK. *Le Muséon* 57:147–55.

———. See also: F. Thureau-Dangin.

Dothan, M. See: B. Mazar.

Dothan, T. See: B. Mazar.

Dougherty, R. P. 1929. *Nabonidus and Belshazzar: A Study of the Closing Events of the Neo-Babylonian Empire*. Yale Oriental Series. Researches, vol. 15. New Haven: Yale Univ. Reprint 1980. New York: AMS.

Doughty, C. 1888. *Travels in Arabia Deserta*. 2 vols. Cambridge: Cambridge Univ. Press.

———. 1891. *Documents épigraphiques recueillis dans le nord de l'Arabie*. Paris: Imprimerie Nationale.

Dresden, M. J. 1971. Middle Iranian. In *Linguistics in South West Asia and North Africa*, ed. T. Sebeok, 26–63. Current Trends in Linguistics, vol. 6. Paris: Mouton.

Dressler, H. H. P. 1979. The Identification of the Ugaritic Dnil with the Daniel of Ezekiel. *VT* 29:152–61.

Drijvers, H. J. W. 1971. Review of *Aramaic Ritual Texts from Persepolis*, by R. A. Bowman. *NedTT* 25:332.

———. 1973. Syriac and Aramaic. In *A Basic Bibliography for the Study of the Semitic Languages*, ed. J. H. Hospers, 283–335. Leiden: Brill.

———. 1973a. Review of *Die aramäische Inschrift von Taxila*, by H. Humbach. *BO* 30:466–67.

Driver, G. R. 1926. An Aramaic Inscription in the Cuneiform Script. *AfO* 3:47–53.

———. 1926a. The Aramaic of the Book of Daniel. *JBL* 45:110–119.

———. 1932. The Aramaic *Papyri* from Egypt: Notes on Obscure Passages. *JRAS*: 77–90.

———. 1932–33. Notes on the Aramaic Inscription from Soudschin. *AfO* 8:203–6.

———. 1935. Problems in Aramaic and Hebrew Texts. In *Miscellanea orientalia dedicata Antonio Deimel*, 46–70. AnOr 12. Rome: Pontifical Biblical Institute.

———. 1937. A Babylonian Tablet With an Aramaic Endorsement. *Iraq* 4:16–18.

———. 1938. Old and New Semitic Texts. *PEQ*: 188–92, pl. XIV.

———. 1939. New Aramaeo-Jewish Names in Egypt. *JEA* 25:175–76.

———. 1945. Brief Notes. *PEQ*: 5–14 + 1 pl.

———. 1948. *Semitic Writing*. The Schweich Lectures of the British Academy. 3rd rev. ed., 1976. London: Oxford Univ. Press.

———. 1949. New Aramaic Documents on Leather. In *Actes du XXIe Congrès International des Orientalistes* 108. Paris: Société Asiatique.

———. 1954. *Aramaic Documents of the Fifth Century B.C., Transcribed and Edited With Translation and Notes*. Oxford: Clarendon.
Reviews: D. Diringer 1955; T. Jansma 1954: *BO* 11:214–15; J. Lewy 1955; J. T. Milik 1954.

———. 1955. Corrections. *Syria* 32:99–100.

———. 1955a. Review of *The Brooklyn Museum Aramaic Papyri*, by E. G. Kraeling. *PEQ*:91–94.

———. 1955b. Hebrew Seals. *PEQ*:183.

———. 1957. *Aramaic Documents of the Fifth Century B.C: Abridged and Revised Edition*. Oxford: Clarendon.
Reviews: T. Jansma 1958: *BO* 15:46; O. Eissfeldt 1958.

———. 1957a. Aramaic Names in Accadian Texts. *RSO* 32:41–57.

Driver, S. R. 1890. *Notes on the Hebrew Text of the Books of Samuel*. Oxford: Clarendon. 2nd ed. 1913.

———. 1900. *The Book of Daniel*. The Cambridge Bible for Schools and Colleges. Cambridge: Cambridge Univ. Press.

———. 1908. An Aramaic Inscription from Syria. *Expositor* 7/5:481–90.

———. 1929. *An Introduction to the Literature of the Old Testament*. 9th ed. Edinburgh: Clark.

Drouin, E. 1889. La numismatique araméene sous les Arsacides et en Mésopotamie. *JA* 8/13:376–401.

Dubberstein, W. H. See: G. R. Hughes.

Dumbrell, W. J. 1971. The Tell el-Maskhuṭa Bowls and the "Kingdom" of Qedar in the Persian Period. *BASOR* 203:33–44.

Dumm, D. R. 1967. Ahikar (Achior). In *New Catholic Encyclopedia*, ed. W. J. McDonald et al., 1:222–23. New York: McGraw-Hill.

Dunand, M. 1939. Stèle araméenne dédiée à Melqart. *BMB* 3:65–76, pl. XIII.

———. 1942–43. A propos de la stèle de Melqart du Musée d'Alep. *BMB* 6:41–45.

———. See also: F. Thureau-Dangin.

Dunayevsky, I. See: B. Mazar.

Dupont-Sommer, A. 1941–45. Un ostracon araméen inédit d'Éléphantine adressé à Aḥuṭab. *Revue des études sémitiques*: 65–75.

———. 1942–44. La tablette cunéiforme araméenne de Warka. *RA* 39:35–62.

———. 1943. Séance du 22 octobre. *CRAIBL*: 465–66.

———. 1943–45. La tablette cunéiforme araméenne de Warka. *JA* 234:455.

———. 1944. Un contrat de métayage égypto-araméen de l'an 7 de Darius I. *MPAIBL* 14/2:51–106.

———. 1944a. 'Bêl et Nabû, Šamaš et Nergal' sur un ostracon araméen inédit d'Eléphantine. *RHR* 128:28–39.

———. 1944–45. L'ostracon araméen d'Assour. *Syria* 24:24–61.

———. 1945. Séance du 1er Juin. *CRAIBL*: 260–62.

———. 1945a. Un texte araméen d'époque perse en écriture démotique. *RHR* 129:183–84.

———. 1945b. Le syncrétisme religieux des Juifs d'Eléphantine d'après un ostracon araméen inédit. *RHR* 130:17–28.

———. 1945–46. Un ostracon araméen inédit de Larsa. *RA* 40:143–47.

———. 1946–47. Séance du 14 mars 1947. *JA* 235:190–91.

———. 1946–47a. 'Maison de Yahvé' et vêtements sacrés à Eléphantine d'après un ostracon araméen du Musée du Caire. *JA* 235:79–87.

———. 1946–47b. Sur la fête de la Pâque dans les documents araméens d'Eléphantine. *REJ* 107:39–51.

———. 1947. Une inscription araméenne inédite de l'Ouâdi Ḥammâmât. *RA* 41:105–10.

———. 1947a. 'Yahô' et 'Yahô-Ṣeba'ôt' sur des ostraca araméens inédits d'Eléphantine. *CRAIBL*: 175–91.

———. 1948. Ostraca araméens d'Eléphantine (Clermont-Ganneau 16; *CIS* II. 137). *ASAE* 48:109–33.

———. 1948a. Une inscription nouvelle du roi Kilamou et le dieu Rekoub-el. *RHR* 133:19–33.

———. 1948b. Un papyrus araméen d'époque saïte découvert à Saqqarah. *Sem* 1:43–68.

———. 1949. La collection des ostraca araméens recueillis par Clermont-Ganneau à Eléphantine. In *Actes du XXIe Congrès Internationale des Orientalistes* 109–111. Paris: Société Asiatique.

———. 1949a. *Les Araméens*. L'Orient ancien illustré. Paris: Maisonneuve.

———. 1949b. L'ostracon araméen du Sabbat (Clermont-Ganneau 152). *Sem* 2:29–39.

———. 1950–51. Deux nouvelles inscriptions sémitiques trouvées en Cilicie. *JfKF* 1:43–47, pl. IV.

———. 1950–51a. Fragment d'inscription araméenne découvert à Bahadirli (Cilicie). *JfKF* 1:108, pl. IV/5.

———. 1953. Aramaic Inscription on an Altar. In *Lachish III: The Iron Age*, ed. O. Tufnell, 1.226, 1.358–59, pls. 2.49/3, 2.68/1. Wellcome-Marston Archaeological Research Expedition to the Near East 3. London: Oxford Univ. Press.

———. 1953b. Les autels à encens de Lakish. *Annuaire de l'Institut de philologie et d'histoire orientales et slaves (Mélanges Isidore Lévy)* 13:135–52.

———. 1954. Sur les débuts de l'histoire araméenne. In *Congress Volume Copenhagen 1953*, 40–49. VTSup 1. Leiden: Brill.

———. 1956. Une stèle araméenne d'un prêtre de Ba'al trouvée en Egypte. *Syria* 33:79–87.

———. 1957. Un ostracon araméen inédit d'Eléphantine (Collection Clermont-Ganneau n° 186). In *Scritti in onore di Giuseppe Furlani*, 403–9. RSO 32. Rome: G. Bardi.

———. 1957a. Une stèle araméenne inédite de Sfiré (Syrie) du VIIIe siècle avant J.-C. *CRAIBL*: 245–48.

———. 1958. Un traité araméen du VIII siècle av. J.-C. *CRAIBL*: 177–82.

———. 1959. Une stèle araméenne inédite de Sfiré (Syrie), du VIIIe siècle avant J.-C. In *Akten des vierundzwanzigsten Internationalen Orientalisten-Kongresses München—28. August bis 4. September 1957*, ed. H. Franke, 238–41. Wiesbaden: Deutsche Morgenländische Gesellschaft.

———. 1959a. Une inscription nouvelle en grec et en araméen du roi Asoka. *RHR* 155:136–38.

———. 1960. Une inscription gréco-araméenne du roi Asoka récemment découverte en Afghanistan. In *Proceedings of the IXth International Congress for the History of Religions: Tokyo and Kyoto, 1958*, 617–23. Tokyo: Maruzen.

———. 1960a. Sabbat et Parascève à Eléphantine d'après des ostraca araméens inédits. *MPAIBL* 15:67–88.

———. 1960b. Trois stèles araméennes provenant de Sfiré: un traité de vassalité du VIIIe siècle avant J.-C. *AASyr* 10:21–54, pls. I–X.

———. 1961. Une inscription araméenne inédite de Cilicie et la déesse Kubaba. *CRAIBL*: 19–23, pl. p. 20.

———. 1962. Sur la déesse Kubaba, à propos d'une inscription araméenne récemment découverte en Cilicie. In *Proceedings of the 25th International Congress of Orientalists, Moscow, 9–16 August 1960, Vol. 1, 336–37. Moscow: Izdatel'stvo Vostochnoi Literatury*.

———. 1963. Un ostracon araméen inédit d'Eléphantine (Collection Clermont-Ganneau N° 44). In *Hebrew and Semitic Studies: Presented to Godfrey Rolles Driver*, ed. D. Winton Thomas and W. D. McHardy, 53–58 + 1 pl. Oxford: Clarendon.

———. 1964. Note sur le mot TQM dans les ostraca araméens d'Éléphantine. *Sem* 14:71–72.

———. 1964a.   Trois inscriptions araméennes inédites sur des bronzes de Luristan: Collection de M. Foroughi. *Iranica antiqua* 4:109–18, pls. XXXIII-XXXVII.

———. 1965.   Une inscription araméene inédite de Bahadirli (Cilicie). *Anadolu Araştirmalari* II:200–209, pls. XX–XXI.

———. 1966.   L'inscription araméenne de Daskyleion. *Annual of the Archaeological Museums of Istanbul* 13–14:112–17, pl. VII/15.

———. 1966a.   Une inscription araméenne inédite d'époque perse trouvée à Daskyléion (Turquie). *CRAIBL*: 44–57.

———. 1966b.   Une nouvelle inscription araméenne d'Asoka découverte à Kandahar (Afghanistan). *CRAIBL*: 440–51.

———. 1967.   Observations sur les papyrus araméens d'époque perse provenant d'Hermopolis. *CRAIBL*: 302–4.

———. 1970.   Une nouvelle inscription araméenne d'Asoka trouvée dans la vallée du Laghman (Afghanistan). *CRAIBL*: 158–73.

———. 1974.   La stèle trilingue récemment découverte au Lêtôon de Xanthos: Le texte araméen. *CRAIBL*: 132–49.

———. 1979.   L'inscription araméenne. In *Fouilles de Xanthos, Tome VI: La stèle trilingue de Létôon*, ed. H. Metzger, 129–78, pls. XVI–XXIII. Institut français d'études anatoliennes. Paris: C. Klincksieck.
Reviews: R. Contini 1981; P. Frei 1981.

———. 1979a.   Note sur le fragment araméen A (No. 5627) découvert dans le Létôon de Xanthos. *Sem* 29:101–3.

Dupont-Sommer, A., and J. Starcky. 1956 [appeared 1958].   Une inscription araméenne inédite de Sfiré. *BMB* 13:23–41, pls. I–VI.
Reviews: P. Mouterde 1958.

———. 1960 [appeared 1958].   *Les inscriptions araméennes de Sfiré (stèles I et II)*. MPAIBL 15, 197–351. Paris: Imprimerie Nationale.
Reviews: J. J. Koopmans 1960; D. Winton Thomas 1960.

Dupont-Sommer, A., and L. Robert. 1964.   Une inscription araméenne et la déesse Kubaba. In *La déesse de Hiérapolis Castabala (Cilicie)* 7–15, pls. I–II. Bibliothèque archéologique et historique de l'Institut Français d'archéologie d'Istanbul 16. Paris: Maisonneuve.
Review: G. Ryckmans 1965.

Dupont-Sommer, A. See also: E. Benveniste, D. Schlumberger.

Durand, J.-M. See: A. Lemaire.

Durand, M. See: F. Thureau-Dangin.

Dussaud, R. 1908.   Le royaume de Hamat et de Lou'ouch au VIIIᵉ siècle avant J.-C. *RArch* IVᵉ ser. 11:222–35.

———. 1911.   Les papyrus judéo-araméens d'Éléphantine publiés par M. Sachau. [Review article: E. Sachau, *Aramäische Papyrus und Ostraka aus einer jüdischen Militärkolonie zu Elephantine*.] *RHR* 64:343–53.

———. 1922.   La stèle araméenne de Zakir au Musée du Louvre. *Syria* 3:175–76.

————. 1927. *Topographie historique de la Syrie antique et médiévale*. Paris: Geuthner.

————. 1928. Torse de statuette de Sefiré. *Syria* 9:170–71.

————. 1930. Séance du 20 juin. *CRAIBL*: 155–58.

————. 1931. Nouvelles inscriptions araméennes de Sefiré, près d'Alep. *CRAIBL*: 312–21.

————. 1932. Inscriptions araméennes de Sefiré (Soudjin). *Syria* 13:401–2.

————. 1932a. Review of *Arslan Tash*, by F. Thureau-Dangin, et al. *Syria* 13:388–90.

————. 1934. Découverte de tablettes à Persépolis. *Syria* 15:298.

————. 1945. Séance du 23 mars. *CRAIBL*: 173–76.

————. 1949. Yahô chez les Juifs d'Éléphantine. [Review article: A. Dupont-Sommer, *'Yahô' et 'Yahô-Seba'ôt' sur des ostraca araméens inédits d'Eléphantine*.] *Syria* 26:390–91.

————. 1949a. Un papyrus araméen d'epoche saïte découvert à Saqqarah, dans *Semitica*, I (1948), p. 43–68 avec une planche. *Syria* 26:152–53.

————. 1949b. Anciens bronzes du Louristan et cultes iraniens. *Syria* 26:196–229.

————. 1950. Un nouveau lot de papyrus judéo-araméens d'Éléphantine. *Syria* 27:200.

Duval, R. 1884. Le passif dans l'araméen biblique et la palmyrénien. *REJ* 8:57–63.

————. 1888. La Dîme à Teima. *RA* 2:1–3.

Ebeling, E. 1913. אלוד=i-lu-mi-ir. *OLZ* 16:254.

————. 1925. *Ein Beschwörungstext in aramäisch-akkadischer Mischsprache*. Berliner Beiträge zur Keilschriftforschung II/2. Berlin: Erich Ebeling.

————. 1972. *Das aramäisch-mittelpersische Glossar Frahang-i-pahlavik im Lichte der assyriologischen Forschung*. MAOG 14/1. Osnabrück: Zeller.

Eberharter, A. 1912–13. Die aramäischen Schriftdenkmäler aus Elefantine und ihre Bedeutung für die alttestamentliche Wissenschaft. *Theologisch-praktische Monatsschrift* 23:265–75.

Edzard, D. O. 1964. Mari und Aramäer? *ZA* 56:142–49.

Eerdmans, B. D. 1908. Een nieuwe Jahwe-Tempel. *Theologisch Tijdschrift* 42:72–81.

————. 1932. Origin and Meaning of the Aramaic Part of Daniel. In *Actes du XVIIIe Congrès International des Orientalistes*, 198–202. Leiden: Brill.

Eggermont, P. H. L. 1956. *The Chronology of the Reign of Aśoka Morya: A Comparison of the Data of the Asoka Inscriptions and the Data of the Tradition*. Leiden: Brill.

————. 1959. Review of *Un editto bilingue greco-aramaico di Aśoka*, by G. Pugliese-Carratelli, et al. *BO* 16:159–60.

————. 1965–66. New Notes on Aśoka and His Successors. *Persica* 2:27–70.

————. 1969. New Notes on Aśoka and His Successors, II. *Persica* 4:77–120.

Eggermont, P. H. L., and J. Hoftijzer. 1962. The Greco-Aramaic Inscription of Kandahar. In *The Moral Edicts of King Aśoka* 42–46. Textus Minores 29. Leiden: Brill.

Ehrlich, A. B. 1914. *Randglossen zur Hebräischen Bibel. Textkritisches, sprachliches und sachliches. 7. Band: Hohes Lied, Ruth, Klaglieder, Koheleth, Esther, Daniel, Ezra, Nehemia, Könige, Chronik: Nachträge und Gesamtregister*, 126–55 (Daniel), 156–82 (Ezra). Leipzig: Hinrichs.

Eichner, H. 1983. Etymologische Beiträge zum Lykischen der Trilingue vom Letoon bei Xanthos. *Or* 52:48–66.

Eichrodt, W. 1959. Zum Problem des Menschensohnes. *EvT* 19:1–3.

Eilers, W. 1954–56. Neue aramäische Urkunden aus Ägypten. *AfO* 17:322–35.

———. 1957–58. Neue aramäische Urkunden aus Ägypten: Nachträgliche Bemerkungen zu AfO 17, pp. 322–335. *AfO* 18:125–27.

———. 1962. Die altiranische Vorform des Vāspuhr. In *A Locust's Leg: Studies in Honor of S. H. Taqizadeh*, ed. W. B. Henning and E. Yarshater, 55–63. London: Lund Humphries.

———. 1968. Zum altpersischen Relativpronomen. *Zeitschrift für vergleichende Sprachforschung auf dem Gebiet der indogermanischen Sprachen* 83:63–68.

———. 1988. Euphonisches *i* und der aramäische Emphaticus auf *yā*. In *A Green Leaf: Papers in Honour of Professor J. P. Asmussen*, 109–23. Acta Iranica 28/2: Hommages et opera minora 12. Leiden: Brill.

Eisen, G. A. 1940. *Ancient Oriental Cylinder and Other Seals with a Description of the Collection of Mrs. William H. Moore.* OIP 47. Chicago: Univ. of Chicago Press.

Eissfeldt, O. 1930. Der Gott Bethel. *Archiv für Religionswissenschaft 18:1–30.*

———. 1932. Baal Zaphon, Zeus Kasios und der Durchzug des Israeliten durchs Meer. In *Beiträge zur Religions-Geschichte des Altertums* 1:25–27. Halle (Saale): Niemeyer.

———. 1951. Die Menetekel-Inschrift und ihre Deutung. *ZAW* 22:105–14.

———. 1955. El und Jahwe. In *Proceedings of the Twenty-Third International Congress of Orientalists*, ed. D. Sinor, 94–95. London: Royal Asiatic Society.

———. 1958. Review of *Aramaic Documents of the Fifth Century B.C.*, by G. R. Driver. *OLZ* 53:559–60.

———. 1959. Review of *Un edito bilingue greco-aramaico di Aśoka*, by G. P. Carratelli and G. Levi della Vida. *OLZ* 54:465–66.

———. 1963. "Juda" in II Könige 14,28 und "Judäa" in Apostelgeschichte 2,9. *Wissen. Zeits. Halle* 12:229–38.

———. 1964. "Juda" und "Judäa" als Bezeichnungen nordsyrischer Bereiche. *Forschungen und Fortschritt* 38:20–25.

Eitan, I. 1927–30. Hebrew and Semitic Particles. *AJSL* 44:177–205, 254–260, 45:48–63, 130–45, 197–211, 46:22–51.

———. 1941. Biblical Studies. *HUCA* 14:1–22.

Elat, M. 1977. *Economic Relations in the Lands of the Bible c. 1000–539 B.C.* Jerusalem : Mosad Bialik & the Israel Exploration Society.

Elhorst, H. J. 1912. Nieuw licht uit Elephantine. *Nieuw theologisch tijdschrift* 1:19–34.

———. 1912a. The Passover Papyrus from Elephantine. *JBL* 31:147–49.

Ellenbogen, M. 1962. *Foreign Words in the Old Testament: Their Origin and Etymology.* London: Luzac.

Elliger, K. 1947. Sam'al und Hamat in ihrem Verhältnis zu Hattina, Unqi und Arpad: Ein Beitrag zur Territorialgeschichte der nordsyrischen Staaten im 9. und 8. Jahrhundert v. Chr. In *Festschrift: Otto Eissfeldt zum 60. Geburtstage —1. September 1947*, ed. J. Fück,

69–108. Halle (Saale): Niemeyer.

Emerton, J. A. 1958.   The Origin of the Son of Man Imagery. *JTS* 9:225–42.

———. 1960.   The Participles in Daniel v.12. *ZAW* 31:262–63.

———. 1986.   Review of *The Balaam Text from Deir 'Alla,* by J. A. Hackett. *JTS* 37:476–78.

Engberg, R. M. See: G. R. Hughes.

Eph'al, I. 1973.   חפירות ומחקרים; מוגש In .לאבחנת גולי ישראל ויהודה בממלכת אשור לפרופסור שמואל ייבין, ed. Y. Aharoni, 201–3. Publications of the Institute of Archaeology 1. Tel Aviv: Archeological Institute, Univ. of Tel-Aviv.

———. 1978.   The Western Minorities in Babylonia in the 6th–5th Centuries B.C.: Maintenance and Cohesion. *Or* 47:74–90.

Eph'al, I., and J. Naveh. 1989.   Hazael's Booty Inscriptions. *IEJ* 39:192–200.

Epstein, J. N. 1912.   Glossen zu den "aramäischen Papyrus und Ostraka." *ZAW* 32:128–38.

———. 1912a.   Jahu, AŠMbēthēl und ANTbēthēl. *ZAW* 32:139–45.

———. 1913.   Weitere Glossen zu den "aramäischen Papyrus und Ostraka." *ZAW* 33:138–50, 222–35.

———. 1913a.   Nachträge und Berichtigungen zu meinen Glossen in Jahrgang 1912 und 1913. *ZAW* 33:310–12.

———. 1916.   Eine Nachlese zu den Aḥiqarpapyri. *OLZ* 19:204–9.

———. 1942.   Notes on the Sujin Pact. *Kedem* 1:37–43.

———. 1960.   דקדוק ארמית בבלית. Jerusalem: Magnes.

Epstein, L. M. 1927.   *The Jewish Marriage Contract: A Study in the Status of the Woman in Jewish Law.* New York: Jewish Theological Seminary.

Erdmann, K. 1960.   Review of *Persepolis,* by E. F. Schmidt. *BO* 17:79–86.

Eshel, H. 1988.   ממצאים ממערה ותעודות בכתף-יריחו. *Qadmoniot* 21:18–23.

Eshel, H., and H. Misgav. 1986–87.   תעודה מן המאה הרביעי לפסה"נ. *Tarbiz* 56:461–77.

———. 1988.   A Fourth Century B.C.E. Document from Ketef Yeriḥo. *IEJ* 38:158–76.

Eskhult, M. 1981.   Hebrew and Aramaic ᵃlōqīm. *OS* 30:137–39.

Euler, K. F. 1937.   Die Bedeutung von *spr* in der Sudschin-Inschrift im Lichte des ATlichen Gebrauchs von *sepaer*. *ZAW* 55:281–91.

Euting, J. 1871.   Punische Steine. *Mémoires de l'Académie impériale des sciences de St. Pétersbourg* 7/17, 3:1–37, pls. I–XLVI.

———. 1885.   *Nabatäische Inschriften aus Arabien.* Berlin: G. Reimer.

———. 1885a.   Epigraphische Miscellen. *SPAW* 21:669–88.

———. 1887.   Epigraphische Miscellen. *SPAW* 23:407–22.

———. 1903.   Notice sur un papyrus égypto-araméen de la Bibliothèque Impériale de Strasbourg. *MPAIBL* 11:297–311 + photo.

———. 1914.   *Tagbuch einer Reise in Inner-Arabien.* 2 vols., ed. E. Littmann. Leiden: Brill.

———. See also: R. Lepsius.

Ewald, H. 1856. Erklärung der grossen phönikischen Inschrift von Sidon und einer ägyptisch-aramäischen mit den zuverlässigen Abbildern beider. *AbhKGWG* 7:3–68.

———. 1856a. Übersicht der 1855–1856 erschienenen Schriften zur biblischen Wissenschaft. *Jahrbücher d. bibl. Wiss.* 8:118–273.

———. 1856–57. Über eine neulichst gefundene ägyptisch-aramäische Inschrift. *AbhKGWG* 7:52–63.

Eybers, I. H. 1966. Relations between Jews and Samaritans in the Persian Period. In *Biblical Essays: Proceedings of the Ninth Meeting of "Die OuTestamentiese Werkgemeenskap in Suid-Afrika,"* 72–89. Stellenbosch: Stellenbosch Univ. Press.

Faber, A. 1987. On the Etymology and Use of Yaudi *mt. ZDMG* 137:278–84.

———. 1988. Indefinite Pronouns in Early Semitic. In *Fucus: A Semitic/Afrasian Gathering in Remembrance of Albert Ehrman,* ed. Y. L. Arbeitman, 221–38. Current Issues in Linguistic Theory 58. Amsterdam/Philadelphia: Benjamins.

Fabricy, G. 1803. *De Ioannis Hyrcani Hasmonaei Iudaeorum summi pontificis hebraeo-samaritico numo.* Vol. 1. Rome.

Fāḍil, 'A. 1958. 'Arabī, Arāmā, 'Ibrī. *Sumer* 14:180–88.

Fales, F. M. 1973. Remarks on the Neirab Texts. *OrAnt* 12:131–42.

———. 1974. West Semitic Names from the Governor's Palace. *Annali della Facoltà di Lingue e Letterature straniere di Ca' Foscari* 13/3 (sez. or. 5):179–88.

———. 1976. Sulla tavoletta aramaica A.O. 25.341. *AION* 36:541–47.

———. 1977. On Aramaic Onomastics in the Neo-Assyrian Period. *OrAnt* 16:41–68.

———. 1978. L'onomastica aramaica in età neo-assira: Raffronti tra il corpus alfabetico e il materiale cuneiforme. In *Atti del 1. Convegno italiano sul Vicino Oriente antico (Roma, 22–24 Aprile 1976),* 199–229. Orientis Antiqui Collectio 13. Rome: Centro per le Antichità e la Storia dell'Arte del Vicino Oriente.

———. 1978a. Una diffida relativa a fuorusciti mesopotamici in aramaico. *AION* 38:273–82.

———. 1978b. A Cuneiform Correspondence to Alphabetic ﬠ in West Semitic Names of the I Millennium B. C. *Or* 47:91–98.

———. 1979. A List of Assyrian and West Semitic Women's Names. *Iraq* 41:55–73.

———. 1980. Accadico e aramaico: Livelli dell'interferenza linguistica. *VO* 3:243–67.

———. 1982. Note di semitico nordoccidentale. *VO* 5:75–83.

———. 1982a. Massimo sforzo, minima resa: Maledizioni divine da Tell Fekheriye all'Antico Testamento. *Annali della Facoltà di Lingue e Letterature straniere di Ca' Foscari* 21/3:1–12.

———. 1983. Le double bilinguisme de la statue de Tell Fekherye. *Syria* 60:233–50.

———. 1984. Assyro-Aramaica: Three Notes. *Or* 53:66–71.

———. 1985. Assiro e aramaico: Filologia e interferenza linguistica. *Atti del sodalizio glottologico milanese* 25:21–30.

———. 1986. *Aramaic Epigraphs on Clay Tablets of the Neo-Assyrian Period.* Dipartimento di Studi Orientali. Studi Semitici n.s. 2. Rome: Università degli studi "La Sapienza."

————. 1986a.   Review of *Les inscriptions araméennes de Sfiré et l'Assyrie de Shamshi-Ilu*, by A. Lemaire and J.-M. Durand. *RA* 80:88–93.

————. 1987.   Aramaic Letters and Neo-Assyrian Letters: Philological and Methodological Notes. *JAOS* 107:451–69.

————. 1987a.   La tradizione assira ad Elefantina d'Egitto. *Dialoghi di Archeologia* 5:36–70.

————. 1987b.   Materiali per il lessico aramaico del I millennio a.C. In *Atti della 4a Giornata di Studi Camito-Semitici e Indoeuropei*, ed. G. Bernini, 77–83. Milan: Unicopli.

————. 1989.   Nuovi dati sull'onomastica aramaica in cuneiforme neo-assiro. *Atti del sodalizio glottologico milanese* 27:75–84.

————. 1990.   Istituzioni a confronto tra mondo semitico occidentale e Assiria nel I millennio a.C.: il trattato di Sefire. In *I trattati nel mondo antico. Forma, ideologia, funzione*, ed. L. Canfora et al., 149–73. Rome.

Falk, Z. W. 1954.   The Deeds of Manumission in Elephantine. *JJS* 5:114–17.

————. 1958.   Manumission by Sale. *JSS* 3:127–28.

————. 1959.   Ezra VII 26. *VT* 9:88–89.

Farzat, H. 1967.   Encore sur le mot TQM dans les documents araméens d'Eléphantine. *Sem* 17:77–80.

Fassberg, S. E. 1989.   The Origin of the Ketib/Qere in the Aramaic Portions of Ezra and Daniel. *VT* 39:1–12.

Feldmann, F. 1909.   Die Papyri von Elefantine und der Pentateuch. *ThGl* 1:288.

Fellman, J. 1980.   Sociolinguistic Notes on the History of Aramaic. *JNSL* 8:15–16.

Fellows, C. 1841.   *An Account of Discoveries in Lycia, Being a Journal Kept During a Second Excursion in Asia Minor*. London: J. Murray.

Fennelly, J. M. 1980.   The Persepolis Ritual. *BA* 43:135–62.

Fensham, F. C. 1962.   Malediction and Benediction in Ancient Near Eastern Vassal-Treaties and the Old Testament. *ZAW* 74:1–9.

————. 1962a.   Salt as Curse in the Old Testament and the Ancient Near East. *BA* 25:48–50.

————. 1963.   Common Trends in Curses of the Near Eastern Treaties and *kudurru*-Inscriptions compared with Maledictions of Amos and Isaiah. *ZAW* 75:155–75.

————. 1963a.   The Wild Ass in the Aramean Treaty between Bar-Ga'ayah and Mati'el. *JNES* 22:185–86.

————. 1963b.   Clauses of Protection in Hittite Vassal-Treaties and the Old Testament. *VT* 13:133–43.

————. 1964.   The Treaty between Israel and the Gibeonites. *BA* 27:96–100.

————. 1967.   Covenant, Promise and Expectation in the Bible. *TZ* 23:305–22.

Ferch, A. J. 1980.   Daniel 7 and Ugarit: A Reconsideration. *JBL* 99:75–86.

————. 1983.   The Book of Daniel and the "Maccabean Thesis." *AUSS* 21:129–41.

Feuillet, A. 1953.   Le Fils de l'Homme de Daniel et la tradition biblique. *RB* 60:170–202; 321–46.

Février, J.-G. 1959. *Histoire de l'écriture*. 2nd ed. Paris: Payot.

Filliozat, H. 1961–62. Graeco-Aramaic Inscription of Aśoka near Kandahar. *Epigraphica Indica* 34:1–8.

Fischer, L. 1913. Zur Erklärung des Papyrus F von Assuan. *OLZ* 16:306–8.

Fish, T. See: W. von Soden.

Fisher, C. S. See: G. A. Reisner.

Fitzmyer, J. A. 1957. The Syntax of *kl, kl'* in the Aramaic Texts From Egypt and in Biblical Aramaic. *Bib* 38:170–84. Reprinted as "The Syntax of כל, כלא, 'All' in Aramaic Texts from Egypt and in Biblical Aramaic" in Fitzmyer 1979, 205–17.

———. 1958. The Aramaic Suzerainty Treaty from Sefire in the Museum of Beirut. *CBQ* 20:444–76.

———. 1961. The Aramaic Inscriptions of Sefire I and II. *JAOS* 81:178–222.

———. 1962. The Padua Aramaic Papyrus Letters. *JNES* 21:15–24. Reprinted in Fitzmyer 1979, 219–30.

———. 1965. The Aramaic Letter of King Adon to the Egyptian Pharaoh. *Bib* 46:41–55. Reprinted in Fitzmyer 1979, 231–42.

———. 1967. *The Aramaic Inscriptions of Sefire*. BibOr 19. Rome: Pontifical Biblical Institute.
Reviews: Z. Ben-Hayyim 1972–73; W. Beuken 1968; S. P. Brock 1968; J. Coppens 1968; M. Delcor 1968; O. Eissfeldt 1970: *OLZ* 65:366; J. C. Greenfield 1968; P. Grelot 1968; L. F. Hartman 1968; H. H. Rowley 1968–69; J. A. Soggin 1968; J.-L. Vesco 1968.

———. 1967a. Aramaeans; Aramaic Language, Ancient. In *New Catholic Encyclopedia*, ed. W. J. McDonald, et al., 1:735–37. New York: McGraw-Hill.

———. 1969. A Further Note on the Aramaic Inscription Sefire III 22. *JSS* 14:197–200.

———. 1970. Review of *Altaramäische Grammatik der Inschriften des 10.–8. Jh.v.Chr.*, by R. Degen. *Or* 39:580–84.

———. 1971. A Re-Study of an Elephantine Aramaic Marriage Contract (*AP* 15). In *Near Eastern Studies in Honor of William Foxwell Albright*, ed. H. Goedicke, 137–68. Baltimore: Johns Hopkins. Reprinted in Fitzmyer 1979, 243–71.

———. 1973. Review of *Lexicon linguae aramaicae Veteris Testamenti documentis antiquis illustratum*, by E. Vogt. *Bib* 54:131–35.

———. 1974. Some Notes on Aramaic Epistolography. *JBL* 93:201–25. Reprinted as "Aramaic Epistolography" in Fitzmyer 1979, 183–204, and with revisions in *Studies in Ancient Letter Writing*, ed. J. L. White (Semeia 22; Chico, Cal.: Scholars Press), 25–57.

———. 1975. Review of *Documents araméens d'Égypte*, by P. Grelot. *Bib* 56:254–56.

———. 1976. Review of *La langue de Yaudi*, by P.-E. Dion. *CBQ* 38:98–100.

———. 1977. Review of *Textbook of Syrian Semitic Inscriptions II*, by J. C. L. Gibson. *JBL* 96:425–27.

———. 1977a. Review of *Studies in Aramaic Inscriptions and Onomastics I*, by E. Lipiński. *CBQ* 39:262–63.

———. 1978. Review of *Aramaic Texts from Deir 'Alla*, by J. Hoftijzer and G. van der Kooij. *CBQ* 40:93–95.

————. 1979. *A Wandering Aramean: Collected Aramaic Essays.* SBL Monograph Series 25. Missoula, Mont.: Scholars Press.
Reviews: Le Déaut 1981.

————. 1979a. The Phases of the Aramaic Language. In Fitzmyer 1979, 57–84.

————. 1984. Review of *La statue de Tell Fekherye*, by A. Abou Assaf et al. *JBL* 103:265–67.

————. 1986. Review of *Aramaic Texts from North Saqqâra*, by J. B. Segal. *CBQ* 48:541–44.

Flusser, D. 1972. The four empires in the Fourth Sibyl and in the Book of Daniel. *IOS* 2:148–75.

Fohrer, G. 1975. Review of *La langue de Ya'udi*, by P.-E. Dion. *ZAW* 87:98–100.

Forbes, A. D. See: F. I. Andersen.

Fotheringham, J. K. 1908–9. Calendar Dates in the Aramaic Papyri from Assuan. *MNRAS* 69:12–20, 470.

————. 1909. Note on the Regnal Years in the Elephantine Papyri. *MNRAS* 69:446–48, 542.

————. 1910–11. A Reply to Professor Ginzel on the Calendar Dates in the Elephantine Papryi. *MNRAS* 71:661–63.

————. 1913. Dates in the Elephantine Papyri. *JTS* 14:570–75.

Fowler, J. D. 1988. *Theophoric Personal Names in Ancient Hebrew: A Comparative Study.* *JSOT* Supplement Series 49. Sheffield: Sheffield Academic Press.

Fowler, H. N. 1905. Agatcha-Kalé. *AJA* 2/9:344.

Fox, M. 1973. *Ṭôb* as Covenant Terminology. *BASOR* 209:41–42.

Fraenkel, S. 1886. *Die aramäischen Fremdwörter in Arabischen.* Leiden: Brill. Reprint Hildesheim: G. Olms, 1962.

————. 1907. Review of *Drei aramäische Papyrusurkunden aus Elephantine*, by E. Sachau. *TLZ* 32:657–59.

————. 1908. Zu den Papyri von Elephantine. *ZA* 21:240–43.

Fraikin, D. See: P.-E. Dion.

Frank, R. M. 1959. The Description of the "Bear" in Dn 7,5. *CBQ* 21:505–7.

Franken, H. J. 1967. Texts from the Persian Period from Tell Deir 'Allā. *VT* 17:480–81.

————. 1976. The Problem of Identification in Biblical Archaeology. *PEQ* 108:3–11.

————. 1979. The Identity of Tell Deir 'Allā, Jordan. *Akkadica* 14:11–15.

————. 1991. Deir 'Alla Re-Visited. In *BTDAR*, 3–15.

Franken, H. J., and M. M. Ibrahim. 1977–78. Two Seasons of Excavations at Tell Deir 'Alla, 1976–1978. ADAJ 22:57–79.

Frankena, R. 1965. The Vassal-Treaties of Esarhaddon and the Dating of Deuteronomy. *OTS* 14:122–54.

Frankfort, H. 1939. *Cylinder Seals.* London: Macmillan.

Fraser, J. 1923. The Lydian Language. In *Anatolian Studies presented to Sir William Mitchell Ramsay* 139–50. Manchester: Manchester Univ. Press.

Freedman, D. N. 1957. The Prayer of Nabonidus. *BASOR* 145:31–32.

Freedman, D. N., and F. I. Andersen. 1989. The Spelling of Samaria Papyrus 1. In *To Touch the Text: Biblical Studies in Honor of Joseph A. Fitzmyer, S.J.*, ed. M. P. Horgan and P. J. Kobelski, 15–32. New York: Crossroad.

Freedman, D. N. See also: F. I. Andersen, F. M. Cross.

Frei, P. 1976–77. Die Trilingue vom Letoon, die lykischen Zahlzeichen und das lykische Geldsystem. *Schweizerische numismatische Rundschau* 55:5–16; 56:66–78.

———. 1981. Review of *Fouilles de Xanthos, Tome VI: La stèle trilingue de Létôon*, ed. H. Metzger. *BO* 38:354–71.

Frei, P., and V. Shevoroshkin. 1978. Sull'interpretazione delle righe 20–21 della trilingue di Xanthos. *Incontri linguistici* 4:235–39.

Freund, L. 1907. Bemerkungen zu Papyrus G. des Fundes von Assuan. *WZKM* 21:169–77.

Freydank, H. 1975. Eine aramäische Urkunde aus Assur. *Altorientalische Forschungen* 2:133–35.

———. See also: L. Jakob-Rost.

Friedrich, J. 1922. Der Schwund kurzer Endvokale im Nordwestsemitischen. *ZS* 1:3–14.

———. 1930. Zu den kleinasiatischen Personnennamen mit dem Element *muwa*. In *Kleinasiatische Forschungen*, ed. F. Sommer and H. Ehelof, 359–78. 1/3. Weimar: Böhlau.

———. 1932. *Kleinasiatische Sprachdenkmäler*. KlT 163. Berlin: De Gruyter.

———. 1936. Kein König פלמה in der Stele von Sudschin. *ZA* 9:327–28.

———. 1940. Denkmäler mit westsemitischer Buchstabenschrift. In *Die Inschriften vom Tell Halaf: Keilschrifttexte und aramäische Urkunden aus einer assyrischen Provinzhauptstadt*, ed. J. Friedrich et al., 69–78. *AfO* Beiheft 6. Berlin: Selbstverlag des Herausgebers.

———. 1951. *Phönizisch-punische Grammatik*. AnOr 32. Rome: Pontifical Biblical Institute.

———. 1957. Zur Bezeichnung des langes ā in den Schreibweisen des Aramäischen. *Or* 26:37–42.

———. 1957a. In aller Kürze. *AfO* 18:61.

———. 1957b. Zur passivischen Ausdrucksweise im Aramäischen. *AfO* 18:124–25.

———. 1957c. Eine aramäische und eine punische Datierung. *AfO* 18:108.

———. 1957–58. Das bildhethitische Siegel des Br-Rkb von Sam'al. *Or* 26:345–47; 27:111.

———. 1965. Zur Stellung des Jaudischen in der nordwestsemitischen Sprachgeschichte. In *Studies in Honor of Benno Landsberger on his Seventy-fifth Birthday, April 21, 1965*, 425–29. Assyriological Studies, vol. 16. Chicago: Univ. of Chicago Press.

———. 1966. Zu der altaramäischen Stele des ZKR von Hamat. *AfO* 21:83.

Friedrich, J., and B. Landsberger. 1933. Zu der altaramäischen Stele von Sudschin. *ZA* 41:313–18.

Fronzaroli, P. 1985. Le lingue della Siria antica: Dall'eblaita all'aramaico. In *Da Ebla a Damasco: Diecimila anni di archeologia in Siria*, ed. G. Garroni and E. Parcu, 56–61.

Milan: Electa.

Frye, R. N. 1982. The "Aramaic" Inscription on the Tomb of Darius. *Iranica Antiqua* 17:85–90.

Fuhs, H. F. 1977. *Ḥzh* einem angeblichen Aramaismus im Hebräischen. *BN* 2:7–12.

Fuller, J. M. 1885. The Book of Daniel in the Light of Recent Research and Discoverys. *Expositor* 3/1:217–25; 431–38.

Funk, S. 1909. Die Papyri von Assuan als älteste Quelle einer Halacha. *JJLG* 7:378–79.

———. 1924. Die Sprache des Scheidebriefes. *JJLG* 16:123–35.

Furlani, G. 1948. Aram. גזרין = scongiuratori. *AANL Rendiconti* ser. 8, vol. 3:177–96.

Fürst, J. 1835. *Lehrgebäude der aramäischen Idiome mit Bezug auf die indo-germanischen Sprachen.* Leipzig: Tauchnitz.

Furtwängler, A. 1900. *Die antiken Gemmen.* 3 vols. Leipzig: Giesecke & Devrient.

Fussman, G. 1972. Intailles et empreintes indiennes du Cabinet des Médailles de Paris. *Revue numismatique* VIe série 14:21–48.

Fuye, A. de la. 1919. Le monnaies de l'Élymaïde. *Revue numismatique* 4e ser. 22:45–84.

Gabra, S. 1945–46. Lettres araméennes trouvées à Touna el Gebel (Hermoupolis Ouest). *BIE* 28:161–62 + 2 pls.

———. 1947. Fouilles de l'Université Fouad Ier, à Hermopolis Ouest Tounah el-Gabal et Meir, saison 1946–1947. *Bulletin of the Faculty of Arts* (L'Université Fouad Ier) 9/1:131–34.

Gai, A. 1986. The Non-Active Participles in the Ancient Semitic Languages. *ZDMG* 136:8–14.

Gall, A. F. von. 1926. Βασιλεία τοῦ Θεοῦ. Heidelberg: C. Winter.

Gallavotti, C. 1959. The Greek Version of the Kandahār Bilingual Inscription of Aśoka. *EAW* 10:185–91.

———. 1959a. Il manifesto di Asoka nell'Afghanistan. *Rivista di cultura classica e medioevale* 1:113–26.

Galling, K. 1938. Denkmäler zur Geschichte Syriens und Palästinas unter der Herrschaft der Perser. *Palästinajahrbuch des Deutschen evangelischen Instituts für Altertumswissenschaft des Heiligen Landes zu Jerusalem* 34:59–79.

———. 1941. Beschriftete Bildsiegel des ersten Jahrtausends v. Chr. vornehmlich aus Syrien und Palestina. *ZDPV* 64:121–202.

———. 1948. Review of *Die Kleinfunde von Sendschirli*, by F. von Luschan. *BO* 5:115–20.

———. 1950. A Note on the Gold Sheath of Zendjirli and Ecclesiastes 12:11. *BASOR* 119:15–18.

———. 1953. Archäologisch-historische Ergebnisse einer Reise in Syrien und Liban im Spätherbst 1952. *ZDPV* 69:181–87.

———. 1954. *Die Bücher der Chronik, Esra, Nehemia.* Das Alte Testament Deutsch. Göttingen: Vandenhoeck & Ruprecht.

———. 1954a. Die 62 Jahre des Meders Darius in Dan 6,1. *ZAW* 25:152.

———. 1956. Der Ehrenname Elisas und die Entrückung Elias. *Zeits. f. Theologie und Kirche* 53:129–48.

————. 1963. Eschmunazar und der Herr der Könige. *ZDPV* 79:140–51.

————. 1967. Miscellanea Archaeologica 4: Das Salben der Mutterbrust (Sfire I A 21f.) *ZDPV* 83:123–35.

Galter, H. D. 1986. Review of *Les inscriptions araméennes de Sfiré et l'Assyrie de Shamshi-Ilu*, by A. Lemaire and J.-M. Durand. *BO* 43:445–47.

Garbini, G. 1956. Note aramaiche. 1: *p > b* in yaudico. *Antonianum* 31:310–11.

————. 1956a. L'Aramaico antico. *AANL Memorie* Series 8, 7:235–86.
Reviews: S. Moscati 1956; P. Nober 1958.

————. 1956b. Sul nome Y'dy. *RSO* 31:31–35.

————. 1957. La congiunzione semitica **pa-*. *Bib* 38:419–27.

————. 1957a. Note aramaiche. 2–4. *Antonianum* 32:427–30.

————. 1958. Israele e gli Aramei di Damasco. *RivB* 6:199–209.

————. 1958a. Considerazioni sulla parola ebraica *peten*. *RivB* 6:263–65.

————. 1959. Unité et varieté des dialectes araméens anciens. In *Akten des vierundzwanzigsten internationalen Orientalistenkongresses*, ed. H. Franke, 242–44. Wiesbaden: Steiner.

————. 1959a. Nuovo materiale per la grammatica dell'aramaico antico. *RSO* 34:41–54.

————. 1960. 'Atar dio aramaico? *RSO* 35:25–28.

————. 1960a. *Il semitico di nord-ovest*. Quaderni della sezione linguistica degli Annali, I. Naples: Istituto universitario orientale di Napoli.
Reviews: G. Buccellati 1962; F. Cantera 1961; P. Nober 1960; M. H. Pope 1961; G. Rinaldi 1962; W. Röllig 1962.

————. 1961. Sefīre I A, 28. *RSO* 36:9–11.

————. 1961a. Review of *A Grammar of Biblical Aramaic*, by F. Rosenthal. *RSO* 36:307–10.

————. 1962. The Dating of Post-Exilic Stamps. In Y. Aharoni 1962a, 61–68.

————. 1964. The Aramaic Section of the Kandahar Inscription. *Istituto italiano per il medio ed estremo oriente: Serie orientale Roma* 29:1–22.

————. 1965. Sull'iscrizione aramaica di Bahadirli. *RSO* 40:135–37.

————. 1967. Un nuovo sigillo aramaico-ammonita. *AION* 27:251–56 + 1 pl.

————. 1967a. Appunti di epigrafia aramaica. *AION* 27:89–96.

————. 1969. I dialetti dell'aramaico antico e lo yaudico. *AION* 29:1–8.

————. 1969a. Le matres lectionis e il vocalismo nell'aramaico antico. *AION* 29:8–15.

————. 1970. Review of *Altaramäische Grammatik der Inschriften des 10.–8. Jh. v. Chr.*, by R. Degen. *AION* 30:275–77.

————. 1971. Qualche considerazioni sull'aramaico della tavoletta cuneiforme di Warka. *HomAD-S*, 27–36.

————. 1974. Sul nome 'Athtar/'Ashtar. *AION* 34:409–10.

————. 1976. La lingua di Ya'udi. [Review of *La langue de Ya'udi*, by P.-E. Dion.] *AION* 36:123–32. Reprinted in Garbini 1988, 69–80.

———. 1976a. Review of *Textbook of Syrian Semitic Inscriptions II*, by J. C. L. Gibson. *OrAnt* 15:351–54.

———. 1977. Osservazioni sul testo aramaico della trilingue di Xanthos. *Studi micenei ed egeo-anatolici* 18:269–72.

———. 1977a. Review of *Altaramäische Grammatik*, by S. Segert. *AION* 37:274–76. Reprinted in Garbini 1988, 148–52.

———. 1977b. Review of *Studies in Aramaic Inscriptions and Onomastics I*, by E. Lipiński. *AION* 37:276–77.

———. 1977c. Note epigrafiche. *AION* 37:482–83.

———. 1978. Scarabeo con iscrizione aramaica dalla necropoli di Macchiabate. *ParPass* 183:424–26.

———. 1979. L'iscrizione di Balaam Bar-Beor. *Henoch* 1:166–88.

———. 1979a. Nuovi documenti epigrafici dalla Palestina—1976. *Henoch* 1:396–400.

———. 1980. Il bilinguismo dei Giudei. *VO* 3:209–23.

———. 1985. Aramaico $g^e m\bar{\imath}r$ (Esdra 7,12). In *Studi in onore di Edda Bresciani*, ed. S. F. Bondì, S. Pernigotti, F. Serra, and A. Vivian, 227–29. Pisa: Giardini.

———. 1988. *Il Semitico nordoccidentale: Studi di storia linguistica*. Rome: Università degli Studi "La Sapienza."

———. See also: G. Pugliese-Carratelli.

García Daris, L. 1980. El universalismo en Ashoka. *Oriente-Occidente* 1:87–96.

García-Treto, F. O. 1967. Genesis 31[44] and "Gilead." *ZAW* 79:13–17.

Garelli, P. 1971. Nouveau coup d'oeil sur Muṣur. *HomAD-S*, 37–48. Paris: Maisonneuve.

———. 1986. Les archives inédites d'un centre provincial de l'empire assyrien. *Cuneiform Archives and Libraries: Papers read at the 30ᵉ Rencontre assyriologique internationale, Leiden, 4–8 July 1983*, ed. K. R. Veenhof, 241–46. Leiden: Nederlands Instituut voor het Nabije Oosten.

Garr, W. R. 1985. *Dialect Geography of Syria-Palestine, 1000–586 B.C.E.* Philadelphia: Univ. of Pennsylvania Press.
Reviews: J. Huehnergard 1987; B. S. J. Isserlin 1988; A. R. Millard 1991: *JSS* 36.1.

———. 1990. On the Alternation Between Construct and *Dī* Phrases in Biblical Aramaic. *JSS* 25:213–31.

Gehman, H. S. 1924. Notes on the Persian Words in the Book of Esther. *JBL* 43:321–28.

Geiger, A. 1867. Eine aramäische Inschrift auf einem babylonisch-assyrischen Gewichte. *ZDMG* 21:466–68.

———. 1868. Derenbourg's *Notes épigraphiques et mélanges sémitiques*. *JZ* 6:156–58.

Geiss, G. 1961. *Auf Messers Schneide: Eine Auslegung von Daniel 6–12*. Neukirchen: Erziehungsverein.

Gelb, I. J. 1962. Review of *The Vassal-Treaties of Esarhaddon*, by D. J. Wiseman. *BO* 19:159–62.

Gelderen, C. van. 1912. Samaritaner und Juden in Elephantine-Syene. *OLZ* 15:337–44.

Gelin, A. 1953. *Le Livre de Esdras et Néhémie*. La Sainte Bible. Paris: Cerf.

Geller, M. J. 1977.   The Elephantine Papyri and Hosea 2,3: Evidence for the Form of the Early Jewish Divorce Writ. *JSJ* 8:139–48.

Gemser, B. 1924.   *De beteekenis der persoonsnamen voor onze kennis van het leven en denken der oude Babyloniërs en Assyriërs.* Wageningen: Veenman en Zonen.

Genge, H. 1979.   *Nordsyrisch-südanatolische Reliefs.* 2 vols. Det Kongelige Danske Viden-skabernes Selskab: Hist.-filos. meddelelser 49. Copenhagen: Munksgaard.

Geraty, L. T. 1972.   Third Century B. C. Ostraca from Khirbet el-Kom. Ph.D. diss., Harvard Univ.

———. 1975.   The Khirbet el-Kôm Bilingual Ostracon. *BASOR* 220:55–61.

———. 1978.   Review of *Textbook of Syrian Semitic Inscriptions II*, by J. C. L. Gibson. *BASOR* 229:76–78.

———. 1981.   Recent Suggestions on the Bilingual Ostracon from Khirbet el-Kôm. *AUSS* 19:137–40.

———. 1983.   The Historical, Linguistic, and Biblical Significance of the Khirbet el-Kôm Ostraca. In *The Word of the Lord Shall Go Forth: Essays in Honor of David Noel Freed-man in Celebration of His Sixtieth Birthday*, ed. C. L. Meyers and M. O'Connor, 545–48. Winona Lake, Ind.: Eisenbrauns.

Gerstenberger, E. 1965.   Covenant and Commandment. *JBL* 84:38–51.

Gesenius, W. 1833.   *Lexicon manuale Hebraicum et Chaldaicum in Veteris Testamenti libros.* Leipzig: Fr. Chr. Guil. Vogel.

———. 1837.   Monumentum Carpentoractense. In *Scripturae linguaeque phoeniciae monu-menta quotquot supersunt.* Leipzig: F. Chr. Guil. Vogel.

Gevirtz, S. 1957.   On the Etymology of the Phoenician Particle 'š. *JNES* 16:124–27.

———. 1961.   West-Semitic Curses and the Problem of the Origins of Hebrew Law. *VT* 11:137–158.

Gibson, J. C. L. 1961.   Observations on Some Important Ethnic Terms in the Pentateuch. *JNES* 20:217–38.

———. 1975.   *Textbook of Syrian Semitic Inscriptions: Volume II, Aramaic Inscriptions Including Inscriptions in the Dialect of Zenjirli.* Oxford: Clarendon.
     Reviews: S. P. Brock 1977; J. A. Fitzmyer 1977; W. J. Fulco 1979: *Or* 48:289–90; G. Garbini 1976; L. T. Geraty 1978; J. C. Greenfield 1978; D. Pardee 1978; S. Wagner 1984.

———. 1975a.   Review of *Studies in Aramaic Inscriptions and Onomastics I*, by E. Lipiński. *PEQ* 109:59–60.

Gilkey, C. W.   See: R. A. Bowman.

Ginsberg, H. L. 1933–34.   Aramaic Dialect Problems. *AJSL* 50:1–9.

———. 1935–36.   Aramaic Dialect Problems. II. *AJSL* 52:95–103.

———. 1939–40.   A Further Note on the Aramaic Contract Published by Bauer and Meiss-ner. *JAOS* 59:105.

———. 1940.   "King of Kings" and "Lord of Kingdoms." *AJSL* 57:71–74.

———. 1942.   Aramaic Studies Today. *JAOS* 62:229–38.

———. 1945.   Psalms and Inscriptions of Petition and Acknowledgement. In *Louis Ginzberg Jubilee Volume*, ed. S. Lieberman et al., 159–71 (Eng. Section). New York: American

Academy for Jewish Research.

———. 1948. *Studies in Daniel: Text and Studies of the Jewish Theological Seminary of America.* XI. New York: Jewish Theological Seminary.
Reviews: F. Rosenthal 1949.

———. 1948a. An Aramaic Contemporary of the Lachish Letters. *BASOR* 111:24–27.

———. 1954. The Brooklyn Museum Aramaic Papyri. [Review article: E. G. Kraeling, *The Brooklyn Museum Aramaic Papyri*.] *JAOS* 74:153–62.

———. 1959. Notes on Some Old Aramaic Texts. *JNES* 18:143–49.

———. 1960. Ezra 1:4. *JBL* 79:167–69.

———. 1961. Review of *A Grammar of Biblical Aramaic*, by F. Rosenthal. *JBL* 80:386–87.

———. 1969. Aramaic Papyri from Elephantine; Aramaic Letters. In *ANESTP*, 548–9; 633.

———. 1970. The Northwest Semitic Languages. In *World History of the Jewish People, Vol. II: Patriarchs*, ed. B. Mazar, 102–24. New Brunswick, N.J.: Rutgers Univ. Press.

———. 1971. Ben-Hadad. In *Encyclopaedia Judaica*, 4:515–17 + 1 pl.

Ginzel, F. K. 1911–14. *Handbuch der mathematischen und technischen Chronologie.* 3 vols. Leipzig.

Giveon, R. 1958. Notes on the Nimrud and Palestine Ivories. *Yediot* 22:55–61.

———. 1961. Two New Hebrew Seals and their Iconographic Background. *PEQ*:38–42.

Glueck, N. 1938. The First Campaign at Tell el-Kheleifeh (Ezion-Geber). *BASOR* 71:3–17.

———. 1940–41. Ostraca from Elath. *BASOR* 80:3–10, 82:3–11.

———. 1971. Tell el-Kheleifeh Inscriptions. In *Near Eastern Studies in Honor of William Foxwell Albright*, ed. H. Goedicke, 225–42. Baltimore: Johns Hopkins Univ. Press.

———. 1971a. מזבחות קטורת. *EI (Z. Shazar Volume)* 10:120–25.

Goeje, M. J. de. 1894. Mededeeling over de opgravingen te Sendjirli. *Verslagen en Mededeelingen der Koninklijke Akademie van Wetenschappen te Amsterdam, Afdeeling Letterskunde* III, reek 5/10:(32)–(39). Amsterdam: Noord-Hollandsche Uit-geversmaatschappij.

Goetze, A. 1944. Three Achaemenian Tags. *Berytus* 8:97–101.

———. 1962. Cilicians. *JCS* 16:48–58.

Goff, B. L. 1960. Observations on Barnett's *A Catalogue of the Nimrud Ivories*. *JAOS* 80:340–47.

Goldingay, J. 1988. "Holy Ones on High" in Daniel 7:18. *JBL* 107:495–7.

Goldwasser, O., and J. Naveh. 1976. The Origin of the Ṭet-Symbol. *IEJ* 26:15–19.

Golomb, D. 1975. The Date of a New Papyrus from Elephantine. *BASOR* 217:49–53.

González Nuñez, A. 1965. El rito de la Alianza. *EstBib* 24:217–38.

Gonzalez, M. I. See: L. A. Schökel.

Gooding, D. W. 1981. The Literary Structure of the Book of Daniel and its Implications. *Tyndale Bulletin* 32:43–79.

Goodman, A. E. 1958. The Words of Ahikar. *DOTT*, 270–75. London: T. Nelson.

Göpner W. See: T. Nöldeke.

Gordis, R. 1952. Koheleth—Hebrew or Aramaic? *JBL* 71:93–109. Reprinted in *The Word and the Book: Studies in Biblical Language and Literature* (New York: Ktav,1976), 263–79.

Gordon, C. H. 1937–39. The Aramaic Incantation in Cuneiform. *AfO* 12:105–17.

———. 1939. Western Asiatic Seals in the Walters Art Gallery. *Iraq* 6:3–34, pls. II–XV.

———. 1940. The Cuneiform Aramaic Incantation. *Or* 9:29–38.

———. 1941. *The Living Past*. New York: John Day.

———. 1955. The Origin of the Jews in Elephantine. *JNES* 14:56–58.

———. 1985. On Making Other Gods. In *Biblical and Related Studies Presented to Samuel Iwry*, ed. A. Kort and S. Morschauser, 77–79. Winona Lake, Ind.: Eisenbrauns.

Görg, M. 1979. Namenstudien III: Zum Problem einer Frühbezeugung von Aram. *BN* 9:7–10.

Gotō, K. 1973. A Sherd Inscribed with Aramaic Scripts Unearthed at Tell Zeror. *Orient* 9:1–29 + 1pl.

Gottlieb, I. 1980. *N'BṢN ZY 'BN ŠŠ* "Alabaster Vessels" (Kraeling 7:18). *JAOS* 100:512–13.

———. 1981. Succession in Elephantine and Jewish Law: Brooklyn Museum Aramaic Papyrus 2. *JSS* 26:193–203.

Goyon, G. 1957. *Nouvelles inscriptions rupestres du Wadi Ḥammamat*. Paris: Maisonneuve.

———. 1985. L'abécédaire araméen découvert dans le desert arabique égyptien (Wadi Hammamat). In *Pharaonic Egypt: The Bible and Christianity*, ed. S. Israelit-Groll, 65–71. Jerusalem: Magnes.

Grabbe, L. L. 1988. Another Look at the *Gestalt* of "Darius the Mede." *CBQ* 50:198–213.

———. 1988a. The Belshazzar of Daniel and the Belshazzar of History. *AUSS* 26:59–66.

Graf, D. F. 1982. Letter to the Readers. *BA* 45:132.

Gray, G. B. 1903. Notes on the Names in the Papyrus. *PSBA* 25:259–63.

———. 1914. Children Named after Ancestors in the Aramaic Papyri from Elephantine and Assuan. *BZAW* 27:161–76.

Gray, G. B. See also: A. Cowley.

Gray, L. H. 1913. Iranian Miscellanies: On the Aramaic Version of the Behistān Inscriptions. *JAOS* 33:281–94.

———. 1930. Lydian Notes on the Second Singular Imperative and on Hipponax. *JRAS* 62:625–27.

———. 1951. Review of R. G. Kent, *Old Persian Grammar*. *American Journal of Philology* 73:325–28.

Grayson, A. K. 1987. Akkadian Treaties of the Seventh Century B. C. *JCS* 39:127–60.

Greenfield, J. C. 1960. "Le bain des brebis": Another Example and a Query. *Or* 29:98–102.

———. 1962. Studies in Aramaic Lexicography I. *JAOS* 82:290–99.

———. 1964–65. בחינות לשוניות בכתובת ספירה. *Leš* 27–28:303–13.

———. 1965. Studies in West Semitic Inscriptions, I: Stylistic Aspects of the Sefire Treaty Inscriptions. *AcOr* 29:1–18.

————. 1966. Three Notes on the Sefire Inscription. *JSS* 11:98–105.

————. 1967. Ugaritic Lexicographical Notes. *JCS* 21:89–93.

————. 1967a. Some Aspects of Treaty Terminology in the Bible. In *Proceedings of the Fourth World Congress of Jewish Studies*, 1:117–19. Jerusalem: World Union of Jewish Studies.

————. 1967–68. קווים דיאלקטיים בארמית הקדומה. *Leš* 32:359–68.

————. 1968. Review of *The Aramaic Inscriptions of Sefîre*, by J. A. Fitzmyer. *JBL* 87:240–41.

————. 1969. The "Periphrastic Imperative" in Aramaic and Hebrew. *IEJ* 19:199–210.

————. 1970. *HAMARAKARA > 'AMARKAL*. In *W. B. Henning Memorial Volume*, ed. M. Boyce and I. Gershevitch, 180–86. London: Lund Humphries.

————. 1971. The Background and Parallel to a Proverb of Ahiqar. *HomAD-S*, 49–59.

————. 1971a. The Zakir Inscription and the Danklied. In *Proceedings of the Fifth World Congress of Jewish Studies*, 1:174–91. Jerusalem: World Union of Jewish Studies.

————. 1971b. Scripture and Inscription: The Literary and Rhetorical Element in Some Early Phoenician Inscriptions. In *Near Eastern Studies in Honor of William Foxwell Albright*, ed. H. Goedicke, 253–68. Baltimore: Johns Hopkins Univ. Press.

————. 1973. Un rite religieux araméen et ses parallèles. *RB* 80:46–52.

————. 1974. Iranian Vocabulary in Early Aramaic. *Acta iranica* 2:245–46.

————. 1974a. Standard Literary Aramaic. In *Actes du premier congrès international de linguistique sémitique et chamito-sémitique*, ed. A. Caquot and D. Cohen, 280–89. Janua Linguarum, ser. Practica, vol. 159. The Hague: Mouton.

————. 1974b. The *Marzeaḥ* as a Social Institution. AAASH 22:451–55.

————. 1975. Iranian or Semitic? In *Monumemtum H. S. Nyberg*, 311–16. Acta Iranica. Hommages et Opera Minora I. Leiden: Brill.

————. 1976. A New Corpus of Aramaic Texts of the Achaemenid Period from Egypt. *JAOS* 96:131–35.

————. 1976a. The Aramean God Rammān/Rimmōn. *IEJ* 26:195–98.

————. 1976b. Aramaic. *IDB Supplement* 39–44.

————. 1977. On Some Iranian Terms in the Elephantine Papyri: Aspects of Continuity. AAASH 25/1–4:113–18.

————. 1977a. The Prepositions '*ad*/'*al* in Aramaic and Hebrew. *BSOAS* 40:371–72.

————. 1977b. *našû-nadānu* and its Congeners. In *Essays on the Ancient Near East in Memory of Jacob Joel Finkelstein*, ed. M. de Jong Ellis, 87–91. Memoirs of the Connecticut Academy of Arts and Sciences 19. Hamden, Conn.: Archon.

————. 1978. The Dialects of Early Aramaic. *JNES* 37:93–99.

————. 1978a. Review of *Textbook of Syrian Semitic Inscriptions II*, by J. C. L. Gibson. *IEJ* 28:287–89.

————. 1978b. Aramaic and Its Dialects. In *Jewish Languages: Theme and Variations*, ed. H. H. Paper, 29–43. Cambridge, Mass.: Association for Jewish Studies.

————. 1978c. Some Reflections on the Vocabulary of Aramaic in Relationship to the Other

Semitic Languages. In *Atti del secondo congresso internazionale di linguistica camito-semitica*, ed. P. Fronzaroli, 151–56. Quaderni di semitistica 5. Florence: Istituto di linguistica e di lingue orientali.

———. 1979.   Early Aramaic Poetry. *JANES (M. M. Bravmann Memorial Volume)* 11:45–51.

———. 1979a.   The Root *šql* in Akkadian, Ugaritic and Aramaic. *UF* 11:325–27.

———. 1980.   Review of *Aramaic Texts from Deir 'Alla,* by J. Hoftijzer and G. van der Kooij. *JSS* 25:248–52.

———. 1981.   Aḥiqar in the Book of Tobit. In *De la Tôrah au Messie: Études d'exégèse et d'herméneutique bibliques offertes à Henri Cazelles pour ses 25 années d'enseignement à l'Institut catholique de Paris, octobre 1979,* ed. M. Carrez, J. Doré and P. Grelot, 329–36. Paris: Desclée.

———. 1981a.   Aramaic Studies and the Bible. In *Congress Volume Vienna 1980,* ed. J. A. Emerton, 110–30. VTSup 32. Leiden: Brill.

———. 1982.   שתי מקראות לאור תקופתן — יחזקאל טז 30 ומלאכי ג 17. *EI (Orlinsky Volume)* 16:56–61.

———. 1982a.   Babylonian-Aramaic Relationships. In *Mesopotamien und seine Nachbarn: Akten des XXV R.A.I.,* ed. H.-J. Nissen and J. Renger, 471–82. Berlin: Reimer.

———. 1982b.   Some Notes on the Arsham Letters. In *Irano-Judaica,* ed. S. Shaked, 4–11. Jerusalem: Ben-Zvi Institute.

———. 1983.   Aramaic *hnṣl* and Some Biblical Passages. In *Meqor Ḥajjim: Festschrift für Georg Molin zu seinem 75 Geburtstag,* ed. I. Seybold, 115–19. Graz: Akademische Druck und Verlagsanstalt.

———. 1983a.   סיבת ציון—ימי שלטון פרס. In הלשון הארמית בתקופה הפרסית, ed. H. Tadmor et al., 224–28. ההיסטוריה של עם ישראל, vol. 1:6. Jerusalem: Alexander Peli.

———. 1984.   A Touch of Eden. In *Orientalia J. Duchesne-Guillemin emerito oblata,* Acta Iranica 2/9, 219–24. Leiden: Brill.

———. 1984a.   *ana urdūti kabāšu* = כבש לעבד. *Studia orientalia* 55/11:257–63.

———. 1984–86.   Notes on the Early Aramaic Lexicon. *OS* 33–35:149–55.

———. 1985.   [Section VI: Discussion.] *BAT,* 369–70.

———. 1985a.   The Meaning of *Tkwnh.* In *Biblical and Related Studies Presented to Samuel Iwry,* ed. A. Kort and S. Morschauser, 81–85. Winona Lake, Ind.: Eisenbrauns.

———. 1985b.   Aramaic in the Achaemenian Empire. In *The Cambridge History of Iran* 698–713. Cambridge: Cambridge Univ. Press.

———. 1986.   An Ancient Treaty Ritual and Its Targumic Echo. In *Salvación en la palabra: Targum-Derash-Berith en memoria del profesor Alejandro Díez Macho,* ed. D. Muñoz León, 391–97. Madrid: Cristiandad.

———. 1986a.   Aspects of Archives in the Achaemenid Period. In *Cuneiform Archives and Libraries,* ed. K. R. Veenhof, 289–95. Publications de l'Institut historique-archéologique néerlandais de Stamboul, 57. Leiden: Nederlands Instituut voor het Nabije Oosten.

———. 1987.   To Praise the Might of Hadad. In *La vie de la Parole: De l'Ancien au Nouveau Testament: Etudes d'exégèse et d'herméneutique bibliques offertes à Pierre Grelot professeur à l'Institut Catholique de Paris* 3–12. Paris: Desclée.

———. 1987a. Aspects of Aramean Religion. In *Ancient Israelite Religion: Essays in Honor of Frank Moore Cross*, ed. P. D. Miller et al., 67–78. Philadelphia: Fortress.

———. 1989. Idiomatic Ancient Aramaic. In *To Touch the Text: Biblical Studies in Honor of Joseph A. Fitzmyer, S.J.*, ed. M. P. Horgan and P. J. Kobelski, 47–51. New York: Crossroad.

———. 1990. Two Proverbs of Ahiqar. In *Lingering Over Words: Studies in Ancient Near Eastern Literature in Honor of William L. Moran*, ed. T. Abusch et al., 195–201. Harvard Semitic Studies 37. Atlanta: Scholars Press.

———. 1990a. The Aramaic Legal Texts of the Achaemenid Period. *Transeuphratène* 3:85–92.

———. 1991. Philological Observations on the Deir 'Alla Inscription. In *BTDAR*, 109–20.

Greenfield, J. C., and A. Shaffer. 1983. Notes on the Akkadian-Aramaic Bilingual Statue from Tell Fekherye. *Iraq* 45:109–16.

———. 1983a. *qlqlt'*, *tubkinnu*, Refuse Tips and Treasure Trove. *Anatolian Studies* 33:123–29.

———. 1985. Notes on the Curse Formulae of the Tell Fekherye Inscription. *RB* 92:47–59.

Greenfield, J. C., and B. Porten. 1974. מכתבי הרמופוליס. *Qadmoniot* 7:121–22.

———. 1982. *The Bisitun Inscription of Darius the Great: Aramaic Version*. Corpus inscriptionum iranicarum I/5. London: Lund Humphries.
Reviews: M Sokoloff 1989.

Greenfield, J. C. See also: J. Naveh, B. Porten, F. Rosenthal, A. Schaffer.

Greengus, S. 1959. The Aramaic Marriage Contracts in the Light of the Ancient Near East and the Later Jewish Materials. M. A. thesis, Univ. of Chicago.

Greenspahn, F. 1988. Review of *Aramaic Texts from North Saqqâra,* by J. B. Segal. *JQR* 78:308–9.

Grelot, P. 1954. Etudes sur le "Papyrus Pascal" d'Éléphantine. *VT* 4:349–84.

———. 1955. Le papyrus pascal d'Éléphantine et le problème du Pentateuque. *VT* 5:250–65.

———. 1956. On the Root עבק/עבצ in Ancient Aramaic and in Ugaritic. *JSS* 1:202–5.

———. 1961. Les proverbes araméens d'Ahiqar. *RB* 68:178–94.

———. 1962. La racine *hwn* en Dt. i 41. *VT* 12:198–201.

———. 1962a. Review of *A Grammar of Biblical Aramaic*, by F. Rosenthal. *RB* 69:280–84.

———. 1964. L'huile de ricin à Éléphantine. *Sem* 14:63–70.

———. 1967. Sur la stèle de Carpentras. *Sem* 17:73–75.

———. 1967a. Le papyrus pascal d'Éléphantine: Nouvel examen. *VT* 17:114–17.

———. 1967b. Le papyrus pascal d'Éléphantine: Essai de restauration. *VT* 17:201–7.

———. 1967c. Le papyrus pascal d'Éléphantine et les lettres d'Hermopolis. *VT* 17:481–83.

———. 1967d. La reconstruction du temple juif d'Éléphantine. *Or* 36:173–77.

———. 1967e. Review of "Le lettere aramaiche di Hermopoli," by E. Bresciani and M. Kamil. *RB* 74:432–37.

———. 1968. Review of *The Aramaic Inscriptions of Sefîre*, by J. A. Fitzmyer. *RB* 75:280–86.

———. 1970. Post Scriptum. *Sem* 20:21–22.

———. 1970a. La communauté juive d'Éléphantine. [Review article: B. Porten, *Archives from Elephantine: The Life of an Ancient Jewish Military Colony*.] *CdE* 45:120–31.

———. 1970b. Essai de restauration du papyrus A.P. 26. *Sem* 20:23–31.

———. 1970c. Le waw d'apodose en araméen d'Égypte. *Sem* 20:33–39.

———. 1971. Études sur les textes araméens d'Éléphantine. *RB* 78:515–44.

———. 1971a. Notes d'onomastique sur les textes araméens d'E'gypte. *Sem* 21:95–117.

———. 1972. *Documents araméens d'Égypte*. Littératures anciennes du Proche-Orient. Paris: Cerf.
Reviews: E. Bresciani 1975; R. Degen 1975: *WO* 8:136; J. A. Fitzmyer 1975; S. A. Kaufman 1973; E. Lipiński 1974; G. Nahon 1974; S. Segert 1975; J. Teixidor 1976; P. Zivie 1978.

———. 1972a. Review of *Lexicon linguae aramaicae Veteris Testamenti documentis antiquis illustratum*, by E. Vogt. *RB* 79:614–17.

———. 1973. Sur un nom de mesure employé en araméen d'Egypte. *Sem* 23:103–11.

———. 1973a. Review of *Aramaic Ritual Texts from Persepolis*, by R. A. Bowman. *RB* 80:595–98.

———. 1974. La Septante de Daniel IV et son substrat sémitique. *RB* 81:5–23.

———. 1974a. Le chapitre V de Daniel dans la Septante. *Sem* 24:45–66.

———. 1975. Review of *Jews of Elephantine and Arameans of Syene (Fifth Century B.C.E.)*, by B. Porten in collaboration with J. C. Greenfield. *RB* 82:288–92.

———. 1977. Review of *Altaramäische Grammatik*, by S. Segert. *RB* 84:448–53.

———. 1978. Daniel VII, 9–10 et le livre d'Hénoch. *Sem* 28:59–83.

———. 1979. L'orchestre de Daniel iii 5, 7, 10, 15. *VT* 29:23–38.

———. 1985. L'Écriture sur le mur (Daniel 5). In *Mélanges bibliques et orientaux en l'honneur de M. Mathias Delcor*, ed. A. Caquot, et al., 199–207. AOAT 215.

———. 1986. Eléphantine: Araméens et Juifs en Egypte. *MDB* 45:32–35.

———. 1986a. Review of *Textbook of Aramaic Documents from Ancient Egypt I: Letters*, by B. Porten and A. Yardeni. *RB* 95:294–99.

Gressmann, H., et al. 1926. *Altorientalische Texte zum Alten Testament*. Altorientalische Texte und Bilder zum Alten Testament. 2d ed. Berlin/Leipzig: De Gruyter.

Grill, S. 1953. Die drei Männer im Feuer (Dan 3). *Oberrheinisches Pastoralblatt* 54:22–27.

Grimme, A. 1914. Review of *Zur Geschichte der Juden von Elephantine*, by H. Anneler. *OLZ* 17:406–7.

Grimme, H. 1909. Review of *Inscriptions sémitiques de la Syrie, de la Mésopotamie, et de la région de Mossoul*, by H. Pognon. *OLZ* 12:13–18.

———. 1911. Die jüdische Kolonie von Elephantine in neuer Beleuchtung. *ThGl* 3:793–800.

———. 1911a. Bemerkungen zu den aramäischen Achikarsprüchen. *OLZ* 14:529–40.

———. 1912. Die Jahotriade von Elephantine. *OLZ* 15:11–17.

Grintz, J. M. 1966. The Treaty of Joshua with the Gibeonites. *JAOS* 86:113–26.

Gropp, D. 1986. The Samaria Papyri from Wâdi ed–Dâliyeh: The Slave Sales. Ph.D. diss., Harvard Univ.

———. 1990. The Language of the Samaria Papyri: A Preliminary Study. In *Sopher Mahir: Northwest Studies Presented to Stanislav Segert*, ed. E. M. Cook, 169–87 (= *Maarav* 5–6). Winona Lake, Ind.: Eisenbrauns.

Gropp, D., and T. J. Lewis. 1985. Notes on Some Problems in the Aramaic Text of the Hadd-Yith'i Bilingual. *BASOR* 259:45–61.

Grossfeld, B. 1979. The Relationship between Biblical Hebrew ברח and נוס and Their Corresponding Aramaic Equivalents in the Targumim אזל, אפך, ערק: A Preliminary Study in Aramaic-Hebrew Lexicography. *ZAW* 91:107–23.

Grossmann, P. 1980. *Elephantine II: Kirche und spätantike Hausanlagen im Chnum-tempelhof—Beschreibung und typologische Untersuchung.* Archäologische Veröffentlichungen 25. Mainz: P. von Zabern.

Grotefund, G. F. 1839. Urkunden in babylonischer Keilschrift, zweiter Beitrag. *Zeits. f. d. Kunde d. Morgenlandes* 2:177–324.

Gruenthaner, M. J. 1946. The Four Empires of Daniel. *CBQ* 8:72–82; 201–12.

———. 1949. The Last King of Babylon. *CBQ* 11:406–27.

Gubel, E. 1990. Le sceaux de Menaḥem et l'iconographie royale sigillaire. *Sem* 38/1:167–70; pl. xxvi.

———. See also: P. Bordreuil.

Guglielmo, A. de. 1949. Dan. 5:25—An Example of a Double Literal Sense. *CBQ* 11:202–6.

Guillaume, A. 1920–21. Isaiah xliv. 5 in the Light of the Elephantine Papyri. *ExpTim* 32:377–79.

Gunkel, H. 1895. *Schöpfung und Chaos in Urzeit und Endzeit.* Göttingen: Vandenhoeck & Ruprecht.

———. 1911. The Jâhû Temple in Elephantine. Translated by M. Gurney. *Expositor* 8/1:20–39.

Gunneweg, A. H. J. 1982. Die aramäische und die hebräische Erzählung über die nachexilische Restauration — ein Vergleich. *ZAW* 94:299–302.

Gusmani, R. 1975. In margine alla trilingue licio-greco-aramaica di Xanthos. *Incontri linguistici* 2:61–75.

———. 1977. Randbemerkungen zur Trilingue von Xanthos. In *XIX. Deutscher Orientalistentag . . .*, ed. W. Voigt, 52–54. *ZDMG* Supplement 3/1. Wiesbaden: Steiner.

———. 1979. Su due termini della trilingue di Xanthos. In *Mediterranea studia Piero Meriggi dicata*, 225–34. Pavia: Aurora Edizioni.

Gutesmann, S. 1907. Sur le calendrier en usage chez les Israélites au ve siècle avant notre ère. *REJ* 53:194–200.

Gutmann, J. 1928–34. Elephantine. In *Encyclopaedia Judaica: Das Judentum in Geschichte und Gegenwart*, ed. J. Klatzkin, 6:446–52 + 1 pl. Berlin: Verlag Eschkol A.-G.

————. 1971–72. Ahikar, Book of. In *Encyclopaedia Judaica*, 2:460–61.

Guyard, S. 1879. Notes de lexicographie assyrienne. *JA* 7/13:435–55.

Haag, E. 1987. Die drei Männer im Feuer nach Dan 3, 1–30. *Trier theologische Zeitschrift* 96:21–50.

Habachi, L. 1975–86. Elephantine. In *Lexikon der Ägyptologie*, ed. W. Helck and E. Otto, 1217–25. Wiesbaden: Harrassowitz.

Habel, N. C. 1972. "Yahweh, Maker of Heaven and Earth": A Study in Tradition Criticism. *JBL* 91:321–37.

Hackett, J. 1984. The Dialect of the Plaster Text from Tell Deir ʿAlla. *Or* 53:57–65.

————. 1984a. *The Balaam Text from Deir ʿAllā*. HSM 31. Chico, Cal.: Scholars Press.
Reviews: G. I. Davies 1986; J. A. Emerton 1986; W. J. Fulco 1986: *CBQ* 48:109–10. W. Hermann 1986; A. Lemaire 1984.

————. 1986. Some Observations on the Balaam Tradition at Deir ʿAllā. *BA* 49:216–22.

————. 1991. Response to Baruch Levine and André Lemaire. In *BTDAR*, 73–84.

Haddad, G. 1953. Ḥikmat al wazīr Aḥîqār [The wisdom of the vizier Ahikar]. *Les annales archéologiques de Syrie: Revue d'archéologie et d'histoire syriennes* 3:11–28.

Hager, J. 1801. Dissertation on the newly discovered Babylonian Inscriptions. London: n.p. German translation, 1982. Weimar: Comtoirs.

Hahn, I. 1981. Periöken und Periökenbesitz in Lykien. *Klio* 63:51–61.

Haines, B. L. 1967. A Paleographical Study of Aramaic Inscriptions Antedating 500 B.C.. Ph.D. diss., Harvard Univ.

Halévy, J. 1874. *Mélanges d'épigraphie et d'archéologie sémitiques*. Paris: Imprimerie Nationale.

————. 1878. Aus einem Briefe des Hrn. J. Halévy an Prof. Fleischer. *ZDMG* 32:206–7.

————. 1884. [Report]. *CRAIBL*: 332.

————. 1884a. Découvertes épigraphiques en Arabie. *REJ* 9:1–20.

————. 1885. Séance du 11 décembre 1885. *JA* 8/6:551–52.

————. 1886. Encore un mot sur l'inscription de Teima. *REJ* 12:111–13.

————. 1890. Notes sur quelques textes araméens du Corpus. *REJ* 21:224–40.

————. 1891. Procès-verbal de la séance générale du 26 juin 1891. *JA* 8/18:5–9.

————. 1893. Deux inscriptions sémitiques de Zindjîrlî. *RevSém* 1:77–90.

————. 1893a. Une inscription araméenne de Cilicie. *RevSém* 1:183–86.

————. 1893–94. Les deux inscriptions hétéennes de Zindjîrlî. *RevSém* 1:138–67, 218–58, 319–36; 2:25–60.

————. 1894. Communication faite à la Société Asiatique le 10 novembre 1893. *RevSém* 2:167–71.

————. 1895. Notes épigraphiques. *RevSém* 3:183–87.

————. 1895a. Un bas-relief à inscription araméenne de Barrekoub. *RevSém* 3:392–94.

————. 1895b. La première inscription araméenne de Barrekoub ou A1. *RevSém* 3:394–95.

————. 1896. Les deux stèles de Nerab. *RevSém* 4:279–84.

————. 1896a. La première inscription de Bar-Rekoub revue et corrigée. *RevSém* 4:185–87.

————. 1896b. Nouvelles remarques sur les inscriptions de Nêrab. *RevSém* 4:369–73.

————. 1897. Le texte définitif de l'inscription architecturale araméenne de Barrekoub. *RevSém* 5:84–91.

————. 1897a. Un dernier mot sur les inscriptions de Nêrab. *RevSém* 5:189–90.

————. 1898. Une inscription araméenne d'Arabissos. *RevSém* 6:271–73.

————. 1899. Nouvel Examen des inscriptions de Zindjirli. *RevSém* 7:333–55.

————. 1903. Un document judéo-araméen d'Eléphantine. I. *RevSém* 11:250–58.

————. 1904. Documents judéo-araméens d'Éléphantine. II: Ostraka. *RevSém* 12:55–66.

————. 1904a. Nouvel examen du papyrus égypto-araméen de la Bibliothèque impériale de Strasbourg. *RevSém* 12:67–78.

————. 1906. Encore l'inscription araméenne d'Éléphantine. *RevSém* 14:278–80.

————. 1908. Inscription araméenne d'Éléphantine. *RevSém* 16:95–99, 224–40.

————. 1908a. Inscription de Zakir, roi de Hamat, découverte par M. H. Pognon. *RevSém* 16:243–46.

————. 1908b. Une inscription bornaire araméenne de Cilicie. *RevSém* 16:434–37.

————. 1908c. Bibliographie. *RevSém* 16:255–58.

————. 1908d. Nouvelles remarques sur l'inscription de Zakir. *RevSém* 16:357–76.

————. 1911. Lectures erronées à corriger: Avis aux Suméristes. *RevSém* 19:340–43.

————. 1911a. Les nouveaux papyrus d'Éléphantine. *RevSém* 19:473–97.

————. 1912. Les nouveaux papyrus d'Éléphantine. *RevSém* 20:31–78, 153–77.

————. 1912a. L'inscription du roi Kalumu. *JA* 10/19:408–10.

————. 1912b. Opinion de M. Ed. Meyer sur la version araméenne de l'inscription de Darius Ier. *RevSém* 20:178–84.

————. 1912c. L'inscription de Darius Ier à Behistun: Texte araméen. *RevSém* 20:252–62.

————. 1912d. Un ostracon araméen relatif à la Pâque des Juifs d'Éléphantine. *RevSém* 20:263–64.

————. 1912e. La pâque à Éléphantine. *JA* 10/19:622–23.

————. 1913. Recherches de M. Th. Nöldeke sur le roman d'Achikar. *RevSém* 21:339–49.

Haller, A. von. See: T. Nöldeke.

Haller, M. 1920–21. Das Alter von Daniel 7. *Theologische Studien und Kritiken* 93:83–87.

————. 1925. *Das Judentum: Geschichtsschreibung, Prophetie und Gesetzgebung nach den Exil*. Die Schriften des Alten Testaments in Auswahl neu übersetzt und für die Gegenwart erklärt. Göttingen: Vandenhoeck & Ruprecht.

Hallock, R. T. 1950. New Light from Persepolis. *JNES* 9:237–52.

————. 1969. *Persepolis Fortification Tablets*. OIP 92. Chicago: Univ. of Chicago Press.

Halpern, B. 1987. Dialect Distribution in Canaan and the Deir Alla Inscriptions. In *"Working with No Data": Semitic and Egyptian Studies Presented to Thomas O. Lambdin*, ed. D. M. Golomb and S. T. Hollis, 119–39. Winona Lake, Ind.: Eisenbrauns.

Hamaker, H. A. 1822. *Diatribe philologico-critica.* Leiden: Leichtmans.

———. 1828. *Miscellanea phoenicia.* Leiden: Leichtmans.

Hamilton, G. J. See: W. E. Aufrecht.

Hamilton, R. W. See: R. Campbell Thompson.

Hammershaimb, E. 1955. To nye samlinger aramaiske dokumenter fra 5. årh. f. Kr. [Two new collections of Aramaic documents from the 5th. cent. B.C.] *DTT* 18:129–34.

———. 1957. Some Observations on the Aramaic Elephantine Papyri. *VT* 7:17–34.

———. 1962. Om jødisk bosaettelse uden for Palaestina i gammeltestamentlig tid [About Jewish settlements outside Palestine in Old Testament times]. *DTT* 25:36–47.

———. 1968. Some Remarks on the Aramaic Letters from Hermopolis. *VT* 18:265–67.

———. 1971. De aramaiske papyri frå Hermopolis [The Aramaic papyri from Hermopolis]. *DTT* 34:81–104.

———. 1977. De aramaiske indskrifter frå undgravningerne i Deir 'Allā [The Aramaic inscriptions from the excavations at Deir 'Allā]. *DTT* 40:217–42.

Hammond, P. C. 1957. A Note on Two Seal Impressions from Tell Es-Sulṭan. *PEQ* 89:68–69, pl. XVI.

———. 1957a. Correspondence. *PEQ* 89:145.

———. 1957b. A Note on a Seal Impression from Tell es-Sulṭân. *BASOR* 147:37–39.

Hanfmann, G. M. A. 1966. The New Stelae from Daskylion. *BASOR* 184:10–13.

Hanfmann, G. M. A., ed. 1983. *Sardis from Prehistoric to Roman Times.* Cambridge, Mass: Harvard Univ. Press.

Hanhart, R. 1967. Die Heiligen des Höchsten. In *Hebräische Wortforschung: Festschrift zum 80. Geburtstag von Walter Baumgartner*, ed. B. Hartmann et al., 90–101. VTSup 16.

Hanson, R. S. 1968. Aramaic Funerary and Boundary Inscriptions from Asia Minor. *BASOR* 192:3–11.

Harding, L. See: H. Torczyner.

Harmatta, J. 1954. Elamica I. *Acta Linguistica Hungarica* 4:287–308.

———. 1963. Das Problem der Kontinuität im frühhellenistischen Ägypten. *AAASH* 11:199–213.

Harrington, D. J. 1972. Review of *Lexicon linguae aramaicae Veteris Testamenti documentis antiquis illustratum*, by E. Vogt. *CBQ* 34:394–95.

Harris, J. R., A. S. Lewis, and F. C. Conybeare. 1913. The Story of Aḥiḳar. In *The Apocrypha and Pseudepigrapha of the Old Testament in English*, ed. R. H. Charles, 715–84. Oxford: Clarendon.

Harris, J. R. See also: F. C. Conybeare.

Hartman, L. F. 1968. Review of *The Aramaic Inscriptions of Sefîre*, by J. A. Fitzmyer. *CBQ* 30:256–60.

Hartman, L. F., and A. A. Di Lella. 1978. *The Book of Daniel.* AB 23. Garden City, N. Y.: Doubleday.

Hartmann, M. 1908. אלור. *OLZ* 11:341–42.

Hasel, G. F. 1975. The Identity of "The Saints of the Most High" in Daniel 7. *Bib* 56:173–92.

———. 1981. The Book of Daniel: Evidences Relating to Persons and Chronology. *AUSS* 19:37–49.

———. 1981a. The Book of Daniel and Matters of Language: Evidences Relating to Names, Words, and the Aramaic Language. *AUSS* 19:211–25.

Hawkins, J. D. 1980–83. KTK. In *RlA* 6:254–56.

———. 1982. The Neo-Hittite States in Syria and Anatolia. In *The Cambridge Ancient History*, 2nd ed., ed. I. E. S. Edwards et al., 372–441. Cambridge: Cambridge Univ. Press.

Hayes, J. P., and J. Hoftijzer. 1970. Notae Hermopolitanae. *VT* 20:98–106.

Head, B. V. 1911. *Historia Numorum*. Oxford: Clarendon.

Healey, J. F. 1983. Phoenician and the Spread of Aramaic. In *Atti del I congresso de studi fenici e punici*, 663–66. Rome: Consiglio Nazionale delle Ricerche.

———. 1989. Ancient Aramaic Culture and the Bible. *Aram* 1:31–37.

Healey, J. P. 1984. The Archaic Aramaic Inscriptions from Zinjirli. Ph.D. diss., Harvard Univ.

Helck, W. 1975. Aramäer. In *Lexikon der Ägyptologie*, ed. W. Helck and E. Otto, 1:361. Wiesbaden: Harrassowitz.

Held, M. 1968. The Root *ZBL/SBL* in Akkadian, Ugaritic and Biblical Hebrew. *JAOS* 88:90–96.

Heltzer, M. 1958. Nadpis' Ben-Adada I, carja Damaska i mešdunarodnye otnošenija v perednei Azii v načale IX v. do N. E. [The inscription of Ben-Adad I, ruler of Damascus, and international relations in the Near East at the beginning of the 9th cent. B.C.E.] *Epigrafika Vostoka* 12:16–22.

———. 1971. Some North-west Semitic Epigraphic Gleanings from the XI–VI Centuries B.C. *AION* 31:183–98.

———. 1978. Eighth Century B. C. Inscriptions from Kalakh (Nimrud). *PEQ* 110:3–9.

———. 1981. *The Suteans*. Seminario di studi asiatici ser. minor, vol. 13. Naples: Istituto universitario orientale.

———. 1982. The Inscription on the Nimrud Bronze Bowl No. 5 (BM. 91303). *PEQ* 114:1–6.

———. 1983. An Old-Aramean Seal-Impression and Some Problems of the History of the Kingdom of Damascus. In *Arameans, Aramaic and the Aramaic Literary Tradition*, ed. M. Sokoloff, 9–13. Ramat-Gan: Bar-Ilan Univ. Press.

———. 1989. The Tell el-Mazār Inscription No. 7 and Some Historical and Literary Problems of the Vth Satrapy. *Transeuphratène* 1:111–18.

Hempel, J. 1927. Elephantine-Urkunden. *RGG*[2] 2:100–102.

Hempel, J., and H. Bauer. 1932. Zeitschriftenschau: *Mélanges de l'Université Saint-Joseph*. Beyrouth (Liban) XV (1930). *ZAW* 50:178–83.

Hennequin, L. 1934. Éléphantine (La colonie militaire juive d'). *Dictionnaire de la Bible, Supplément* 2.962–1032 + 2 pls.

Henning, W. 1935. Arabisch ḫarāǧ. *Or* 4:291–93. Reprinted in *Acta iranica (W.B. Henning, Selected Papers I)* 14 (1977): 355–57.

———. 1949–51. The Aramaic Inscription of Asoka Found in Lampāka. *BSOAS* 13:80–88 + 2 pls. Reprinted in *Acta iranica (W.B. Henning, Selected Papers II)* 15 (1977): 331–38.

———. 1958. Mitteliranisch. In *Iranistik*, 20–130. Handbuch der Orientalistik, ed. B. Spuler, part 1, vol. 4/1. Leiden: Brill.

———. 1968. Ein persischer Titel im Altaramäischen. In *In Memoriam Paul Kahle*, ed. M. Black and G. Fohrer, 138–45. BZAW 103. Berlin: Töpelmann. Reprinted in *Acta iranica (W.B. Henning, Selected Papers)* 15 (1977): 659–66.

Henninger, I. 1927. *Hebräische Archäologie*. 3rd ed. Leipzig.

Henshaw, R. A. 1967–68. The Office of Šaknu in Neo-Assyrian Times. *JAOS* 87:517–25; 88:461–83.

Herdner, A. 1946–48. Dédicace araméenne au dieu Melqart. *Syria* 25:329–30.

Hermann, W. 1986. Review of *The Balaam Text from Deir ʿAlla*, by J. A. Hackett. *OLZ* 81:473–75.

Herr, L. G. 1978. *The Scripts of Ancient Northwest Semitic Seals*. HSM 18. Missoula, Mont.: Scholars Press.
Reviews: F. Israel 1986; J. Naveh 1980.

———. 1980. The Formal Scripts of Iron Age Transjordan. *BASOR* 238:21–34.

Herrmann, G. 1989. The Nimrud Ivories, 1: The Flame and Frond School. *Iraq* 51:85–109.

Herz, N. 1907–8. The Elephantinê Papyri. *ExpTim* 19:333.

———. 1907–8a. The New Aramaic Papyri. *ExpTim* 19:522.

———. 1908–9. Aramaic Papyri Discovered at Assuan. *ExpTim* 20:232–33.

Herzfeld, E. 1926. Reisebericht. *ZDMG* 80:225–84.

———. 1927–28. A New Asokan Inscription from Taxila. *Epigraphia indica* 19:251–53.

———. 1933. Summa imis confundere. *AMI* 5:143–48.

———. 1935. *Archaeological History of Iran*. Schweich Lectures for 1934. London: British Academy.

———. 1937. Die Silberschüsseln Artaxerxes' des I. und die goldene Fundamenturkunde des Ariaramnes. *AMI* 8:5–57.

———. 1938. *Altpersische Inschriften*. AMI Ergänzungsband 1. Berlin: D. Reimer.

———. 1947. *Zoroaster and His World*. Princeton: Princeton Univ. Press.

Hestrin, R., and M. Dayagi-Mendels. 1979. *Inscribed Seals: First Temple Period: Hebrew, Ammonite, Moabite, Phoenician, and Aramaic*. Jerusalem: Israel Museum.

Hestrin, R. et al., eds. 1973. *Inscriptions Reveal: Documents from the Time of the Bible, the Mishna and the Talmud*. 2d ed. Jerusalem: Israel Museum.

Hill, G. F. 1900. *Catalogue of the Greek Coins of Lycaonia, Isauria, and Cilicia*. A Catalogue of the Greek Coins in the British Museum 21. London: British Museum, Dept. of Coins and Medals. Reprint: Bologna: Arnaldo Forni, 1964.

———. 1914. *Catalogue of the Greek Coins of Palestine (Galilee, Samaria, and Judaea)*. A Catalogue of the Greek Coins in the British Museum 27. London: British Museum, Dept.

of Coins and Medals. Reprint: Bologna: Arnaldo Forni, 1964.

———. 1922. *Catalogue of Greek Coins of Arabia, Mesopotamia and Persia.* A Catalogue of the Greek Coins in the British Museum 28. London: British Museum, Dept. of Coins and Medals. Reprint: Bologna: A. Forni, 1965.

Hillers, D. R. 1964. *Treaty-Curses and the Old Testament Prophets.* BibOr 16. Rome: Pontifical Biblical Institute.
Reviews: J. M. Wevers 1966: *BO* 23:75–76.

———. 1964a. A Note on Some Treaty Terminology in the Old Testament. *BASOR* 176:46–47.

———. 1971. A Hebrew Cognate of *unuššuΓunt* in Is. 33:8. *HTR* 64:257–59.

———. 1979. Redemption in Letters 6 and 2 from Hermopolis. *UF* 11:379–82.

———. 1985. A Difficult Curse in Aqht (19 [1 Aqht] 3.152–154). In *Biblical and Related Studies Presented to Samuel Iwry*, ed. A. Kort and S. Morschauser, 105–7. Winona Lake, Ind.: Eisenbrauns.

———. 1990. *Rite*: Ceremonies of Law and Treaty in the Ancient Near East. In *Religion and Law: Biblical-Judaic and Islamic Perspectives*, ed. E. B. Firmage et al., 351–64. Winona Lake, Ind.: Eisenbrauns.

Hilprecht, H. V., and A. T. Clay. 1898. *Business Documents of Murashû Sons of Nippur Dated in the Reign of Artaxerxes I.* The Babylonian Expedition of the University of Pennsylvania IX. Philadelphia: Univ. of Pennsylvania Museum.

Hinnells, J. R. 1973. Religion at Persepolis. *Religion* 3:157–60.

Hinz, W. 1960–61. Zu den Persepolis-Täfelchen. *ZDMG* 110:236–51.

———. 1974. Die Behistan-Inschrift des Darius in ihrer ursprünglichen Fassung. *AMI* 7:121–34, pls. 29–30.

———. 1975. Zu den Mörsern und Stosseln aus Persepolis. *Acta Iranica* 4:371–85.

———. 1988. Grosskönig Darius und sein Untertan. In *A Green Leaf: Papers in Honour of Professor J. P. Asmussen*, 473–81. Acta Iranica 28/2: Hommages et opera minora 12. Leiden: Brill.

Hirschberg, A. S. 1921. The Discovery of Papyri at Elephantine and at Syene [in Hebrew]. *Hatkufa* 8:339–68.

Hitti, P. K. 1951. *History of Syria Including Lebanon and Palestine.* New York: Macmillan.

Hitzig, F. 1871. Epigraphische Miscellen. *ZDMG* 25:251–55.

Hoberman, R. D. 1985. The Phonology of Pharyngeals and Pharyngealization in pre-Modern Aramaic. *JAOS* 105:221–31.

Hoffmann, G. 1896. Aramäische Inschriften aus Nêrab bei Aleppo: Neue und alte Götter. *ZA* 11:207–92.

———. 1896a. Zur Bauinschrift des Barrekab. *ZA* 11:317–22.

———. 1907. Bemerkungen zu den Papyrusurkunden aus Elephantine (aus einem Briefe an D. H. Müller). *WZKM* 21:413–15.

Hoftijzer, J. 1957–58. Kanttekeningen bij het Onderzoek van de westsemitische Epigrafie. *JEOL* 15:112–25.

———. 1959. Notae Aramaicae. *VT* 9:312–18.

————. 1962. Ein Papyrusfragment aus El-Hibeh. *VT* 12:341–42.

————. 1964. Review of *Aramäische Chrestomathie*, by J. J. Koopmans. *BO* 21:71–72.

————. 1964a. Review of *Introduction to the Law of the Aramaic Papyri*, by R. Yaron. *BO* 21:220–22.

————. 1973. De ontcijfering van Deir-'Alla Teksten. *Oosters Genootschap in Nederland* 5:111–34.

————. 1976. The Prophet Balaam in a 6th Century Aramaic Inscription. *BA* 39:11–17.

————. 1976a. De aramese teksten uit Deir 'Alla. *Phoenix* 22:84–91, figs. 41–42.

————. 1977–78. Note on a Newly Found Text Fragment on a Bowl from Deir 'Alla. ADAJ 22:69, 79–80, 215, pl. XXIX.

————. 1983. De Hermopolis-Papyri: Arameese brieven uit Egypte (5ᵉ eeuw v. Chr.) In *Schrijvend verleden: Documenten uit het oude Nabije Oosten vertaald en toegelicht*, ed. K. R. Veenhof, 107–19. Leiden: Ex Oriente Lux.

————. 1986. Aramäische Prophetien: Die Inschrift von Deir 'Alla. In *Religiöse Texte*, ed. O. Kaiser, 138–48. TUAT 2. Gütersloh: G. Mohn.

————. 1989. Six Shekels and a Half (Notes on Hermopolis Papyri 2 and 6). *Studi epigrafici e linguistici* 6:117–22.

————. 1991. What Did the Gods Say? Remarks on the First Combination of the Deir 'Alla-Plaster Texts. In *BTDAR*, 121–42.

Hoftijzer, J., and G. van der Kooij. 1976. *Aramaic Texts from Deir 'Alla*. With contributions from H. J. Franken, V. R. Mehra, J. Voskuil, and J. A. Mosk. Documenta et monumenta orientis antiqui 19. Leiden: Brill.

Reviews: J. A. Fitzmyer 1978; J. C. Greenfield 1980; S. A. Kaufman 1980; O. Loretz 1978; J. Naveh 1979; D. Pardee 1979; E. Puech 1985; J. B. Segal 1978; S. Segert 1980; G. Wallis 1978.

Hoftijzer, J., and G. van der Kooij, eds. 1991. *The Balaam Text from Deir 'Alla Re-Evaluated: Proceedings of the International Symposium held at Leiden 21–24 August 1989.* Leiden: Brill.

Hoftijzer, J., and P. W. Pestman. 1962. Hereditary Rights as Laid Down in the Marriage Contract Krael. 2. *BO* 19:216–19.

Hoftijzer, J. See also: P. H. L. Eggermont, C.-F. Jean, J. P. Hayes.

Hogarth, D. G. 1920. *Hittite Seals with Particular Reference to the Ashmolean Collection.* Oxford: Clarendon.

Hogg, H. H. 1901. North-Semitic Epigraphy. [Review article: M. Lidzbarski, *Handbuch der nordsemitischen Epigraphik*.] *AJSL* 18:1–8.

Holma, H. 1918. Zum Verständnis des Pap. Sachau Nr. 2. *OLZ* 21:204.

Holtzmann, O. 1912. Review of *Chronological Notes from the Aramaic Papyri*, by M. Sprengling. *TLZ* 37:166–67.

Homès-Fredericq, D. 1978. The Collections of the Ancient Near East in the Royal Museum of Brussels. *Akkadica* 9:44–45.

————. 1986. Coquillages et glyptique araméenne. In *Insight Through Images: Studies in Honor of Edith Porada*, ed. Marilyn Kelly-Buccellati, 111–18. Malibu, Cal.: Undena.

Hommel, F. 1899. Assyriological Notes. *PSBA* 21:115–39.

Honeyman, A. M. 1960. Two Votaries of Han-'Ilat. *JNES* 19:40–41.

Honigmann, E. 1923–24. Historische Topographie von Nordsyrien im Altertum. *ZDPV* 46:149–93; 47:1–64.

Honroth, W., O. Rubensohn, and F. Zucker. 1909–10. Bericht über die Ausgrabungen auf Elephantine in den Jahren 1906–1908. *ZÄS* 46:14–61 + 9 pls.

Hontheim, J. 1907. Die neu entdeckten jüdisch-aramäischen Papyri von Assuan. *BZ* 5:225–34.

———. 1908. Zu den neuesten jüdisch-aramäischen Papyri aus Elefantine. *BZ* 6:245–61.

Hoonacker, A. van. 1909. Les troubles d'Éléphantine en 411 av. J.C. d'après les papyrus Euting et Sachau. *ZA* 23:187–96.

———. 1909a. Die rechtliche Stellung des jüdischen Tempels in Elephantine gegenüber den Einrichtungen des Alten Testamentes. *ThGl* 1:438–47.

———. 1915. *Une communauté judéo-araméenne à Éléphantine, en Égypte, aux VIe et Ve siècles av. J.-C.* The Schweich Lectures 1914. London: Oxford Univ. Press for the British Academy.

Horn, S. H. 1962. An Early Aramaic Seal with an Unusual Design. *BASOR* 167:16–18.

———. 1968. Where and When Was the Aramaic Saqqara Papyrus Written? *AUSS* 6:29–45.

Horn, S. H., and L. H. Wood. 1954. The Fifth-Century Jewish Calendar at Elephantine. *JNES* 13:1–20 + 1 pl.

Hospers, J. H. 1948. *Twee problemen betreffende het Aramees van het boek Daniël.* [Inaugural Lecture, Rijksuniversiteit te Groningen].

Hrouda, B. 1962. In *Tell Halaf, vierter Band: Die Kleinfunde aus historischer Zeit.* Berlin: De Gruyter.

Huber, C. 1884. Inscriptions recueillies dans l'Arabie centrale 1878–1882. *Bulletin de la Société de Géographie* 7/5:289–303.

Huehnergard, J. 1983. Asseverative *la and Hypothetical *lu/law in Semitic. *JAOS* 103:569–93.

———. 1986. Review of *La statue de Tell Fekherye*, by A. Abou Assaf et al. *BASOR* 61:91–95.

———. 1987. Review of *Dialect Geography of Syria-Palestine, 1000–586 B.C.E.*, by W. R. Garr. *JBL* 106:529–33.

———. 1987a. The Feminine Plural Jussive in Old Aramaic. *ZDMG* 137:266–77.

———. 1991. Remarks on the Classification of the Northwest Semitic Languages. In *BTDAR*, 282–93.

Huffmon, H. B. 1966. The Treaty Background of Hebrew *yāda'*. *BASOR* 181:31–37.

Hug, V. forthcoming. *Altaramäische Grammatik der Texte des 7. und 6. Jr.s v. Chr.* Heidelberger Studien zum Alten Orient 4. Heidelberg: Heidelberger Orientverlag.

Hughes, G. R., R. M. Engberg, and W. H. Dubberstein. 1938. The Oriental Institute Archeological Report on the Near East. *AJSL* 55:319–36.

Hultzsch, E. 1925. *Inscriptions of Asoka.* Corpus Inscriptionum Indicarum 1. Oxford: Clarendon.

Humbach, H. 1969. Additional Notes on the Aramaic Inscription of Taxila. *Münchener Studien zur Sprachwissenschaft* 26:39–42.

———. 1969a. Die aramäische Inschrift von Taxila. *Abhandlungen der Akademie der Wissenschaft und der Literatur, Mainz, Phil.-Hist. Klasse* 1:1–12 + 1 pl.
Reviews: H. J. W. Drijvers 1973.

———. 1971. Indien und Ostiran zur Zeit des Aśoka. *AAASH* 19:53–58.

———. 1972. Late Imperial Aramaic and Early Pahlavi. *Münchener Studien zur Sprachwissenschaft* 30:47–53.

———. 1974. Arameo-Iranian and Pahlavi. In *Commémoration Cyrus: Actes du Congrès de Shiraz 1971 et autres études rédigées à l'occasion du 2500 anniversaire de la fondation de l'empire perse, Hommage Universel, II* 237–43. Acta Iranica 1/2. Leiden: Brill.

———. 1979. Buddhistische Moral in aramäo-iranischem und griechischem Gewande. In *Prolegomena to the Sources on the History of Pre-Islamic Central Asia*, ed. J. Harmatta, 189–96. Budapest: Akadémiai Kiadó.

———. 1981. Die aramäischen Nymphen von Xanthos. *Die Sprache* 27/1:30–32.

———. See also: G. D. Davary.

Hurd, J. C. See: W. E. Aufrecht.

Hurvitz, A. 1968. The Chronological Significance of "Aramaisms" in Biblical Hebrew. *IEJ* 18:234–40.

———. 1969. Review of *Die lexikalischen und grammatikalischen Aramaismen im alttestamentlichen Hebräisch*, by M. Wagner. *IEJ* 19:182–83.

———. 1972. ‏בין לשון ללשון: לתולדות לשון המקרא בימי בית שני‎. Jerusalem: Mosad Bialik.

———. 1982. The History of a Legal Formula: $k\bar{o}l$ $^{a}\check{s}er$- $\d{h}\bar{a}p\bar{e}\d{s}$ $^{c}\bar{a}\acute{s}\bar{a}h$ (Psalms cxv 3, cxxxv 6). *VT* 32:257–67.

———. 1982a. *A Linguistic Study of the Relationship between the Priestly Source and the Book of Ezekiel*. Cahiers de la Revue Biblique, vol. 20. Paris: Gabalda.

Huss, W. 1977. Der 'König der Könige' und der 'Herr der Könige'. *ZDPV* 93:131–40.

Husser, J.-M. 1991. Deux observations à propos des rapports entre le texte de Deir 'Allā (combinaison I) et la Bible. In *BTDAR*, 273–81.

Hyatt, J. P. 1939. The Deity Bethel and the Old Testament. *JAOS* 59:81–97.

Ibrahim, M. M., and G. van der Kooij. 1991. The Archaeology of Deir 'Alla Phase IX. In *BTDAR*, 16–29.

Ibrahim, M. M. See also: H. J. Franken.

Ikeda, Y. 1979. Royal Cities and Fortified Cities. *Iraq* 41:75–87.

Imhoof-Blumer, F., and O. Keller. 1889. *Tier- und Pflanzenbilder auf Münzen und Gemmen des klassischen Altertums*. Leipzig: Teubner.

Ingholt, H. 1940. *Rapport préliminaire sur sept campagnes de fouilles à Hama en Syrie (1932–38)*. Det kgl. Danske Videnskabernes Selskab: Archaeologisk-kunsthistoriske Meddelelser III/1. Copenhagen: Munksgaard.

Israel, F. 1983. L'iscrizione di Tell Fekherye e l'antropologia biblica. In *Atti della settimana: Sangue e antropologia biblica nella letteratura cristiana (Roma, 29 novembre–4 dicembre 1982)*, ed. F. Vattioni, 79–81. Centro studi sanguis Christi 3. Rome: Pia Unione

Preziosissimo Sangue.

———. 1983a. Osservazioni linguistiche all'iscrizione di Tell Fekheriye. *Atti del sodalizio glottologico milanese* 24:78–83.

———. 1986. Observations on Northwest Semitic Seals. [Review article: L. G. Herr 1978.] *Or* 55:70–77.

———. 1987. Les sceaux ammonites. *Syria* 64:141–46.

———. 1991. Reflexions methodologiques sur le classement linguistique de DAPT. In *BTDAR*, 305–17.

Isserlin, B. S. J. 1988. Review of *Dialect Geography of Syria-Palestine, 1000–586 B.C.E.*, by W. R. Garr. *PEQ* 120:72–74.

Itō, G. 1967. On the Iranism Underlying the Aramaic Inscription of Aśoka. In *Yádnáme-ye Jan Rypka*, 21–27. Prague: Academia; The Hague: Mouton.

———. 1976. Syenian *frataraka* and Persian *fratarak*: New Iranian Elements in Ancient Aramaic. *Orient* (Tokyo) 12:47–66.

———. 1977. A New Interpretation of Aśokan Inscriptions, Taxila and Kandahar I. *Studia Iranica* 6:151–61.

———. 1979. Aśokan Inscriptions: Laghmān I and II. *Studia iranica* 8:175–83.

———. 1981. Aramaic Preposition *B* in Parthian (Pahlavica IV). *Orient* 17:59–66.

———. 1981a. Iranological Contributions of Aśokan Aramaic Inscriptions. *Acta iranica (Monumentum Georg Morgenstierne I)* 21:308–15.

Jackson, K. P. 1983. Ammonite Personal Names in the Context of the West Semitic Onomasticon. In *The Word of the Lord Shall Go Forth: Essays in Honor of David Noel Freedman in Celebration of His Sixtieth Birthday*, ed. C. L. Meyers and M. O'Connor, 507–21. Winona Lake, Ind.: Eisenbrauns.

———. 1983a. *The Ammonite Language of the Iron Age*. HSM 27. Chico, Cal.: Scholars Press.

Jahn, G. 1913. *Die elephantiner Papyri und die Bücher Esra-Nehemja: Mit einem Supplement zu meiner Erklärung der hebräischen Eigennamen*. Leiden: Brill.
Reviews: J. W. Rothstein 1913.

———. 1914. Antwort auf die Besprechung meiner Schrift über die elephantiner Papyri durch Prof. J. W. Rothstein ZDMG. 67, 718. *ZDMG* 68:142–48.

Jakob-Rost, L. 1975. *Die Stempelsiegel im Vorderasiatischen Museum*. Berlin: Akademie Verlag.

Jakob-Rost, L., and H. Freydank. 1972. Spätbabylonische Rechtsurkunden aus Babylon mit aramäischen Beischriften. *FuB* 14:7–35.

Jamme, A. See: J. Starcky.

Jampel, S. 1907. Der Papyrusfund von Assuan. *MGWJ* 51:617–34.

———. 1911. Die neuen Papyrusfunde in Elephantine. *MGWJ* 55:641–65.

Janssen, J. M. A. 1955–56. Egyptological Remarks on *The Story of Joseph in Genesis*. *JEOL* 14:63–72.

Janssens, G. 1975–76. The feminine Ending -(a)t in Semitic. *OLP (Miscellanea in honorem Joseph Vergote)*: 6–7:277–84.

Jaritz, H. 1980. *Elephantine III: Die Terrassen vor den Tempeln des Chnum und der Satet.* Archäologische Veroffentlichungen 32. Mainz: P. von Zabern.

Jastrow, M. 1894. The Excavations at Sendschirli, and Some of Their Bearings on the Old Testament. *BW* 3:406–16.

Jaussen, A. J., and R. Savignac. 1909, 1914, 1922. *Mission archéologique en Arabie.* 3 vols. Paris: I–E. Leroux; II & III–Geuthner.

Jean, C.-F., and J. Hoftijzer. 1965. *Dictionnaire des inscriptions sémitiques de l'ouest.* Leiden: Brill.
Reviews: W. Baumgartner 1970: *BO* 27:14; O. Eissfeldt 1967: *TLZ* 92:353; J. Friedrich 1966: *VT* 16:364–66; G. Garbini 1967: *JSS* 12:111–12; R. Meyer 1967: *OLZ* 62:165–66; R. Meyer 1970: *OLZ* 65:158–61; W. Röllig 1969: *WZKM* 62:304–7; S. Segert 1968: *ArOr* 36:164–67.

Jenni, E. 1968. *Das hebräische Piel: Syntaktische-semasiologische Untersuchung einer Verbalform im Alten Testament.* Zurich: EVZ.

———. 1988. Jer 3,17 "nach Jerusalem": ein Aramaismus. *Zeitschrift für Althebraistik* 1:107–11.

Jensen, H. 1958. *Die Schrift in Vergangenheit und Gegenwart.* 2nd ed. Berlin: VEB Deutscher Verlag der Wissenschaften.

Jensen, P. 1926. *Der aramäische Beschwörungstext in spätbabylonischer Keilschrift.* Marburg: A. Ebel.
Reviews: E. Littmann 1929.

Jepsen, A. 1942–43. Israel und Damaskus. *AfO* 14:153–72.

———. 1952–53. Zur Melqart-Stele Barhadads. *AfO* 16:315–17.

———. 1969. Kleine Bemerkungen zu drei westsemitischen Inschriften. *MIO* 15:1–5.

Jerusalmi, I. 1978. *The Aramaic Sections of Ezra and Daniel.* Auxiliary Material for the Study of Semitic Languages 7. 2nd ed. Cincinnati: Hebrew Union College.

Jirku, A. 1912. *Die jüdische Gemeinde von Elephantine und ihre Beziehungen zum Alten Testament.* Biblische Zeit- und Streitfragen ser. 7, vol. 11. Berlin: Runge.

———. 1912a. Die fünf Städte bei Jes. 19, 18 und die fünf Tore des Jahu-Tempels zu Elephantine. *OLZ* 15:247–48.

Johns, A. F. 1963. *A Short Grammar of Biblical Aramaic.* Andrews Univ. Monographs 1. Revised edition 1972. Berrien Springs, Mich.: Andrews Univ. Press.
Reviews: L. Running 1968: *BO* 25:379–80; G. Wallis 1971.

Johns, C. H. W. 1901. *Assyrian Deeds and Documents: Cuneiform Texts, Introduction, Officials, Metrology.* 2 vols. Cambridge: Deighton Bell.

———. 1905. Note on the Aramaic Papyrus from Elephantine. *PSBA* 27:187–88.

———. 1907. The Assuan Aramaic Papyri. *Expositor* 7/3:544–51.

———. 1925–26. Assyrian Deeds and Documents. *AJSL* 42:170–204; 228–75.

Joshi, M. C., and B. M. Pande. 1967. A Newly Discovered Inscription of Aśoka at Bahapur, Delhi. *JRAS* 3–4:96–98, pl. I–II.

Joüon, P. 1927. Notes sur quelques versets araméens de Daniel et d'Esdras. *Bib* 8:182–87.

———. 1930–31. Sémantique des verbes statifs de la forme *qatila (qatel)* en arabe, hébreu et araméen. *MUSJ*:1–32.

————. 1933. Les mots pour 'sur', 'au dessus de', 'en haut' et 'au dessous de', 'en bas' en hébreu, araméen et arabe. *Or* 2:275–80.

————. 1934. Notes grammaticales, lexicographiques et philologiques sur les papyrus araméens d'Égypte. *MUSJ* 18:1–90.

————. 1934a. Notes de lexicographie hébraïque. I. Le substantif 'El "le haut" et ses dérivés en araméen et en hébreu. *Bib* 15:399–401.

————. 1941. Cinq imparfaits (*yiqtul*) remarquables dans l'araméen de Daniel (4, 8. 31. 33; 6, 20; 7, 16). *Bib* 22:21–24.

————. 1941a. Notes de grammaire et de lexicographie araméenne. *Bib* 22:263–68.

Judas, A.-C. 1847. *Étude démonstrative de la langue phénicienne et de la langue libyque*. Paris: F. Klincksieck.

————. 1858–59. Sur l'inscription phénicienne d'un libatoire du Sérapéum de Memphis. *RArch* 15/2:677–96, facs., p. 679.

Kaddari, M. 1969. Construct State and *di*-Phrases in Imperial Aramaic. In *Proceedings of the International Conference on Semitic Studies, 1965*, 102–15. Jerusalem: Israel Academy of Sciences and Humanities.

————. 1983. The Existential Verb *HWH* in Imperial Aramaic. In *Arameans, Aramaic and the Aramaic Literary Tradition*, ed. M. Sokoloff, 43–46. Ramat-Gan: Bar-Ilan Univ. Press.

Kahle, P. 1948–49. Das zur Zeit Jesu in Palästina gesprochene Aramäisch. *TRu* 17:201–16.

Kahle, P., and F. Sommer. 1930. Die lydisch-aramäische Bilingue. *Kleinasiatische Forschungen* 1/1:18–86.

Kamil, M. 1945–46. Papyri araméens découverts à Hermoupolis-Ouest. *BIE* 28:253–57.

————. 1947. Notice on the Aramaic Papyri Discovered at Hermopolis West [in Arabic]. *Revue de l'Histoire juive en Egypte* 1:1–3; 173–72.

————. 1948. An Aramaic Document on Leather from the 5th Century B.C. [in Arabic]. *Bulletin of the Faculty of Arts* (L'Université Fouad Ier) 10:113–30.

————. 1949. The Aramaic Papyri Discovered at Hermopolis West. In *Actes du XXIe Congrès des Orientalistes Paris 23–31 juillet 1948* 106–7. Paris: Imprimerie Nationale.

————. 1952. Les dernières découvertes araméennes en Egypte. In *Studia aegyptiaca I. Mardis de Dar-el-Salam* 189–204.

————. See also: E. Bresciani.

Kamphausen, A. 1896. *The Book of Daniel*. The Sacred Books of the Old Testament. Leipzig: J. C. Hinrichs.

Kaplan, J. 1958. ב-זיתון אבו בתל החפירות. 1957. *Yediot* 22:98–99.

Kataja, L. 1986. On the Rection of Verbs Denoting Motion and Communication in Neo-Assyrian and Aramaic. M.A. thesis, Univ. of Helsinki.

Kaufman, S. A. 1970. Si'gabbar, Priest of Sahr in Nerab. *JAOS* 90:270–71.

————. 1973. Review of *Documents araméens d'Égypte*, by P. Grelot. *CBQ* 35:385–86.

————. 1974. *The Akkadian Influences on Aramaic*. Assyriological Studies 19. Chicago: Univ. of Chicago Press.

Reviews: J. Oelsner 1980; D. Pardee 1977; W. Röllig 1977; W. von Soden 1977; M. Sokoloff 1976;

D. J. Wiseman 1977: *BSOAS* 40:144.

————. 1975. Appendix C: Alphabetic Texts. In *Excavations at Nippur: Eleventh Season*, ed. McGuire Gibson, 151–52. Oriental Institute Communications 22. Chicago: Univ. of Chicago Press.

————. 1977. An Assyro-Aramaic *egirtu ša šulmu*. In *Essays on the Ancient Near East in Memory of Jacob Joel Finkelstein*, ed. M. de Jong Ellis, 119–27. Memoirs of the Connecticut Academy of Arts and Sciences 19. Hamden, Conn.: Archon.

————. 1977a. Review of *Altaramäische Grammatik*, by S. Segert. *BO* 34:92–97.

————. 1978. The Enigmatic Adad-Milki. *JNES* 37:101–9.

————. 1978a. Review of *Lexicon linguae aramaicae Veteris Testamenti documentis antiquis illustratum*, by E. Vogt. *JNES* 37:69–70.

————. 1980. The Aramaic Texts from Deir ʿAllā. [Review article: J. Hoftijzer and B. van der Kooij, *Aramaic Texts from Deir ʿAlla*.] *BASOR* 239:71–74.

————. 1982. Reflections on the Assyrian-Aramaic Bilingual from Tell Fakhariyeh. *Maarav* 3:137–75.

————. 1983. The History of Aramaic Vowel Reduction. In *Arameans, Aramaic and the Aramaic Literary Tradition*, ed. M. Sokoloff, 47–55. Ramat-Gan: Bar-Ilan Univ. Press.

————. 1984. On Vowel Reduction in Aramaic. *JAOS* 104:87–95.

————. 1984a. Review of *La statue de Tell Fekherye*, by A. Abou Assaf et al. *JAOS* 104:571–73.

————. 1985. Review of *Les inscriptions araméennes de Sfiré et l'Assyrie de Shamshi-Ilu*, by A. Lemaire and J.-M. Durand. *CBQ* 47:534–36.

————. 1986. The Pitfalls of Typology: On the Early History of the Alphabet. *HUCA* 57:1–14.

————. 1986a. Review of *The Aramaic Proverbs of Ahiqar*, by J. M. Lindenberger. *JNES* 45:151.

————. 1988. The Classification of the North West Semitic Dialects of the Biblical Period and Some Implications Thereof. In *Proceedings of the Ninth World Congress of Jewish Studies, Jerusalem, 4–12 August 1985: Division D*, 41–57. Jerusalem: World Union of Jewish Studies.

————. 1989. Assyro-Aramaica. [Review article: M. M. Fales *Aramaic Epigraphs on Clay Tablets of the Neo-Assyrian Period*.] *JAOS* 109:97–102.

Kautzsch, E. 1884. *Grammatik des Biblisch-Aramäischen*. Leipzig: F. C. W. Vogel.
    Reviews: T. Nöldeke 1884.

————. 1903. *Die Aramaismen in Alten Testament*. Halle: Niemeyer.
    Reviews: E. Littmann 1903.

Keel, O., M. Shuval, and C. Uehlinger. 1990. *Studien zu den Stempelsiegeln aus Palästina/Israel, III: Die frühe Eisenzeit, ein Workshop*. Freiburg: Universitätsverlag; Göttingen: Vandenhoeck and Ruprecht.

Kees, H. 1931. Syene. In *Pauly-Wissowa*, ser. 2, vol. 4/1, 1018–23. Stuttgart: J. B. Metzler.

Keil, C. F. 1884. *The Book of the Prophet Daniel*. Translated by M. G. Easton. Edinburgh: Clark.

Keller, O. See: F. Imhoof-Blumer.

Kelso, J. A. 1909. The Unity of the Sanctuary in the Light of the Elephantine Papyri. *JBL* 28:71–81.

Kent, R. G. 1953. *Old Persian: Grammar, Texts, Lexicon.* 2nd ed. New Haven: American Oriental Society.

Kienast, B. 1957. Das Possessivsuffix der 3. m. sg. am pluralischen Nomen des Maskulinum im Südostaramäischen. *Münchener Studien zur Sprachwissenschaft* 10:72–76.

———. 1987. É-a und der aramäische "Status emphaticus." In *Ebla 1975–1985. Dieci anni di studi linguistici e filologici. Atti del convegno internazionale (Napoli, 9–11 ottobre 1985),* ed. Luigi Cagni, 37–47. Naples: Istituto Universitario Orientale, Dipartimento di Studi Asiatici.

Kitchen, K. A. 1965. The Aramaic of Daniel. In *Notes on Some Problems in the Book of Daniel,* ed. D. J. Wiseman, 31–79. London: Tyndale.
Reviews: H. H. Rowley 1966.

———. 1965a. A Late Luvian Personal Name in Aramaic. *Revue hittite et asianique* 23, 76:25–28.

———. 1979. Egypt, Ugarit, Qatna and Covenant. *UF* 11:453–64.

Kittel, R. 1925. Der Gott Bet'el. *JBL* 44:125–53.

———. 1926. Zum Gott Bet'el. *ZAW* 44:170–72.

Klíma, O. 1967. *gaiθāma miyama* (Behistun). In *Festschrift Wm. Eilers,* 202–3. Wiesbaden: Harrassowitz.

———. 1979. Review of *La langue de Ya'udi,* by P.-E. Dion. *ArOr* 47:211–12.

———. 1986. Review of *The Aramaic Proverbs of Ahiqar,* by J. M. Lindenberger. *ArOr* 54:193.

Klengel, H. 1965. Der Wettergott von Ḫalab. *JCS* 19:87–93.

Knauer, G. N. 1954. *sarabara. Glotta* 33:100–118.

Knauf, E. A. 1984. Supplementa ismaelitica. *BN* 25:19–26.

———. 1987. Haben Aramäer den Griechen das Alphabet vermittelt? *WO* 18:45–48.

———. 1990. The Persian Administration in Arabia. *Transeuphratène* 2:201–17.

Knevett, E. de. 1909. Une stèle araméenne de Memphis. *Bulletin des Musées Royaux* 2e sér., 2:78–80.

Knobel, E. B. 1907–09. A suggested explanation of the Ancient Jewish Calendar Dates in the Aramaic Papyri translated by Professor A. H. Sayce and Mr. A. E. Cowley. *MNRAS* 68:334–45; 69:8–11.

Knopf, C. S. 1933. Items of Interest from Miscellaneous Neo-Babylonian Documents. *Bulletin of the Southern California Academy of Sciences* 32:50–51.

Knudtzon, J. A. 1912. Der Gottesname יהוה —יהו. *OLZ* 15:486–92.

Köberle, D. 1908. Die Papyri von Assuan und das Alte Testament. *Neue kirchliche Zeitschrift* 19:173–206.

Köbert, R. 1985. Review of *The Aramaic Proverbs of Ahiqar,* by J. Lindenberger. *Or* 54:457–58.

Kochavi, M. 1965. Tel Zeror. *RB* 72:548–51.

————. 1972. Tel Malḥata. *RB* 79:593–96.

Kochman, M. 1982. 'יהוד מדינתא' לאור טביעות 'יהוד'–'פחוא'. *Cathedra* 24:3–30.

Koenig, J. 1981. L'inscription de Deir Alla, Balaam et le prophétisme. *Akkadica* 24:34–35.

————. 1983. La déclaration des dieux dans l'inscription de Deir 'Alla (I,2). *Sem* 33:77–88.

Kohler, J. 1912. Bemerkungen zu den aramäischen Urkunden von Elephantine. *ZVR* 27:142–44.

Koschaker, P. 1935. Keilschriftrecht. *ZDMG* 89:1–39.

Kokovtsov, P. 1899. Drevnearameyskie nadpisi iz Niraba bliz Aleppo [Old Aramaic inscriptions from Nerab near Aleppo]. *ZVO* 12:145–78.

————. 1899a. Nouvel essai d'interprétation de la seconde inscription araméenne de Nirab. *JA* 9/14:432–45.

————. 1900. Imena zhretsov v Nirabskikh Nadpisyakh [The names of the priests in the Nerab inscriptions]. *ZVO* 13:93–97.

————. 1904–5. O novom arameyskom papyryse imperatoskoy Strasburgskoy Biblioteki [Of the new Aramaic papyri of the Imperial Strassburg Library]. *ZVO* 16:xxii–xxvii.

Koldewey, R. 1898. Die Architektur von Sendschirli. In *Ausgrabungen in Sendschirli II*, 103–200. Mittheilungen aus den orientalischen Sammlungen 12. Berlin: W. Spemann.

————. 1900. [Communications], MDOG 4:1–14.

————. 1901. Aus sieben Briefen Dr. Koldewey's. *MDOG* 11:4–13.

————. 1902. [Communication], MDOG 11:10.

————. 1914. *Das wieder erstehende Babylon: Die bisherigen Ergebnisse der deutschen Ausgrabungen.* 3rd ed. Leipzig: J. C. Hinrichs.

König, E. 1901. Mene Mene Tekel. *Neue kirchliche Zeitschrift* 12:957.

————. 1901a. The Emphatic State in Aramaic. *AJSL* 17:209–21.

————. 1913. Jahu, oder Jaho? *OLZ* 16:107–14.

————. 1915. Religionsgeschichtliche Hauptmomente in den Elephantinetexten. *ZAW* 35:110–19.

König, F. W. 1938. *Relief und Inschrift des Königs Dareios I am Felsen von Bagistan.* Leiden: Brill.

Kooij, G. van der. 1986. Deir Alla. *MDB* 46:34–35.

————. 1991. Book and Script at Deir 'Allā. In *BTDAR*, 239–62.

————. See also: J. Hoftijzer, M. M. Ibrahim.

Koopmans, J. J. 1957. De literatuur over het aramees na 1940. *JEOL* 15:125–32.

————. 1957a. *Arameese Grammatica.* Leiden: Nederlands Institut v. h. Nabije Oosten.

————. 1960. Review of *Les inscriptions araméennes de Sfiré*, by A. Dupont-Sommer and J. Starcky. *BO* 17:51–52.

————. 1962. *Aramäische Chrestomathie: Ausgewählte Texte (Inschriften Ostraka und Papyri) bis zum 3. Jahrhundert n. Chr. für das Studium der aramäischen Sprache gesammelt.* 2 vols. Leiden: Nederlands Institut voor het Nabije Oosten.
Reviews: J. Hoftijzer 1964; R. Meyer 1967.

Kopp, U. F. 1817–29. *Palaeographia critica*. Mannheim: n.p.

———. 1821. *Bilder und Schriften der Vorzeit*. Mannheim: privately published.

Körner, J. 1962. Das soziale und religiöse Leben in der Militärkolonie von Elephantine: Eine Interpretation ausgewählter Papyri aus Elephantine als Beitrag zur Religionsgeschichte und Theologie des Alten Testaments. Ph.D. diss., Friedrich Schiller Univ.

———. 1977. Review of *Kanaanäische und Aramäische Inschriften I-III*, by H. Donner and W. Röllig. *OLZ* 72:276–79.

Kornfeld, W. 1967. Aramäische Sarkophage in Assuan. *WZKM* 61:9–16 + 8 pl.

———. 1973. Jüdisch-aramäische Grabinschriften aus Edfu. *AÖAWW* 110:121–37.

———. 1974. Beiträge zur aramäischen Namenforschung. *AÖAWW* 111:374–83 + 1 pl.

———. 1976. Onomastica aramaica und das Alte Testament. *ZAW* 88:105–12.

———. 1978. *Onomastica aramaica aus Ägypten*. Sitzungsberichte der Österreichischen Akademie der Wissenschaften 333. Vienna: Austrian Academy of Sciences.
Reviews: E. Lipiński 1980a.

———. 1978a. Neues über die phönikischen und aramäischen Graffiti in den Tempeln vom Abydos. *AÖAWW* 115:193–204 + 18 pls.

———. 1979. Zu den aramäischen Inschriften aus Edfu. *WZKM* 71:48–52.

Korngruen, P. 1948. ‏מושבות צבאיות של היהודים בימי קדם‎. Tel Aviv: Massada.

Korošec, V. 1961. Quelques traités de l'époque néo-assyrienne. *Romanitas III/3–4: In honorem H. Levy-Bruhl*:261–77.

Kortleitner, F. X. 1927. *De Judaeorum in Elephantine-Syene colonia eiusque rationibus cum vetere testamento intercedentibus*. Commentationes biblicae 2. Innsbruck: F. Rauch.

Kosambi, D. D. 1959. Notes on the Kandahar Edict of Asoka. *JESHO* 2:205–6.

Kottsieper, I. 1988. Anmerkungen zu Pap. Amherst 63 I:12, 11–19 — Eine aramäische Version von Ps 20. *ZAW* 100:217–44.

———. 1990. *Die Sprache der Aḥiqarsprüche*. BZAW 194. Berlin: de Gruyter.

Kraay, C. M. 1962. The Celenderis Hoard. *NC* 7th ser. v.2:1–15.

Kraeling, E. G. 1918. *Aram and Israel; or The Aramaeans in Syria and Mesopotamia*. CUOS 13. New York: Columbia Univ. Press.

———. 1933. Some Babylonian and Iranian Mythology in the Seventh Chapter of Daniel. In *Oriental Studies in Honour of Cursetji Erachji Pavry*, ed. J. D. C. Pavry, 228–31. London: Oxford Univ. Press.

———. 1944. The Handwriting on the Wall. *JBL* 63:11–18.

———. 1952. New Light on the Elephantine Colony. *BA* 15:50–67 + 2 pls.

———. 1953. *The Brooklyn Museum Aramaic Papyri: New Documents of the Fifth Century B.C. from the Jewish Colony at Elephantine*. New Haven: Yale Univ. Press. Reprint: New York: Arno, 1969.
Reviews: B. Couroyer 1954; G. R. Driver 1955; T. Jansma 1954: *BO* 11:215–16; J. T. Milik 1954; J. Reider 1953–54.

———. 1957. Elephantine-Urkunden. *RGG*[3] 2:415–18.

———. 1962. Book of Ahikar. *IDB* 4:68–69.

Krahmalkov, C. R. 1981. The Historical Setting of the Adon Letter. *BA* 44:197–98.

Krappe, A. H. 1941. Is the Story of Aḥikar the Wise of Indian Origin? *JAOS* 61:280–84.

Krückmann, O. 1933. *Neubabylonische Rechts- und Verwaltungstexte*. Texte und Materialien der Frau Prof. Hilprecht Collection of Babylonian Antiquities 2–3. Leipzig: J. C. Hinrichs.

Kruse, H. 1959. Compositio libri Daniel et idea Filii Hominis. *VD* 37:147–61; 193–211.

Kselman, J. S. 1986. Review of *The Aramaic Proverbs of Ahiqar*, by J. M. Lindenberger. *JBL* 105:114–15.

Kuhl, C. 1930. *Die drei Männer im Feuer*. Berlin: Töpelmann.

Kuhn, K. G. 1935. יהוה, יהו, יו: Über die Entstehung des Namens Jahwe. In *Orientalistische Studien: Enno Littmann zu seinem 60. Geburtstag am 16. September 1935*, 25–42. Leiden: Brill.

Kutscher, E. Y. 1942–3. Review of *Die aramaistische Forschung seit Th. Nöldekes Veröffentlichungen*, by F. Rosenthal. *Kiryat Sepher* 19:177–81.

———. 1945. מגלה ארמית מן המאה החמשית לפני ספה"נ. *Kedem* 2:66–74. Reprinted in *Hebrew and Aramaic Studies* (Jerusalem: Magnes,1977), יא-יט.

———. 1950. פרקים מתוך תחביר של יב. M.A. thesis, Hebrew Univ.

———. 1951. הארמית המקראית — ארמית מזרחית היא או מערבית? *Leš* 17:119–22. Reprinted in *World Congress of Jewish Studies (Summer 1947) I* (Jerusalem: Hebrew Univ.,1952), 123–27.

———. 1954. New Aramaic Texts. [Review article: E. G. Kraeling *The Brooklyn Museum Aramaic Papyri*.] *JAOS* 74:233–48. Reprinted in *Hebrew and Aramaic Studies* (Jerusalem: Magnes,1977), 37–52.

———. 1954a. בְעֵל טְעֵם. *EM* 2:293–94.

———. 1957. Review of *Aramaic Documents of the Fifth Century B. C.*, by G. R. Driver. *JBL* 76:336–38.

———. 1960. ארמית. *EM* 1:584–93.

———. 1961. פחוא ואחיותיה. *Tarbiz* 30:112–19. Reprinted in *Hebrew and Aramaic Studies* (Jerusalem: Magnes, 1977), סנט-סו.

———. 1964. של הארמית בעברית (Calque) בבואה. *Tarbiz* 33:118–30. Reprinted in *Hebrew and Aramaic Studies* (Jerusalem: Magnes, 1977), שצד-תו.

———. 1965. Contemporary Studies in North-Western Semitic. [Review article: *Il semitico di nord-ovest*, by G. Garbini.] *JSS* 10:21–51.

———. 1969. Two "Passive" Constructions in Aramaic in the Light of Persian. In *Proceedings of the International Conference on Semitic Studies held in Jerusalem, 19–23 July 1965*, 132–51. Jerusalem: Israel Academy of Sciences and Humanities. Reprinted in *Hebrew and Aramaic Studies* (Jerusalem: Magnes, 1977), 70–89.

———. 1970. Aramaic. In *Linguistics in South West Asia and North Africa*, ed. T. A. Sebeok, 347–412. Current Trends in Linguistics, vol. 6. Paris: Mouton.

———. 1970a. The Genesis Apocryphon of Qumran Cave I. *Or* 39:178–83.

———. 1971. The Hermopolis Papyri. *IOS* 1:103–19.

————. 1972. תולדות הארמית. Jerusalem: Akademon.

Kutscher, E. Y., J. Naveh, and S. Shaked. 1969–70. הכתובות הארמיות של אשוקה. *Leš* 34:125–36.

Kutscher, E. Y. See also: E. L. Sukenik.

Kvanvig, H. S. 1981. An Akkadian Vision as Background for Dan 7? *Studia theologica* 35:85–89.

Kyrieleis, H., and W. Röllig. 1988. Ein altorientalischer Pferdeschmuck aus dem Heraion von Samos. *Mitteilungen des Deutschen Archäologischen Instituts, Athenische Abteilung* 103:37–75.

LaSor, W. S. 1980. Samples of Early Semitic Poetry. In *The Bible World: Essays in Honor of Cyrus H. Gordon*, ed. G. Rendsburg et al., 99–121. New York: Ktav.

Lack, R. 1962. Les origines de ʿElyon, le Très-Haut, dans la tradition culturelle d'Israël. *CBQ* 24:44–64.

Lacocque, A. 1976. *Le livre de Daniel.* Commentaire de l'Ancien Testament 15b. Neuchâtel: Delachaux et Niestlé.
Reviews: E. Lipiński 1978.

Lagarde, P. de. 1878. Zur Erklärung der aramäischen Inschrift von Carpentras. *Nachrichten von der Königl. Gesellschaft der Wissenschaften und der G. A. Universität zu Göttingen*: 357–72.

Lagrange, M.-J. 1904. Bulletin. *RB* 13:130–59.

————. 1905. *Études sur les religions sémitiques.* 2nd ed. Paris: Lecoffre.

————. 1905a. Bulletin. *RB* 14:132–60.

————. 1907. Les papyrus araméens d'Éléphantine. [Review article: A. H. Sayce and A. E. Cowley, *Aramaic Papyri Discovered at Assuan.*] *RB* 4:258–71.

————. 1908. Les fouilles d'Éléphantine. *RB* 5:260–67.

————. 1908a. Les nouveaux papyrus d'Éléphantine. *RB* 5:325–49.

————. 1915. Review of *Une communauté judéo-araméenne à Éléphantine, en Égypte, aux VIe et Ve siècles av. J.-C.*, by A. van Hoonacker. *RB* 12:595–98.

Lajard, F. 1837–49. *Recherches sur le culte, les symboles, les attributs, et les monuments figurés de Vénus, en Orient et en Occident.* Paris: Bourgeois-Maze.

————. 1867. *Recherches sur la culte public et les mystères de Mithra en Orient et Occident.* Paris: Imprimerie Nationale.

Lambdin, T. O. 1971. The Junctural Origin of the West Semitic Definite Article. In *Near Eastern Studies in Honor of W. F. Albright*, ed. H. Goedicke, 315–33. Baltimore: Johns Hopkins Univ. Press.

————. 1985. Philippi's Law Reconsidered. In *Biblical and Related Studies Presented to Samuel Iwry*, ed. A. Kort and S. Morschauser, 135–45. Winona Lake, Ind.: Eisenbrauns.

Lambert, M. 1893. De l'emploi du *lamed* en araméen biblique devant le complément direct. *REJ* 17:269–70.

Lamotte, É. 1958. Nouveaux édits d'Aśoka et bilingue de Kandahār. In *Histoire du bouddhisme indien: Des origines à l'ère Śaka*, 789–98. Bibliothèque du Muséon, vol. 43. Louvain: Publications Universitaires.

Lance, H. D. 1971.   The Royal Stamps and the Kingdom of Josiah. *HTR* 64:315–32.

Lanci, M. A. 1825.   *Osservazioni sul basso-rilievo fenico-egizio che si conserva in Carpentrasso.* Rome: F. Bourlié.
Reviews: E. Rödiger 1828.

———. 1827.   *La sacra scrittura illustrata con monumenti fenico-assyri et egiziani.* Rome: Società Tipografica.

Landels, J. G. 1966.   Ship-Shape and *Sambuca*-Fashion. *JHS* 86:69–77.

Landsberger, B. 1937–39.   Zu den aramäischen Beschwörungen in Keilschrift. *AfO* 12:247–57.

———. 1948.   *Samal: Studien zur Entdeckung der Ruinenstätte Karatepe.* Veröffentlichungen der türkischen historischen Gesellschaft 7/16. Ankara: Turkish Historical Society.

———. See also: J. Friedrich.

Langdon, S. 1933.   Note on the Aramaic Treaty of Bar-Ga'ya and Mati'el. *JRAS*: 23–24.

Lapp, P. W. 1963.   Ptolemaic Stamped Handles from Judah. *BASOR* 172:22–35.

———. 1963a.   The Samaria Papyri. *Archaeology* 16:204–6.

———. 1978.   Bedouin Find Papyri Three Centuries Older than Dead Sea Scrolls. *BARev* 4/1:16–24.

Laroche, E. 1974.   La stèle trilingue récemment découverte au Lêtôon de Xanthos: Le texte Lycien. *CRAIBL*: 115–25.

Larraya, J. A. G. 1963–65.   Ḥāzāēl. *EncBib* 3:1096–98.

Lauer, J. P. 1967.   Recherches et travaux menés dans la nécropole de Saqqarah au cours de la campagne 1966–1967. *CRAIBL*: 493–510 + 4 pls., 4 figs.

Lauth, [J.] 1878.   Aegyptisch-aramäische Inschriften. *SPAW* 2:97–149.

Layard, A. H. 1853.   *Discoveries among the Ruins of Nineveh and Babylon.* New York: Harper, Putnam. Abridged reprint: 1875.

———. 1853a.   *The Monuments of Nineveh, Second Series.* London: J. Murray.

Layton, S. C. 1988.   Old Aramaic Inscriptions. *BA* 51:172–89.

Le Déaut, R. 1981.   Review of *A Wandering Aramean: Collected Aramaic Essays*, by J. A. Fitzmyer. *Or* 50:222–25.

Le Roy, C. 1987.   Araméen, Lycien et Grec: Pluralité des langues et pluralités des cultures. *Hethitica* 8:263–66.

Leander, P. 1912.   Der elephantinische Gottesname יהו. *OLZ* 15:151–53.

———. 1927.   Verbesserungen am aramäischen Teil von Gesenius' Handwörterbuch, 17 Aufl. *ZAW* 45:156–59.

———. 1928.   *Laut- und Formenlehre des Ägyptisch-Aramäischen.* Göteborgs Högskolas Årsskrift 34 (1928:4). Göteborg: Elanders.
Reviews: V. Christian 1929: *WZKM* 36:316–17; J. A. Montgomery 1931.

———. 1930.   Review of *The Aramaic of the Old Testament*, by H. H. Rowley. *OLZ* 33:773–76.

———. See also: H. Bauer.

Leclant, J. 1968. Fouilles et travaux en Egypte et au Soudan, 1966–1967. *Or* 37:94–140.

——. 1969. Fouilles et travaux en Egypte et au Soudan, 1967–1968. *Or* 38:240–307.

——. 1973. Fouilles et travaux en Egypte et au Soudan, 1971–1972. *Or* 42:393–440.

Ledrain, E. 1882. Note sur deux sceaux portant le même nom hébreu. *RArch* 43:285–87.

——. 1882a. Note métrologique de M. Ledrain sur les lions de bronze assyriens. *Revue égyptologique* 2:173–76.

——. 1883. Notes sur quelques monuments à inscriptions sémitiques provenant des pays assyro-babyloniens. *Gazette archéologique* 8:73–77.

——. 1884. Réponse de M. Ledrain. *RA* 1:16–17.

——. 1884a. Mots égyptiens contenus dans quelques stèles araméennes d'Egypte. *RA* 1:18–23.

——. 1884b. Papyrus du Vatican et Papyrus de la Propagande. *RA* 1:23–32.

——. 1884c. Une brique babylonienne inédite, avec un nom propre. *RA* 1:38–39.

——. 1884d. Études sur quelques objets sémitiques. *RA* 1:66–69.

——. 1884e. Étude sur quelques intailles sémitiques du Musée du Louvre. *RA* 1:35–38.

——. 1885. Étude sur quelques inscriptions sémitiques. *RA* 1:162–64.

——. 1888. *Notice sommaire des monuments phéniciens.* Paris: Musée National du Louvre.

——. 1891. Quelques inscriptions sémitiques du Louvre. *RA* 3:143–45.

——. 1892. Quelques inscriptions inédites entrées au Musée du Louvre. *RA* 2:93–95.

Leemhuis, F. 1986. An Early Witness for a Fronted /g/ in Aramaic? The Case of the Tell Fekherye Inscription. In *Scripta signa vocis: Studies about Scripts, Scriptures, Scribes and Languages in the Near East, Presented to J. H. Hospers*, ed. H. L. J. Vanstiphout et al., 133–42. Groningen: Forsten.

Legrain, L. 1925. *The Culture of the Babylonians from Their Seals in the Collection of the Museum.* University Museum Publications of the Babylonian Section 14. Philadephia: University Museum.

——. 1951. *Seal Cylinders.* Ur Excavations 10. Oxford: Oxford Univ. Press.

Leibovitch, J. 1935–36. Quelques égyptianismes contenus dans les textes araméens d'Égypte. *BIE* 18:19–29.

Lemaire, A. 1974. Un nouveau roi arabe de Qedar dans l'inscription de l'autel à encens de Lakish. *RB* 81:63–72.

——. 1975. Un nouvel ostracon araméen du ve siècle av. J.-C. *Sem* 25:87–96, pl. V.

——. 1977. Les inscriptions de Khirbet el-Qôm et l'Ashérah de Yhwh. *RB* 84:595–608.

——. 1978. Abécédaires et exercices d'écolier en épigraphie nord-ouest sémitique. *JA* 266:221–35.

——. 1978a. Le sceau CIS, II, 74 et sa signification historique. *Sem* 28:11–14.

——. 1979. Nouveau sceau nord-ouest sémitique avec un lion rugissant. *Sem* 29:67–69.

——. 1979–84. La langue de l'inscription sur plâtre de Deir 'Alla. *Comptes rendus du GLECS* 24–28:317–40.

————. 1980. Review of *Inscribed Seals: First Temple Period*, by R. Hestrin and M. Dayagi-Mendels. *Syria* 57:496–97.

————. 1981. Le pays d'Eden et le Bît-Adini aux origines d'un mythe. *Syria* 58:313–30.

————. 1981a. Sfiré I A 24 et l'araméen ṣ̌ṭ *Henoch* 3:161–70.

————. 1982. Cinq sceaux araméens inscrits inédits. *Syria* 59:109–16.

————. 1982a. Notes d'épigraphie nord-ouest sémitique 4. Tessons inscrits du territoire de Manassé. *Sem* 32:15–17.

————. 1983. Nouveaux sceaux nord-ouest sémitiques. *Sem* 33:17–31.

————. 1984. Notes d'épigraphie nord-ouest sémitique. *Syria* 61:251–56.

————. 1984a. Qui est Bar Ga'yah roi de KTK? Vers la solution d'une énigme historique. *JA* 272:473–74.

————. 1984b. La stèle araméenne de Barhadad. *Or* 53:337–49.

————. 1984c. Review of *Aramaic Texts from North Saqqâra*, by J. B. Segal. *Syria* 61:340–42.

————. 1984d. Review of *The Balaam Text from Deir 'Allā*, by J. A. Hackett. *Syria* 61:141–44.

————. 1984e. Mari, the Bible and the Northwest Semitic World. *BA* 47:101–8.

————. 1985. L'inscription de Balaam trouvée à Deir 'Alla: Épigraphie. *BAT*, 313–25.

————. 1985a. Le proverbe araméen Ahiqar 12. In *Miscellanea babyloniaca: Mélanges offerts à Maurice Birot*, ed. J.-M. Durand and J.-R. Kupper, 197–200. Paris: Éditions Recherche sur les Civilisations.

————. 1985b. Les inscriptions de Deir 'Alla et la littérature araméenne antique. *CRAIBL*: 270–85.

————. 1985c. Fragments from the Book of Balaam Found at Deir Alla: Text Foretells Cosmic Disaster. *BARev* 11/5:26–39.

————. 1985d. Notes d'épigraphie nord-ouest sémitique. *Syria* 62:31–47 + 3 pls.

————. 1985e. L'incident du *sibbolet* (Jg 12,6): perspective historique. In *Mélanges bibliques et orientaux en l'honneur de M. Mathias Delcor*, ed. A. Caquot, S. Légasse, and M. Tardieu, 273–81. AOAT 215. Neukirchen-Vluyn: Neukirchener.

————. 1985f. Mari, la Bible et le monde nord-ouest sémitique. [Translation of Lemaire 1984e.] *MARI. Annales de Recherches Interdisciplinaires* 4:549–58.

————. 1986. Les ecrits araméens. In *Ecrits de l'Orient ancien et sources bibliques*, ed. A. Paul, 241–69. Petite bibliothèque des sciences bibliques. Paris: Desclée.

————. 1986a. La disposition originelle des inscriptions sur plâtre de Deir 'Alla. *Studi epigrafici e linguistici* 3:79–93.

————. 1986b. Nouveaux sceaux nord-ouest sémitiques. *Syria* 63:305–25.

————. 1986c. Review of *The Bisitun Inscription of Darius the Great, Aramaic Version*, by J. C. Greenfield and B. Porten. *Or* 55:348–49.

————. 1987. Aššur-šarra-uṣur, gouverneur de Qué. *NABU: Nouvelles assyriologiques brèves et utilitaires* 1:5–6.

————. 1987a. Notes d'épigraphie nord-ouest sémitique. *Syria* 64:205–16; *Sem* 37:47–55.

————. 1988. Recherches actuelles sur les sceaux nord-ouest semitiques. *VT* 38:220–30.

————. 1988a. Hadad l'Edomite ou Hadad l'Araméen. *BN* 43:14–18.

————. 1988b. Le Serment en ouest-sémitique, hébreu et araméen, au Ier millénaire av. J.-C. *Droit et Cultures* 15:115–29.

————. 1988c. Aramaic Literature and Hebrew Literature: Contacts and Influences in the First Millennium B.C.E. In *Proceedings of the Ninth World Congress of Jewish Studies, Panel Sessions: Hebrew and Aramaic Languages*, ed. M. Bar-Asher, 9–24. Jerusalem: World Union of Jewish Studies.

————. 1989. Manuscrit, mur et rocher en épigraphie nord-ouest sémitique. In *Le texte et son inscription* 35–42. Paris: CNRS.

————. 1989a. Les inscriptions palestiniennes d'époque perse: Un bilan provisoire. *Transeuphratène* 1:87–104.

————. 1990. Bala'am/Bela' fils de Be'or. *ZAW* 102:180–87.

————. 1990a. *SMR* dans la petite inscription de Kilamuwa (Zencirli). *Syria* 67:323–27.

————. 1990b. Trois sceaux inscrits inédits avec lion rugissant. *Sem* 39:13–21; pl. II.

————. 1991. Les Inscriptions sur plâtre de Deir 'Alla et leur signification historique et culturelle. In *BTDAR*, 33–57.

Lemaire, A., and B. Delavault. 1975. La tablette ougaritique RS 16.127 et l'abreviation "Ṭ" en nord-ouest sémitique. *Sem* 25:31–41.

Lemaire, A., and H. Lozachmeur. 1977. Deux inscriptions araméennes du Vᵉ siècle avant J.-C. *Sem* 27:99–104.

————. 1987. *Bīrāh/birtā'* en araméen. *Syria* 64:261–66.

————. 1987a. Le site archéologique de Meydancikkale (Turquie): Du Royaume de Pirindu à la garnison ptolémaïque. II. Les inscriptions araméennes. *CRAIBL*: 365–77.

Lemaire, A., and J.-M. Durand. 1984. *Les inscriptions araméennes de Sfiré et l'Assyrie de Shamshi-Ilu.* Ecole pratique des hautes études 2, Hautes études orientales 20. Geneva: Droz.
Reviews: P.-E. Dion 1986; F. M. Fales 1986a; H. D. Galter 1986; S. A. Kaufman 1985; W. von Soden 1985; R. Zadok 1984b.

Lemaire, A. See also: P. Bordreuil, F. Bron, A. Caquot.

Lemonnyer, A. 1914[–19]. Achima. *RSPT* 8:289–96.

————. 1920. La déesse Anath d'Éléphantine. *RSPT* 9:581–88.

Lemosín, R. 1984. Algunas observaciones preliminares en una reconsideración del problema del estudio de los ideogramas arameos en iraní medio. *AO* 2:105–11.

Lenormant, F. 1867. Lettre à M. Ernest Renan sur une stèle araméo-égyptienne encore inédite. *JA* 6/10:511–15.

Lentz, W. 1975. Notes on Some Terms used in Connection with the Aramaic Elements in Middle Persian. *Acta Iranica* 3:313–16.

Lenzen, H. J. 1962. *XVIII. vorläufiger Bericht über die von dem Deutschen Archäologischen Institut und der Deutschen Orient-Gesellschaft aus Mitteln der Deutschen Forschungsgemeinschaft unternommenen Ausgrabungen in Uruk-Warka.* Abhandlungen der Deutschen Orient-Gesellschaft 7. Berlin: Gebr. Mann.

Lenzen, H. See: T. Nöldeke.

Lepsius, R. 1849–59. *Denkmäler aus Ägypten und Äthiopien.* Berlin: Nicolaische Buchhandlung.

Lepsius, R., and J. Euting. 1877. Eine ägyptisch-aramäische Stele. *ZÄS* 15:127–32, Tab. I.

Lerner, Y. 1981–82. ‏במסמכי יב‏ /d/ ‏הסבר חילופי ז/ד בייצוג‏. *Leš* 46:57–64.

Lévi, I. 1907. La colonie juive d'Assouan au ve siècle avant l'ère chrétienne. *REJ* 54:35–44.

———. 1907–8. Le temple du dieu Yahou et la colonie juive d'Eléphantine au ve siècle avant l'ère chrétienne. *REJ* 54:153–65; 56:161–68.

———. 1912. Nouveaux papyrus araméens d'Éléphantine. [Review article: E. Sachau, *Aramäische Papyrus und Ostraka aus einer jüdischen Militärkolonie zu Elephantine.*] *REJ* 63:161–84.

Levi della Vida, G. 1964. Review of *KAI. RSO* 39:295–314.

———. 1965. Ancora sull'iscrizione aramaica di Bahadirli. *RSO* 40:203–4.

Levi della Vida, G., and W. F. Albright. 1943. Some Notes on the Stele of Ben-Hadad. *BASOR* 90:30–34.

Levias, C. 1903. Strack's Aramaic Grammar. [Review article: H. Strack, *Grammatik des Biblisch-Aramäischen.*] *AJSL* 19:64.

Levine, B. A. 1964. Notes on an Aramaic Dream Text from Egypt. *JAOS* 84:18–22.

———. 1972. Aramaic Texts from Persepolis [Review article: R. A. Bowman, *Aramaic Ritual Texts from Persepolis*]. *JAOS* 92:70–79.

———. 1975. On the Origins of the Aramaic Legal Formulary at Elephantine. In *Christianity, Judaism and Other Greco-Roman Cults: Studies for Morton Smith at Sixty,* ed. J. Neusner, 37–54. Studies in Judaism in Late Antiquity, vol. 12. Leiden: Brill.

———. 1981. The Deir 'Allā Plaster Inscriptions. *JAOS* 101:195–205.

———. 1982. ‏הבחינה הלשונית‏ — ‏לחקר המקור הכוהני‏. *EI (Orlinsky Volume)* 16:124–31.

———. 1985. The Balaam Inscription from Deir 'Alla: Historical Aspects. *BAT,* 326–39.

———. 1986. Review of *The Balaam Text from Deir 'Alla,* by J. A. Hackett. *JAOS* 106:364–65.

———. 1991. The Plaster Inscriptions from Deir 'Alla: General Interpretation. In *BTDAR,* 58–72.

———. forthcoming. The Plaster Inscriptions from Deir 'Alla: General Interpretation. In *Proceedings of the 10th World Congress of Jewish Studies,* 58–72. Jerusalem: World Union of Jewish Studies.

Levy, B. B. 1984. Review of *Arameans, Aramaic and the Aramaic Literary Tradition,* ed. M. Sokoloff. *JQR* 75:95–7.

Lévy, I. 1927. Inscriptions araméennes de Memphis. *JA:*282–83, 287, 291–92.

Levy, M. A. 1857. Backsteine, Gemmen und Siegel aus Mesopotamien mit phönizischer (altsemitischer) Schrift. In *Phönizische Studien,* vol. 2, 21–41. Breslau: F. E. C. Leuckart.

———. 1857a. Über die aramäische Inschrift auf einer Vase des Serapeum's zu Memphis, und über eine Gemme mit himjarischer Inschrift. *ZDMG* 11:65–74.

————. 1862. *Geschichte der jüdischen Münzen: Gemeinfasslich dargestellt.* Leipzig: Nies'sche Bunddruckerei (Carl B. Lorck).

————. 1862a. Geschichte der jüdischen Münzen. *JZ* 1:196–206.

————. 1868. Von Hrn. Prof. Levy, Breslau, 22. Mai und 21. Juni. *JZ* 6:296.

————. 1869. *Siegel und Gemmen mit aramäischen, phönizischen, althebräischen, himjarischen, nabathäischen und altsyrischen Inschriften.* Breslau: Schletter.

————. 1870. Inschriften aus Abydos in Aegypten. In *Phönizische Studien*, vol. 4, 14–35. Breslau: Schletter.

Lewis, A. S. 1912. Achikar and the Elephantinê Papyri. *Expositor* 8/3:207–12.

————. See also: F. C. Conybeare, J. R. Harris, H. Torczyner.

Lewis, T. J. See also: D. Gropp.

Lewy, J. 1954. The Problems Inherent in Section 70 of the Bisutun Inscription. *HUCA* 25:169–208.

————. 1955. Review of *Aramaic Documents of the Fifth Century B.C.*, by G. R. Driver. *JQR* 46:289–95.

————. 1959. On Some Akkadian Expressions for "Afterwards" and Related Notices. *WO* 2:432–37.

L'Hour, J. 1962. L'alliance de Sichem. *RB* 69:5–36, 161–84, 350–68.

Lidzbarski, M. 1898. *Handbuch der nordsemitischen Epigraphik nebst ausgewählten Inschriften.* 2 vols. Weimar: E. Felber.

————. 1902–15. *Ephemeris für semitische Epigraphik.* 3 vols. Giessen: J. Ricker.

————. 1907. Review of *Drei aramäische Papyrusurkunden aus Elephantine*, by E. Sachau. *Deutsche Literaturzeitung* 28:3160–63.

————. 1908. Review of *Inscriptions sémitiques de la Syrie, de la Mésopotamie, et de la région de Mossoul*, by H. Pognon. *Literarisches Zentralblatt für Deutschland* 59:582–85.

————. 1911. Review of *Aramäische Papyrus und Ostraka aus einer jüdischen Militär-Kolonie zu Elephantine*, by A. Sachau. *Deutsche Literaturzeitung* 29:66–81.

————. 1912. Phönizische und aramäische Krugaufschriften aus Elephantine. *Abhandlungen der preussischen Akademie der Wissenschaften*, phil.-hist. Kl.:Anhang, Abh. I 1–20, pls. I–VI.

————. 1917. Ein aramäischer Brief aus der Zeit Ašurbanipals. *MDOG* 58:50–52.

————. 1917–18. Die lydisch-aramäische Inschrift von Sardes. *ZA* 31:122–30.

————. 1917–18a. Ein aramäischer Brief aus der Zeit Ašurbanipals. *ZA* 31:193–202.

————. 1921. *Altaramäische Urkunden aus Assur.* Wissenschaftliche Veröffentlichung der Deutschen Orient-Gesellschaft 38. Leipzig: J. C. Hinrichs.

————. 1927. Epigraphisches. *OLZ* 30:1043–44.

Lieberman, S. J. 1968. The Aramaic Argillary Script in the Seventh Century. *BASOR* 192:25–31.

Limburg, J. 1969. The Root ריב and the Prophetic Lawsuit Speeches. *JBL* 88:291–304.

Lindenberger, J. M. 1982. The Gods of Ahiqar. *UF* 14:105–17.

————. 1983. *The Aramaic Proverbs of Ahiqar.* The Johns Hopkins Near Eastern Studies. Baltimore: Johns Hopkins Univ. Press.
Reviews: P.-E. Dion 1983; J. A. Emerton 1987: *VT* 37:237; S. A. Kaufman 1986; T. Muraoka 1987; E. Puech 1988.

————. 1985. Ahiqar (Seventh to Sixth Century B.C.): A New Translation and Introduction. In *The Old Testament Pseudepigrapha, Vol. 2*, ed. J. H. Charlesworth, 479–507. Garden City, N. Y.: Doubleday.

Linder, J. 1935. Das Aramäische im Buche Daniel. *Zeit. f. katholische Theologie* 59:503–45.

Lipiński, E. 1971. ʿAttar-hapēš, the Forefather of Bar-Hadad II. *AION* 31:101–04.

————. 1971a. The Assyrian Campaign to Manṣuate, in 786 B.C. and the Zakir Stela. *AION* 31:393–99.

————. 1971b. An Israelite King of Hamat? *VT* 21:371–73.

————. 1972. Le Ben-Hadad II de la Bible et l'histoire. In *Proceedings of the Fifth World Congress of Jewish Studies*, vol. 1, 157–73. Jerusalem: World Union of Jewish Studies.

————. 1973. Obadiah 20. *VT* 23:368–70.

————. 1974. Textes juridiques et économiques araméens de l'époque sargonide. AAASH 22:373–84.

————. 1974a. Review of *Documents araméens d'Egypt*, by P. Grelot. *BO* 31:119–24.

————. 1974b. Review of *Development of the Aramaic Script*, by J. Naveh. *BO* 31:127–28.

————. 1975. Nordsemitische Texte. In *RTAT*, ed. W. Beyerlin, 245–84. Göttingen: Vandenhoeck & Ruprecht.

————. 1975a. *Studies in Aramaic Inscriptions and Onomastics I.* OrLovAn 1. Louvain: Leuven University Press.
Reviews: J. A. Fitzmyer 1977; G. Garbini 1977; J. Gibson 1977; A. Millard 1976; J. Naveh 1976; S. Segert 1980; F. Vattioni 1979; R. Zadok 1976.

————. 1975b. Les tablettes araméennes de Bruxelles. In *Etudes sémitiques* 25–29. Actes du XXIXe Congrès International des Orientalistes. Paris: L'Asiathèque.

————. 1975c. La stèle égypto-araméenne de Tumma', fille de Bokkorinif. *CdE* 50:93–104 + 1 pl.

————. 1976. Review of *La langue de Ya'udi*, by P.-E. Dion. *BO* 33:231–34.

————. 1977. North-West Semitic Inscriptions. [Review article: *Textbook of Syrian Semitic Inscriptions I-II*, by J. C. L. Gibson.] *OLP* 8:81–117.

————. 1977a. Western Semites in Persepolis. AAASH 25:101–12.

————. 1978. La correspondance des sibilantes dans les textes araméens et les textes cunéiformes néo-assyriens. In *Atti del secondo congresso internazionale di linguistica camito-semitica*, ed. P. Fronzaroli, 201–10. Quaderni di semitistica 5. Florence: Istituto di linguistica e di lingue orientali.

————. 1978a. North Semitic Texts from the First Millennium BC. In *NERTOT*, 228–66. Philadelphia: Westminster .

————. 1978b. The Greek-Aramaic Inscription from Aǧac Kale. In *Proceedings of the Xth International Congress of Classical Archaeology*, 267–72. Ankara: Türk Tarih Kurumu.

————. 1978c. Aramäer und Israel. In *Theologische Realenzyklopädie* 3: 590–99. Berlin:

de Gruyter.

———. 1978d.   Review of *Le Livre de Daniel,* by A. Lacocque. *VT* 28:233–41.

———. 1979.   Les temples néo-assyriens et les origines du monnayage. In *State and Temple Economy in the Ancient Near East,* ed. E. Lipiński, 2.565–88. OrLovAn 6.

———. 1979a.   Aram et Israël du Xe au VIIIe siècle av. n. è. AAASH 27:49–102.

———. 1979b.   *nešek* and *tarbīt* in the Light of Epigraphical Evidence. *OLP* 10:133–41.

———. 1980.   Études d'onomastique ouest-sémitique. *BO* 37:3–12.

———. 1980a.   Review of *Onomastica aramaica aus Ägypten,* by W. Kornfeld. *BO* 37:5–10.

———. 1981.   L'esclavage d'après les documents araméens du Ier millénaire av. n.è. *Akkadica* 21:54.

———. 1981a.   The Wife's Right to Divorce in the Light of an Ancient Near Eastern Tradition. *The Jewish Law Annual* 4:9–27.

———. 1982.   Egyptian Aramaic Coins from the Fifth and Fourth Centuries B. C. In *Studia Paulo Naster Oblata* I, ed. S. Scheers, 23–33. OrLovAn 12.

———. 1983.   The God 'Arqû-Rashap in the Samallian Hadad Inscription. In *Arameans, Aramaic and the Aramaic Literary Tradition,* ed. M. Sokoloff, 15–21. Ramat-Gan: Bar-Ilan Univ. Press.

———. 1983a.   Notes d'épigraphie phénicienne et punique. *OLP* 14:129–65.

———. 1984.   Review of *La statue de Tell Fekherye,* by A. Abou Assaf et al. *OLZ* 79:455–57.

———. 1985.   Aramaic-Akkadian Archives from the Gozan-Ḥarran Area. *BAT,* 340–48.

———. 1985a.   Un culte de X^{v}an et de Hathya à Eléphantine au Ve s. av. n. è. *Folia Orientalia* 22:5–11.

———. 1985b.   Review of *The Cambridge History of Judaism I: Introduction. The Persian Period,* eds. W. D Davies and L. Finkelstein. *BO* 42: 160–68.

———. 1986.   Review of *The Bisitun Inscription of Darius the Great, Aramaic Version,* by J. C. Greenfield and B. Porten. *CdE* 61:267–69.

———. 1986a.   Review of *Les inscriptions araméennes de Sfiré et l'Assyrie de Shamshi-ilu,* by A. Lemaire and J.-M. Durand. *BASOR* 264:85–86; *OLZ* 81: 351–54.

———. 1987.   Aram, Araméens; Araméen; Damas. In *Dictionnaire encyclopédique de la Bible,* 125–29, 323–25. Turnhourt: Brepols.

———. 1988.   Nouveaux recueils de textes araméens et phénico-puniques. [Review article of *Aramaic Epigraphs on Clay Tablets of the Neo-Assyrian Period,* by F. M Fales; *Die aramäischen Texte vom Toten Meer,* by K. Beyer; and *Corpus de las inscripciones fenicias, púnicas y neopúnicas de España,* by M. Estañol.] *BO* 45:510–17.

———. 1988a.   Review of *Textbook of Aramaic Documents from Ancient Egypt I: Letters,* by B. Porten and A. Yardeni. *Or* 57:434–36.

———. 1989.   "Celllériers" de la province de Juda. *Transeuphratène* 1: 107–9.

———. 1989a.   "Mon père était un Araméen errant." L'histoire, carrefour des sciences bibliques et orientales. *OLP* 20: 23–47.

————. 1990. Géographie linguistique de la Transeuphratène à l'époque achéménide. *Transeuphratène* 3:95–107.

————. 1990a. Araméen d'Empire. In *La Pensée linguistique* 3, ed. P. Swiggers. Leuven: Peeters.

Littmann, E. 1903. Review of *Die Aramaismen im Alten Testament*, by E. Kautzsch. *AJSL* 19:244–46.

————. 1916. *Lydian Inscriptions.* Sardis VI/I, Publications of the American Society for the Excavation of Sardis. Leiden: Brill.

————. 1929. Review of *Der aramäische Beschwörungstext in spätbabylonischer Keilschrift*, by P. Jensen. *OLZ* 32:464–65.

————. 1930. Review of *Kurzgefasste biblisch-aramäische Grammatik*, by H. Bauer and P. Leander. *OLZ* 33:449–51.

————. 1935. Notes et études d'archéologie orientale. *OLZ* 38:166–68.

Liverani, M. 1961. Bar-Guš e Bar-Rakib. *RSO* 36:185–87.

————. 1962. Antecedenti dell'onomastica aramaica antica. *RSO* 37:65–76.

Livingstone, A., et al. 1983. Taimā': Recent Soundings and New Inscribed Material (1402/1982). *Atlal* 7:102–16, pls. 87–97.

Livingstone, A. See also: K. Beyer.

Livshitz, V. A., and I. Sh. Shifman. 1977. On the Interpretation of the New Aramaic Inscriptions of Aśoka [in Russian]. *VDI* 140:7–24.

Llinas, C. 1974. Araméen, Lycien et Grec: La stèle trilingue du Létôon de Xanthos. *ETR* 49:373–76.

Loewenstamm, S. E. 1955–82. **חזאל, חזהאל**. In *EM* 3, 87–88 + 1 pl.

————. See also: Z. Ben-Ḥayyim.

Lohfink, N. 1983. Die Bedeutungen von Hebr. *jrš qal* und *hif. BZ* 27:14–33.

Löhr, M. 1913. Die weiblichen Eigennamen in Sachaus "Aramäischen Papyrus und Ostraka." *OLZ* 16:15–16, 103–6.

Longpérier, A. de. 1855. Les monuments antiques de l'asie. *JA*:407–34.

Loretz, O. 1966. *berît* — "Band — Bund." *VT* 16:239–41.

————. 1978. Review of *Aramaic Texts from Deir 'Alla*, by J. Hoftijzer et al. *UF* 10:472.

Löw, I. 1881. *Aramäische Pflanzennamen.* Leipzig: W. Engelmann. Reprint. 1973.

————. 1906. Aramäische Fischnamen. In *Orientalische Studien T. Nöldeke . . . gewidmet*, 549–70. Giessen: Töpelmann.

————. 1907. **המונית** in dem Papyrus von Elephantine (aus einem Brief an D. H. Müller). *WZKM* 21:415–16.

————. 1909. Bemerkung zu OLZ. 1909, Sp. 11. *OLZ* 12:115–16.

————. 1915. Zu den aramäischen Papyrus von Elephantine. *OLZ* 18:7.

Lozachmeur, H. 1971. Un ostracon araméen inédit d'Éléphantine (Collection Clermont-Ganneau n° 228). *Sem* 21:81–93, pl. 1, f. 1.

————. 1975. Sur la bilingue gréco-araméenne d'Ağcakale. *Sem* 25:97–102.

———. 1990. Un ostracon araméen d'Eléphantine (Collection Clermont-Ganneau no. 125?). *Sem* 39:29–37.

———. See also: A. Lemaire.

Luckenbill, D. D. 1925. Azariah of Judah. *AJSL* 41:217–32.

Lund, H. V. 1879–80. Oprindelsen til ordet *munk* (μοναχός) [The origin of the word "monk"]. *Nordisk tidskrift for filologi* 4:213–22 + 1 pl.

Luria, B. Z. 1985–86. ‏מיהו בלעם בן-בעור?‏. *BM* 31:1–5.

Luschan, F. von. 1893. *Fünf Bildwerke aus Gerdschin*. Ausgrabungen in Sendschirli, I. Mittheilungen aus den orientalischen Sammlungen, vol. 11. Berlin: W. Spemann.

———. 1911. Bildwerke und Inschriften. In *Ausgrabungen in Sendschirli, IV*, 325–80. Mittheilungen aus den orientalischen Sammlungen, vol. 14. Berlin: G. Reimer.

———. 1943. *Die Kleinfunde von Sendschirli: Ausgrabungen in Sendschirli, V*. Mitteilungen aus den orientalischen Sammlungen, vol. 15. Berlin: De Gruyter.
Reviews: K. Galling 1948.

Lust, J. 1978. Daniel 7,13 and the Septuagint. *ETL* 54:62–69.

Luynes, M. le duc de. 1855. Inscription phénicienne sur une pierre à libation du Sérapéum du Memphis. *Bulletin archéologique de l'Athenaeum français* 8:69–74; 9:77–81.

Lyon, D. G. See: G. A. Reisner.

Macalister, R. A. S. 1907. Fifteenth Quarterly Report on the Excavation of Gezer. *PEFQS*:254–68.

———. 1909. Twentieth Quarterly Report on the Excavation of Gezer. *PEFQS*:13–25.

———. 1912. *The Excavation of Gezer 1902–1905 and 1907–1909*. Vol. 2. London: J. Murray.

Macalister, R. A. S., and J. G. Duncan. 1926. *Excavations on the Hill of Ophel, Jerusalem, 1923–1925*. London: Palestine Exploration Fund.

MacDonald, E. M. 1931. *The Position of Women as Reflected in Semitic Codes of Law*. Univ. of Toronto Studies: Oriental Series 1. Toronto: Univ. of Toronto Press.

MacDowall, D. W. 1965. The Dynasty of the Later Indo-Parthians. *NC* 7/5:137–48 + 1 pl.

MacLaurin, E. C. B. 1968. Date of the Foundation of the Jewish Colony at Elephantine. *JNES* 27:89–96.

Macuch, R. 1965. *Handbook of Classical and Modern Mandaic*. Berlin: de Gruyter.

———. 1971. Gesprochenes Aramäisch und aramäische Schriftsprache. In *Christentum am Roten Meer*, ed. F. Altheim and R. Stiehl, 537–57. Berlin: De Gruyter.

———. 1973. A "Revised Reading" of an Aramaic Papyrus. *JAOS* 93:58–60.

———. 1984–86. Hermeneutische Akrobatik aufgrund phonetischen Lautwandels in aramäischen Dialekten. *OS* 33–35:269–83.

———. 1990. Some Orthographico-Phonetic Problems of Ancient Aramaic and the Living Aramaic Pronunication. In *Sopher Mahir: Northwest Semitic Studies Presented to Stanislav Segert*, ed. E. M. Cook (= *Maarav* 5–6), 221–37.

Madden, F. W. 1864. *History of Jewish Coinage and of Money in the Old and New Testament*. London: B. Quaritch. Reprint. New York: Ktav, 1967.

————. 1881. *Coins of the Jews*. The International Orientalia 2. London: Trübner.

Mahler, E. 1912. Die Doppeldaten der aramäischen Papyri von Assuan. *ZA* 26:61–76.

Mai, A. 1825. *Catalogo de' papiri egiziani della biblioteca Vaticana e notizia piu estesa di uno d'essi con breve previo discorso e con susseguenti riflessioni*. Rome: Tipi Vaticani.

Maigret, A. de. 1979. *La cittadella aramaica di Hama: Attività, funzioni e comportamento*. Orientis antiqui collectio 15. Rome: Istituto per l'Oriente.

Malamat, A. 1949–50. The New Aramaic Saqqârah Papyrus from the Time of Jeremiah [in Hebrew]. *BJPES* 15:34–39.

————. 1949–50a. The Tell Ḥalâf (Gozan) Texts [in Hebrew]. *BJPES* 15:99–102.

————. 1950. The Last Wars of the Kingdom of Judah. *JNES* 9:218–27.

————. 1953. Amos 1:5 in the Light of the Til Barsip Inscriptions. *BASOR* 129:25–26.

————. 1956. A New Record of Nebuchadrezzar's Palestinian Campaigns. *IEJ* 6:246–56.

————. 1958. The Kingdom of David and Solomon in its Contact with Egypt and Aram Naharaim. *BA* 21:96–102.

————. 1973. The Aramaeans. In *Peoples of Old Testament Times*, ed. D. J. Wiseman, 134–55. Oxford: Clarendon.

————. 1976. A New Proposal for the Identification of KTK in the Sefire Inscriptions. In *Census Lists and Genealogies and Their Historical Implications*, ed. S. Bendor, vii–xi. Haifa: University of Haifa.

Mallowan, M. E. L. 1966. *Nimrud and Its Remains*. 3 vols. London: Collins.

Malone, J. L. 1971. Wave Theory, Rule Ordering and Hebrew-Aramaic Segolation. *JAOS* 91:44–66.

Mann, A. M. 1985. *The Jewish Marriage Contracts from Elephantine: A Study of Text and Marriage*. Ph.D. diss., New York Univ.

Manson, T. W. 1949–50. The Son of Man in Daniel, Henoch and the Gospels. *BJRL* 32:171–93.

Maraqten, M. 1988. *Die semitischen Personnamen in den alt- und reichsaramäischen Inschriften aus Vorderasien*. Texte und Studien zur Orientalistik 5. Hildesheim: Olms.

Marblestone, H. 1985. Syrus in Tiberim defluxit Orontes. *Mnemosyne* 38:156–58.

Margain, J. 1979–84. A propos d'un phénomène de nounation en hébreu et en araméen. De 'Maryam' à 'Maria'. *Comptes rendus du GLECS* 24–28:81–84.

Margalit, B. 1980. Interpreting the Story of Aqht: A Reply to H. H. P. Dressler, VT 29, (1979), pp. 152–61. *VT* 30:361–65.

Margoliouth, D. S. 1907. The New Papyri of Elephantine. *Expositor* 7/4:481–94.

————. 1912. The Elephantinê Papyri. *Expositor* 8/3:69–85.

————. 1912a. Note on the Elephantinê Papyri. *Expositor* 8/3:351–54.

Margolis, M. L. 1911–12. The Elephantine Documents. *JQR* 2:419–43.

Margueron, J., and J. Teixidor. 1983. Un objet à légende araméenne provenant de Meskéné-Emar. *RA* 77:75–80 + 4 photos + 4 figs.

Maricq, A. 1958. Classica et Orientalia: 5. Res gestae divi Saporis. *Syria* 35:295–360.

Mariette, A. 1880. Lettre à M. Desjardins sur deux stèles d'Abydos et une stèle de Saqqârah, nouvellement découvertes. *CRAIBL* 4/7:121–33.

Marquart, J. 1907. Untersuchung zur Geschichte von Eran. *Philologus* Supplementband 10:1–258.

Marshall, J. 1951. *Taxila.* 3 vols. Cambridge: Cambridge Univ. Press.

Martínez Borobio, E. 1982. Libro arameo de Ajicar. In *Apócrifos del Antiguo Testamento*, ed. A. Díez Macho, 167–87. Madrid: Cristiandad.

Marti, K. 1896. *Kurzgefasste Grammatik der biblisch-aramäischen Sprache.* Porta Linguarum Orientalium XVIII. 3rd edition, 1925. Berlin: Reuther & Reichard.
Reviews: G. Bergsträsser 1912.

————. 1909. Zu Urkunde I. der drei von Ed. Sachau herausgegebenen aramäischen Papyri aus Elephantine. *ZAW* 29:74.

Martin, M. F. 1964. Six Palestinian Seals. *RSO* 39:203–10, I–III.

Mashkur, M. J. 1968. *Farhang-e huzvārešha-ye pahlavi. The Huzvāreš Dictionary. A Collection of (Aramaic) Ideograms in Pahlavi Writing.* Entešārāt-e bonyād-e farhang-e Irān. Tehrān: Iranian Cultural Foundation.

Maspero, G. 1883. *Guide du visiteur au musée de Boulaq.* Boulaq: Au Musée.

Mastin, B. A. 1973. Daniel 2.46 and the Hellenistic World. *ZAW* 85:80–93.

Mateos, J. See: L. A. Schökel.

May, H. G. 1936. The Relation of the Passover to the Festival of Unleavened Cakes. *JBL* 55:65–82.

Mayrhofer, M. 1974. Ein neuer Beleg zu der indogermanischen Sippe für Halsschmuck. In *Antiquitates indogermanicae*, ed. M. Mayrhofer et al., 289–91. Innsbruck: Institut für Sprachwissenschaft.

————. 1978. Alt-neue Iraniernamen aus Persepolis. In *Studia in honorem Veselini Beševliev*, ed. V. Georgiev et al., 56–60. Sofia: Academia litterarum bulgarica.

————. 1979. Die iranischen Elemente im aramäischen Text. In *Fouilles de Xanthos, Tome VI: La stèle trilingue du Létôon*, ed. H. Metzger, 179–85. Institut Français d'Etudes Anatoliennes. Paris: C. Klincksieck.

Mazar (Maisler), B. 1940–41. בית טוביה. *Tarbiz* 12:109–23.

————. 1948. The Historical Background of the Samaria Ostraca. *JPOS* 21:117–33.

Mazar, B. 1956. בן-טבאל ובית טוביה. *EI (Ben-Zvi Volume)* 4:249–51.

————. 1957. The Tobiads. *IEJ* 7:137–45, 229–38.

————. 1962. The Aramean Empire and Its Relations with Israel. *BA* 25:98–120. Reprinted in *The Biblical Archaeologist Reader* (Garden City, N. Y.: Doubleday Anchor, 1964), 127–51.

————. 1962a. Ein Gev. *RB* 69:399–401.

————. 1967. En-gedi. In *Archaeology and Old Testament Study*, ed. D. Winton Thomas, 223–30. Oxford: Clarendon.

————. 1986. The Aramean Empire and Its Relations with Israel. In *The Early Biblical Period: Historical Studies*, ed. S. Aḥituv and B. A. Levine, 151–72. Jerusalem: Israel Exploration Society.

Mazar, B., A. Biran, M. Dothan, and I. Dunayevsky. 1964. 'Ein Gev: Excavations in 1961. *IEJ* 14:1–49.

Mazar, B., and I. Dunayevsky. 1964. En-Gedi: Third Season of Excavations, Preliminary Report. *IEJ* 14:123–30.

————. 1965. Engeddi. *IEJ* 15:258–59.

Mazar, B., T. Dothan, and I. Dunayevsky. 1963. The Excavations at Tel Goren (Tell el-Jurn) [in Hebrew]. *BIES* 27:20–82; *fig. 12*.

————. 1966. *En-Gedi Excavations*. Jerusalem: Dept. of Antiquities and Museums, Ministry of Education and Culture.

McCarter, P. K., Jr. 1980. The Balaam Texts from Deir 'Allā: The First Combination. *BASOR* 239:49–60.

————. 1991. The Dialect of the Deir 'Alla Texts. In *BTDAR*, 87–99.

McCarthy, D. J. 1963. *Treaty and Covenant: A Study in Form in the Ancient Oriental Documents and in the Old Testament*. AnBib 21. Rome: Pontifical Biblical Institute.

————. 1972. *Old Testament Covenant: A Survey of Current Opinions*. Growing Points in Theology. Richmond: John Knox.

————. 1979. Ebla, ὅρκια τέμνειν, *ṭb, šlm*: Addenda to *Treaty and Covenant*. *Bib* 60:247–53.

————. 1982. Covenant "Good" and an Egyptian Text. *BASOR* 245:63–64.

McCown, C. C. 1947. *Tell en-Naṣbeh Excavated Under the Direction of the Late William Frederic Badè*. Berkeley: Palestine Institute of the Pacific School of Religion; New Haven: ASOR.

————. 1957. The 'Araq el-Emir and the Tobiads. *BA* 20:63–76.

McCurdy, J. F. 1908. Aram, Arameans, and the Aramaic Language. In *The New Schaff-Herzog Encyclopedia of Religious Knowledge*, 254–57. New York: Funk and Wagnalls.

McEwan, G. 1983. The First Seleucid Document from Babylonia. *JSS* 30:169–80.

McKane, W. 1970. Ahikar. In *Proverbs: A New Approach*, 156–82. The Old Testament Library. Philadelphia: Westminster.

McNamara, M. 1957. De populi Aramaeorum primordiis. *VD* 35:129–42.

Meissner, B. 1917. *Das Märchen vom weisen Achiqar*. Der alte Orient, vol. 16, pt. 2. Leipzig: J. C. Hinrichs.

————. 1941. *Kaṣâru* oder *qaṣâru*? *AfO* 14:202–3.

————. See also: H. Bauer.

Melkman, J. 1939. Daniël V. *Nieuw Theologisch Tijdschrift* 28:143–50.

Mellink, M. 1965. Archaeology in Asia Minor. *AJA* 69:133–49.

Mellink, M., and R. S. Young. 1966. Art Treasures of Turkey. *Archaeology* 19:190–98.

Meltzer, U. 1924. West- und ostaramäische Formen in Mittelpersischen. *ZS* 3:296–305.

————. 1925. Die aramäischen Zeitwörter im Mittelpersischen. *WZKM* 32:225–54.

————. 1927. Zur Aussprache der aramäischen Wörter im Mittelpersischen. *ZS* 5:312–38.

Menant, J. 1886. *Les pierres gravées de la haut-Asîe: Recherches sur la glyptique orientale*, vol. 2. Paris: Maisonneuve.

Menasce, J. de. 1954. Mots d'emprunt et noms propres iraniens dans les nouveaux documents araméens. *BO* 11:161–62.

———. 1972. A propos d'une inscription araméenne d'Aśoka. *IOS* 2:290–92.

Mendecki, N. 1986. Filistyni, Aramejczycy i Kanaejczycy w drugiej polowie drugiego tysiclecia przed Chr. [The Philistines, the Arameans and the Canaanites in the second half of the Second Millennium before Christ]. *Collectanea theologica* 56:43–46.

———. 1987. Izraelici a Kananejczycy i Aramejczycy [Israel in relation to the Canaanites and the Arameans]. *Collectanea theologica* 57:41–44.

Mendelsohn, I. 1949. *Slavery in the Ancient Near East*. New York: Oxford Univ. Press.

Mentz, A. 1922. Zur Schrift und Sprache der Lyder. *OLZ* 25:489–92.

Menzel, B. 1981. *Assyrische Tempel*. 2 vols. Studia Pohl: Series Maior, vol. 10. Rome: Pontifical Biblical Institute.

Meriggi, P. 1934–36. Die erste Person Singularis im Lydischen. *Revue hittite et asianique* 3:69–116.

Mertens, A. 1971. *Das Buch Daniel im Lichte der Texte vom Toten Meer*. SBM 12. Stuttgart: Katholisches Bibelwerk.

Merx, A. 1865. *Cur in libro Danielis iuxta Hebraeam Aramaea adhibita sit dialectus explicatur*. Jena: Ratii.

———. 1868. Bemerkungen über bis jetzt bekannte aramäische Inschriften. *ZDMG* 22:674–99.

Meshorer, Y. 1989. The Mints of Ashdod and Ascalon during the Late Persian Period [in Hebrew]. *EI* (Yadin Volume) 20:287–91.

Mesnil du Buisson, R. du. 1930. Compte rendu de la mission de Khan Sheikhoun et de Souran, au nord de Hama (Syrie). *CRAIBL*: 320–31.

———. 1963. Origine et évolution du panthéon de Tyr. *RHR* 164:133–63.

———. 1970. *Études sur les dieux phéniciens hérités par l'empire romain*. Études préliminaires aux religions orientales dans l'empire romain 14. Leiden: Brill.

Messina, G. 1934. L'antico arameo. In *Miscellanea Biblica* 69–103. Vol. 2. Rome: Pontifical Biblical Institute.

———. 1936. Nota aramaica. *Bib* 17:102–3.

Metheny, J. R. 1907. Road Notes from Cilicia and North Syria. *JAOS* 28:155–63.

Metzger, H. 1974. La stèle trilingue récemment découverte au Létoon de Xanthos: Le texte grec. *CRAIBL*: 82–93.

Metzger, H., ed. 1980. *Actes du colloque sur la Lycie antique*. Bibliothèque de l'Institut français d'études anatoliennes d'Istanbul 27. Paris: Maisonneuve.

Metzler, D. 1984. Aḥīqar in Trier. In ΘΙΑΣΟΣ ΤΩΝ ΜΟΥΣΩΝ: *Studien zu Antike und Christentum—Festschrift für Josef Fink zum 70. Geburtstag*, ed. D. Ahrens, 97–107. Cologne: Böhlau.

———. See also: F. Altheim.

Meyer, E. 1911. Zu den aramäischen Papyri von Elephantine. *SPAW* 47:1026–53.

———. 1912. *Der Papyrusfund von Elephantine: Dokumente einer jüdischen Gemeinde aus der Perserzeit und das älteste erhaltene Buch der Weltliteratur*. 2nd ed. Leipzig: J. C.

Hinrichs.

———. 1915. Ägyptische Dokumente aus der Perserzeit. *SPAW* 51:287–311.

———. 1953. *Geschichte des Altertums.* 5 vols. 3rd ed. Stuttgart: Cotta.

Meyer, G. R. 1965. *Altorientalische Denkmäler im Vorderasiatischen Museum zu Berlin.* Leipzig: Seemann.

Meyer, R. 1954. Ein aramäischer Papyrus aus den ersten Jahren Nebukadnezars II. In *Festschrift für Friedrich Zucker zum 70. Geburtstage,* ed. W. Müller, 251–62. Berlin: Akademie Verlag.

———. 1967. Review of *Aramäische Chrestomathie,* by J. J. Koopmans. *OLZ* 62:473–75.

Michaud, H. 1961. Review of *A Grammar of Biblical Aramaic,* by F. Rosenthal. *Syria* 38:327–30.

Michelini Tocci, F. 1962. Un frammento di stele aramaica da Tell Sifr. *OrAnt* 1:21–22, pl. II.

Mikaya, A. 1981. Earliest Aramaic Inscription Uncovered in Syria. *BARev* 7/4:52–53.

Mildenberg, L. 1979. Yehud:A Preliminary Study of the Provincial Coinage of Judaea. In *Greek Numismatics and Archaeology, Essays in Honor of Margaret Thompson,* ed. O. Mørkholm and N. M. Waggoner, 183–96. Wetteren.

Milik, J. T. 1954. Review of *The Brooklyn Museum Aramaic Papyri,* by E. G. Kraeling. *RB* 61:247–51.

———. 1954a. Review of *Aramaic Documents of the Fifth Century B. C.,* by G. R. Driver. *RB* 61:592–95.

———. 1958–59. Nouvelles inscriptions sémitiques et grecques du pays de Moab. *SBFLA* 9:330–58.

———. 1960. Lettre araméenne d'el-Hibeh. *Aeg* 40:79–81.

———. 1960a. Inscriptions au pays de Moab. *RB* 67:243–44.

———. 1967. Les papyrus araméens d'Hermopoulis et les cultes syro-phéniciens en Egypte perse. *Bib* 48:546–622.

Millard, A. R. 1962. Alphabetic Inscriptions on Ivories from Nimrud. *Iraq* 24:41–51.

———. 1965. The Assyrian Royal Seal Type Again. *Iraq* 27:12–16.

———. 1970. "Scriptio continua" in Early Hebrew: Ancient Practice or Modern Surmise? *JSS* 15:2–15.

———. 1971. Baladan, the Father of Merodach-Baladan. *Tyndale Bulletin* 22:125–26.

———. 1972. Some Aramaic Epigraphs. *Iraq* 34:131–38.

———. 1972a. ^F*ša ekalli*—*šgl*—^d*sagale.* *UF* 4:161–62.

———. 1973. Adad-Nirari III, Aram, and Arpad. *PEQ* 105:161–64.

———. 1975. A Decree of a Persian Governor. *Buried History* 11:84–91.

———. 1976. Assyrian Royal Names in Biblical Hebrew. *JSS* 21:1–14.

———. 1976a. Review of *Studies in Aramaic Inscriptions and Onomastics I,* by E. Lipiński. *JSS* 21:174–78.

———. 1976b. The Canaanite Linear Alphabet and its Passage to the Greeks. *Kadmos* 15:130–44.

————. 1977. Daniel 1–6 and History. *Evangelical Quarterly* 49:67–73.

————. 1977a. The Persian Names in Esther and the Reliability of the Hebrew Text. *JBL* 96:481–88.

————. 1978. Epigraphic Notes, Aramaic and Hebrew. *PEQ* 110:23–26.

————. 1980. A Wandering Aramean. *JNES* 39:153–55.

————. 1982. In Praise of Ancient Scribes. *BA* 45:143–53.

————. 1983. Assyrians and Arameans. *Iraq* 45:101–8.

————. 1984. The Etymology of Eden. *VT* 34:103–6.

————. 1984a. Review of *Early History of the Alphabet*, by J. Naveh. *PEQ*:75–76.

————. 1985. Daniel and Belshazzar in History. *BARev* 11/3:72–78.

————. 1985a. An Assessment of the Evidence for Writing in Ancient Israel. *BAT*, 301–12.

————. 1985b. La prophétie et l'écriture: Israël, Aram, Assyrie. *RHR* 202:125–45.

————. 1987. The Etymology of *Nebraštā'*, Daniel 5:5. *Maarav* 4:87–92.

————. 1988. Ebla Personal Names and Personal Names of the First Millennium B.C. in Syria and Palestine. In *Eblaite Personal Names and Semitic Name-Giving: Papers of a Symposium held in Rome July 15–17, 1985*, ed. A. Archi, 159–64. Rome: Università degli Studi di Roma "La Sapienza," Missione Archeologia Italiana in Siria.

————. 1988a. Inscribed Seals. In *Catalogue of Ancient Near Eastern Seals in the Ashmolean Museum. Volume II: The Iron Age Stamp Seals (c. 1200–350 BC)*, by B. Buchanan and P. R. S. Moorey, 44–46. Oxford: Clarendon.

————. 1988b. Review of *Catalogue des sceaux ouest-sémitiques inscrits de la Bibliothèque Nationale, du Musée du Louvre et du Musée Biblique de Bible et Terre Sainte*, by P. Bordreuil and *Hebrew Bullae from the Time of Jeremiah*, by N. Avigad. *PEQ* 120:69–71.

————. 1989. Please Speak Aramaic. *Buried History* 25:67–73.

————. 1989a. Note on Two Seal Impressions on Pottery. *Levant* 21:60–61.

————. 1989b. Mari'. *RlA* 7/5–6:418–19.

————. 1989c. The Homeland of Zakkur. *Sem* 39:60–66.

————. 1990. Israelite and Aramean History in the Light of Inscriptions. *Tyndale Bulletin* 41:261–275.

Millard, A. R., and P. Bordreuil. 1982. A Statue from Syria with Assyrian and Aramaic Inscriptions. *BA* 45:135–41.

Millard, A. R., and H. Tadmor. 1973. Adad-Nirari III in Syria: Another Stele Fragment and the Dates of His Campaigns. *Iraq* 35:57–64 + 1 pl.

Millard, A. See also: A. Abou Assaf.

Miller, F. 1897. Die semitischen Elemente der Pahlawi-Sprache. *SKAWW*, 136/10:1–12.

Miller, J. M. 1969. Geshur and Aram. *JNES* 28:60–61.

Miller, J. M. See also: J. A. Dearman.

Misgav, H. See: H. Eshel.

Mitchell, L. A. 1984. *A Student's Vocabulary for Biblical Hebrew and Aramaic*. Grand Rapids, Mich.: Zondervan.

Mitchell, T. C. 1967. Philistia. In *Archaeology and Old Testament Study: Jubilee Volume for SOTS 1917–1967*, ed. D. Winton Thomas, 405–27. Oxford: Clarendon.

Mittwoch, E. 1912. Der Wiederaufbau des jüdischen Tempels in Elephantine — Ein Kompromiss zwischen Juden und Samaritanern. In *Judaica: Festschrift zu Hermann Cohens siebzigstem Geburtstage*, 227–33. Berlin: Bruno Cassirer.

———. 1939. Neue aramäische Urkunden aus der Zeit der Achämenidenherrschaft in Ägypten. *MGWJ* 83:93–100.

Mode, R. H. 1907. The Assuan Aramaic Papyri. *BW* 29:305–9.

Montfaucon, B. de. 1724. *Supplement au livre de l'antiquité expliquée et représentée en figures*. 5 vols. Paris: Le Veuvel Delaulne et al.

Montgomery, J. A. 1907. Report on an Aramaic Boundary Inscription in Cilicia. *JAOS* 28:164–67 + 1 pl.

———. 1908. An Aramaic Ostracon from Nippur and the Greek Obolos. *JAOS* 29:204–9.

———. 1909. Some Gleanings from Pognon's ZKR Inscription. *JBL* 28:57–70.

———. 1912. Some Notes on Sachau's Aḥiḳar Papyri. *OLZ* 15:535–36.

———. 1912–13. Some Correspondences between the Elephantinê Papyri and the Gospels. *ExpTim* 24:428–29.

———. 1917. Babylonian *niš* "oath" in West-Semitic. *JAOS* 37:329–30.

———. 1923. Adverbial *kúlla* in Biblical Aramaic and Hebrew. *JAOS* 43:391–95.

———. 1927. *A Critical and Exegetical Commentary on the Book of Daniel*. ICC. New York: Scribner. 2nd ed. Edinburgh: Clark, 1950.

———. 1931. Review of *Grammatik des Biblisch-Aramäischen*, by H. Bauer and P. Leander; *Kurzgefasste Grammatik des Biblisch-Aramäischen*, by H. Bauer and P. Leander; *Laut- und Formenlehre des Ägyptisch-Aramäischen*, by P. Leander; *The Aramaic of the Old Testament*, by H. H. Rowley; *A Critical and Exegetical Commentary on the Book of Daniel*, by R. H. Charles. *JAOS* 51:317–27.

———. 1934. Notes on Early Aramaic Inscriptions. *JAOS* 54:421–25.

———. 1940–41. Rosenthal's Review of Recent Studies in the Aramaic Field. [Review of *Die aramaistische Forschung seit Th. Nöldekes Veröffentlichungen*, by F. Rosenthal] *JQR* 31:411–12.

Moor, J. C. de. 1988. Narrative Poetry in Canaan. *UF* 20:149–71.

Moortgat, A. 1926. Hellas und die Kunst der Achaemeniden, MAOG II/1. Leipzig: E. Pfeiffer.

———. 1940. *Vorderasiatische Rollsiegel: Ein Beitrag zur Geschichte der Steinschneidekunst*. Berlin: Gebr. Mann.

Moortgat-Correns, U. 1955. Altorientalische Rollsiegel der staatlichen Münz-Sammlung München. *Münchener Jahrbuch der bildenden Kunst* 6:7–27.

Morag, S. 1962. *The Vocalization Systems of Arabic, Hebrew, and Aramaic: Their Phonetic and Phonemic Principles*. Janua Linguarum 13. The Hague: Mouton.

———. 1964. Biblical Aramaic in Geonic Babylonia. In *Studies in Egyptology and Linguistics in honour of H. J. Polotsky*, ed. H. B. Rosén, 117–31. Jerusalem: Israel Exploration Society.

————. 1973. *The Book of Daniel: A Babylonian-Yemenite Manuscript.* Jerusalem: Kirjath Sepher.

————. 1974. כתב-יד בבלי-תימני של ספר דניאל. In *Sepher Zikaron leḤanok Yalon,* ed. E. Kutscher et al., 221–74. Ramat-Gan: Bar-Ilan Univ. Press.

Moran, W. L. 1963. A Note on the Treaty Terminology of the Sefîre Stelas. *JNES* 22:173–76.

————. 1963a. The Ancient Near Eastern Background of the Love of God in Deuteronomy. *CBQ* 25:77–87.

Mordtmann, A. D. 1860. Aus Briefen des Hrn. Dr. Mordtmann an Prof. Brockhaus. *ZDMG* 14:555–56.

Morenz, S. 1951. Das Tier mit den Hörnern, ein Beitrag zu Dan 7.7f. *ZAW* 63:151–54.

Morgan, J. de. 1896. Recherches archéologiques. In *Mission scientifique en Perse* 298. Paris: E. Leroux.

Morgenstern, J. 1924. The Three Calendars of Ancient Israel. *HUCA* 1:13–78.

Moriya, A. 1980. *'dy kō* (On *'dy*) [in Japanese]. *Kyūsh–Kyōritsu-Daigaku Kiyō* 15:165–76.

————. 1985. The Functions of the Gods in the Aramaic Inscriptions of Sefire. *Oriento* 25/2:38–54.

Mørkholm, O. 1962. Some Cappodocian Problems. *NC* 7/2:407–11 + 1 pl.

————. 1964. Some Cappodocian Die-Links. *NC* 7/4:21–25.

Morrow, W. S., and E. G. Clarke. 1986. The *Ketib/Qere* in the Aramaic Portions of Ezra and Daniel. *VT* 36:406–22.

Mosca, P. G. 1986. Ugarit and Daniel 7: A Missing Link. *Bib* 67:496–517.

Moscati, S. 1951. *L'epigrafia ebraica antica, 1935–1950.* BibOr 15. Rome: Pontifical Biblical Institute.

————. 1951a. Sulle origini degli Aramei. *RSO* 26:16–22.

————. 1954. Il plurale esterno maschile nelle lingue semitiche. *RSO* 29:28–52.

————. 1956. Review of "L'Aramaico antico," by G. Garbini. *RSO* 31:316–17.

————. 1956a. Sulla posizione linguistica del semitico nord-occidentale. *RSO* 31:229–34.

————. 1956b. Il Semitico di Nord-Ovest. In *Studi orientalistici in onore di Giorgio Levi della Vida* 202–21. Pubblicazioni dell'Istituto per l'Oriente 52. Rome: Giovanni Bardi.

————. 1959. The Aramaean Aḥlamū. *JSS* 4:303–07.

————. 1962. Lo stato assoluto dell'aramaico orientale. *AION* 22:79–83.

Mouterde, P. 1939. Review of *Die aramaistische Forschung seit Th. Nöldekes Veröffentlichungen,* by F. Rosenthal. *MUSJ* 22:221–23.

————. 1958. Review of A. Dupont-Sommer and J. Starcky 1956 and J. A. Fitzmyer 1958. *MUSJ* 35:242–45.

Mowinckel, S. 1923. Die vorderasiatischen Königs- und Fürsteninschriften. Eine stilistische Studie. In *Eucharistērion: Hermann Gunkel zum 60. Geburtstag* 278–322. Forschungen zur Religion und Literatur des Alten und Neuen Testaments 11. Göttingen: Vandenhoeck & Ruprecht.

———. 1965. *Studia theologica* 19:130–35.

Mudarres, J. 1974. Syria and Lebanon in Antiquity. *Berytus* 23:105–25.

Muffs, Y. 1969. *Studies in the Aramaic Legal Papyri from Elephantine.* Studia et Documenta ad Iura Orientis Antiqui Pertinentia 8. Leiden: Brill.
Reviews: E. Vogt 1975.

———. 1973. Two Comparative Lexical Studies. *JANES* 5:287–98.

———. 1982. Abraham the Noble Warrior: Patriarchal Politics and Laws of War in Ancient Israel. *JJS* 33:81–107.

Muilenburg, J. 1960. The Son of Man in Daniel and the Ethiopic Apocalypse of Enoch. *JBL* 79:197–209.

Mukherjee, B. N. 1984. *Studies in the Aramaic Edicts of Asoka.* Calcutta: Indian Museum.

Mulder, M. J. 1980. Der Gott Hadad im nordwestsemitischen Raum. In *Interaction and Acculturation in the Mediterranean*, ed. J. G. P. Best and N. M. W. de Vries, 1:69–83. Amsterdam: Grüner.

Müller, C. See: G. Dankwarth.

Müller, D. H. 1884. Review of *Altaramäische Inschriften aus Teimâ*, by T. Nöldeke. *Oesterreichische Monatsschrift für den Orient* 10:209–10, 278–79.

———. 1891. Glossen zum Corpus Inscriptionum Semiticarum II. *WZKM* 5:1–8.

———. 1892. Sitzung der philosophisch–historischen Klasse vom 19. Oktober. *Anzeiger d. kaiserl. Akad. d. Wiss. zu Wien* 29/20–21:85–86.

———. 1893. Die altsemitischen Inschriften von Sendschirli. *WZKM* 7:33–70, 113–40.

———. 1894. The Excavations at Sendschirli. *The Contemporary Review* 65:563–75.

———. 1896. Die Bauinschrift des Barrekub. *WZKM* 10:193–97 + 1 pl.

———. 1907. Die Korrespondenz zwischen der Gemeinde von Elephantine und den Söhnen Sanaballaṭs. *WZKM* 21:416–19.

Müller, F. 1897. Die semitischen Elemente der Pahlawi-Sprache. *SKAWW* 136/10:1–12.

Müller, H.-P. 1978. Einige alttestamentliche Probleme zur aramäischen Inschrift von Der 'Allā. *ZDPV* 94:56–67.

———. 1982. Die aramäische Inschrift von Deir Allā und die älteren Bileamsprüche. *ZAW* 94:214–44.

———. 1986. Aramaisierende Bildungen bei Verba Mediae Geminatae—Ein Irrtum der Hebraistik? *VT* 36:423–37.

———. 1991. Die Funktion divinatorischen Redens und die Tierbezeichnungen der Inschrift von Tell Deir 'Allā. In *BTDAR*, 185–205.

Müller, M. 1972. *Messias og "Menneskesøn" i Daniels Bog, Første Enoksbog og Fjerde Ezrabog.* Tekst og tolkning, vol. 3. Copenhagen: Gad.

———. 1984. Betydningen af *br'nš* i Dan. 7, 13. *DTT* 3:177–86.

Müller, R. 1935. Der Name der Nil-Insel Elephantine. *Zeitschrift für Ortsnamenforschung* 11:183–84.

Müller, W. 1980. Die Papyrusgrabung auf Elephantine 1906–1908: Das Grabungstagebuch der 1. und 2. Kampagne. *FuB* 20–21:75–88.

———. See also: R. Degen.

Müller, W. M. 1907. Ein aramäischer Siegelstein. *OLZ* 10:151–52.

Muraoka, T. 1966. Notes on the Syntax of Biblical Aramaic. *JSS* 11:151–67.

———. 1976. Segolate Nouns in Biblical and Other Aramaic Dialects. *JAOS* 96:226–35.

———. 1983–84. The Tell-Fekherye Bilingual Inscription and Early Aramaic. *Abr-Nahrain* 22:79–117.

———. 1987. Review of *The Aramaic Proverbs of Ahiqar*, by J. M. Lindenberger. *JSS* 32:186–89.

Murray, M. A. 1904. *The Osireion at Abydos*. Egyptian Research Account, Ninth Year, 1903. London: B. Quaritch.

Murray, R. 1984. The Origin of Aramaic 'îr, Angel. *Or* 53:303–17.

Murtonen, A. 1960–61. Review of *A Grammar of Biblical Aramaic*, by F. Rosenthal. *Abr-Nahrain* 2:72–76.

Muscarella, O. W. 1981. *Ladders to Heaven, Art Treasures from Lands of the Bible*. Toronto: McClelland and Stewart.

Muuss, R. 1916. Der Jahwetempel in Elephantine. *ZAW* 36:81–107.

Myers, J. M. 1965. *Ezra, Nehemiah*. The Anchor Bible, vol. 14. Garden City, N. Y.: Doubleday.

Na'aman, N. 1977–78. Looking for KTK. *WO* 9:220–39.

Nahon, G. 1971. Review of *Archives from Elephantine*, by B. Porten. *REJ* 130:103.

———. 1974. Review of *Documents araméens d'Égypte*, by P. Grelot. *REJ* 133:342–43.

Narkiss, M. 1936–38. מטבעות ארץ ישראל. 2 vols. Jerusalem: Mosad Bialik.

Naster, P. 1968. Note d'épigraphie monétaire de Perside: *fratakara*, *frataraka* ou *fratadāra*? *Iranica antiqua* 8:74–80.

Nau, F. N. 1909. *Histoire et sagesse d'Ahikar l'Assyrien (fils d'Anaël, neveu de Tobie): Traduction des versions syriaques avec les principales différences des versions arabes, arménienne, grecque, néo-syriaque, slave et roumaine*. Documents pour l'étude de la Bible. Paris: Letouzey et Ané.

———. 1911. Juifs et Samaritains à Éléphantine. *JA* 10/18:660–62.

———. 1912. Le denier du cult juif à Éléphantine au ve siècle avant notre ère. *Revue de l'orient chrétien* 17:100–104.

———. 1912a. Ahiqar et les papyrus d'Éléphantine. *RB* 9:68–79.

———. 1914–15. Préceptes anonymes et histoire d'Ahikar d'après le ms. syriaque de Berlin Sachau 162. *Revue de l'orient chrétien* 19:209–14.

———. 1918–19. Documents relatifs à Ahikar. *Revue de l'orient chrétien* 21:92–96, 287–307, 358–400.

———. 1918–19a. Histoire et sagesse d'Ahikar d'après le ms. de Berlin 'Sachau 162' fol. 86 s. *Revue de l'orient chrétien* 21:148–60.

———. 1920. *Documents relatifs à Ahikar: Textes syriaques édités et traduits*. Paris: Librairie A. Picard.

Naudé, J. A. 1990.   Die toepasbaarheid van GB-teorie op nie-lewende tale: Evidensie oor die interpretasie van klitiekverskynsels in Bybelse Aramees. *Journal for Semitics* 2:22–43.

Naveh, J. 1964–65.   (1960–1964) כתובות ארמיות קדומות. *Leš* 29:183–97.

———. 1965–66.   (1964–1960) כתובות כנעניות ועבריות. *Leš* 30:65–80.

———. 1965–66a.   תוספת לכתובות הארמיות. *Leš* 30:157–60.

———. 1966.   Old Aramaic Inscriptions (1960–65). *AION* 26:19–36.

———. 1966a.   על כתבם של שני אוסטרקנים מאילת. *Yediot* 30:39–44.

———. 1966b.   The Scripts of Two Ostraca from Elath. *BASOR* 183:27–30.

———. 1967.   The Date of the Deir ʿAllā Inscription in Aramaic Script. *IEJ* 17:256–58.

———. 1967–68.   כתובות ארמיות מפוקפקות. *Leš* 32:326–32.

———. 1968.   Dated Coins of Alexander Janneus. *IEJ* 18:20–25.

———. 1968a.   Aramaica Dubiosa. *JNES* 27:317–25.

———. 1970.   The Scripts in Palestine and Transjordan in the Iron Age. In *Near Eastern Archaeology in the Twentieth Century: Essays in Honor of Nelson Glueck*, ed. J. A. Sanders, 277–83. Garden City, N. Y.: Doubleday.

———. 1971.   Hebrew Texts in Aramaic Script in the Persian Period? *BASOR* 203:27–32.

———. 1971a.   The Palaeography of the Hermopolis Papyri. *IOS* 1:120–22.

———. 1971b.   An Aramaic Ostracon from Ashdod. *Atiqot* 9–10:200–201, pl. XIII:1.

———. 1971c.   *The Development of the Aramaic Script*. Proceedings of the Israel Academy of Sciences and Humanities, vol. 5. Israel Academy of Sciences and Humanities: Jerusalem.
Reviews: J. Oelsner 1974; O. Klíma 1973: *ArOr* 41:388; B. Peckham 1971; J. Teixidor 1972.

———. 1972.   שני אוסטרקונים ארמיים מן התקופה הפרסית. In *The Bible and Jewish History: Studies in Bible and Jewish History Dedicated to the Memory Of Jacob Liver*, ed. B. Uffenheimer, 184–89. Tel Aviv: Tel Aviv Univ.

———. 1972a.   טביעות החותם הארמיות יהוד. In *Proceedings of the Fifth World Congress of Jewish Studies 1969*, vol. 1, 98–100. Jerusalem: World Union of Jewish Studies.

———. 1972–73.   "פחלץ" באוסטרקון ארמי חדש. *Leš* 37:270–74.

———. 1973.   Word Division in West Semitic Writing. *IEJ* 23:206–08.

———. 1973a.   The Aramaic Ostraca. In *Beer Sheba I. Excavations at Tel Beer-Sheba. 1969–71 Seasons.*, ed. Y. Aharoni, 79–82. Publications of the Institute of Archaeology 2. Tel Aviv: Tel Aviv University Institute of Archaeology.

———. 1975.   אוסטרקונים ארמיים מתל באר-שבע. *Shnaton* 1:189–95, xvi, 4 pls.

———. 1975a.   האוסטרקונים הארמיים מתל ערד. In *Arad Inscriptions*, ed. Y. Aharoni, 165–204. Jerusalem: The Bialik Institue and the Israel Exploration Society. Reprinted in English in *Arad Inscriptions*, ed. Y. Aharoni, 153–76. Jerusalem: Israel Exploration Society, 1981.

———. 1976.   Review of *Studies in Aramaic Inscriptions and Onomastics I*, by E. Lipiński. *IEJ* 26:148–9.

———. 1978.   The Titles "ʿd/šhd" and "mnḥm" in Jewish Epigraphical Finds. In מחקרים במקרא ובמזרח הקדמון מוגשים לשמואל א. ליונשטם במלאת לו שבעים שנה, ed. Y. Avishur and

J. Blau, 303–7. Jerusalem: Rubinstein.

———. 1978a.   Review of *Aramaic Texts from Deir 'Alla*, by J. Hoftijzer et al. *IEJ* 29:33–36.

———. 1979.   Graffiti and Dedications. *BASOR* 235:27–30.

———. 1979a.   The Aramaic Ostraca from Tel Beer-Sheba (Seasons 1971–76). *Tel Aviv* 6:182–98.

———. 1979b.   Review of *Aramaic Texts from Deir 'Alla*, by J. Hoftijzer and G. van der Kooij. *IEJ* 29:133–36.

———. 1979–80.   The Ostracon from Nimrud: An Ammonite Name-List. *Maarav* 2:163–71.

———. 1980.   Review of *The Scripts of Ancient Northwest Semitic Seals*, by L. G. Herr. *BASOR* 239:75–76.

———. 1981.   כתובות מתקופת המקרא. In *Thirty Years of Archaeology in Eretz-Israel, 1948–1978*, ed. B. Mazar, 75–85. Jerusalem: Israel Exploration Society.

———. 1981–82.   זמנה של הכתובת מתל פחריה: ניתוח פליאוגראפי של הנוסח הארמי. *Shnaton* 5–6:131–40.

———. 1982.   *Early History of the Alphabet: An Introduction to West Semitic Epigraphy and Palaeography*. Jerusalem: Magnes.

———. 1984.   Inscriptions of the Biblical Period. In *Recent Archaeology in the Land of Israel*, ed. H. Shanks and B. Mazar, 59–68. Washington: Biblical Archaeology Society.

———. 1985.   Writing and Scripts in Seventh-Century B.C.E. Philistia: The New Evidence from Tell Jemmeh. *IEJ* 35:8–21.

———. 1985a.   Published and Unpublished Aramaic Ostraca. *Atiqot* 17:114–21.

———. 1985b.   [Response to A. R. Millard, B. Levine, and A. Lemaire]. *BAT*, 354.

———. 1985c.   Review of *Aramaic Texts from North Saqqâra*, by J. B. Segal. *IEJ* 35:210–12.

———. 1987.   Proto-Canaanite, Archaic Greek, and the Script of the Aramaic Text on the Tell Fakhariyah Statue. In *Ancient Israelite Religion: Essays in Honor of Frank Moore Cross*, ed. P. D. Miller, Jr. et al., 101–13. Philadelphia: Fortress.

Naveh, J., and H. Tadmor. 1968.   Some Doubtful Aramaic Seals. *AION* 28:448–52 + 3 pls.

Naveh, J., and J. C. Greenfield. 1984.   Hebrew and Aramaic in the Persian Period. In *The Cambridge History of Judaism*, ed. W. D. Davies and L. Finkelstein, 115–29. Cambridge: Cambridge Univ. Press.

Naveh, J., and S. Shaked. 1971.   A Recently Published Aramaic Papyrus. *JAOS* 91:379–82.

———. 1973.   Ritual Texts or Treasury Documents? *Or* 42:445–57.

Naveh, J. See also: I. Eph'al, O. Goldwasser, E. Y. Kutscher, S. Shaked.

Nelis, J. T. 1954.   De vier wereldrijken in het Boek Daniëel. *Bijdragen* 15:349–62.

Neubauer, A. 1885.   On Some Newly-Discovered Temanite and Nabataean Inscriptions. *Studia biblica* 1:209–32.

———. 1885a.   The God ṣlm. *The Athenaeum* 2992 (28 Feb.):280.

Neufeld, E. 1944.   *Ancient Hebrew Marriage Laws with Special References to General Semitic Laws and Customs*. London: Longmans, Green.

————. 1953–54. The Rate of Interest and the Text of Nehemiah 5.11. *JQR* 44:194–204.

Neuffer, J. 1968. The Accession of Artaxerxes I. *AUSS* 6:60–87.

Newell, E. T. 1926. Some Unpublished Coins of Eastern Dynasts. *Numismatic Notes and Monographs* 30:17.

Niebuhr, C. 1898. Zum historischen Ergebnis der Sendschirli-Texte. *OLZ* 1:345–50, 375–81.

Nims, C. F., and R. C. Steiner. 1983. A Paganized Version of Psalm 20:2–6 from the Aramaic Text in Demotic Script. *JAOS* 103:261–74.

Nims, C. F. See also: R. C. Steiner.

Nober, P. 1957. El significado de la palabra aramea 'āsparna en Esdras. *EstBib* 16:393–401.

————. 1958. Review of "L'Aramaico antico," by G. Garbini. *VD* 36:309.

————. 1958a. אדרזדא (Esdras 7,23). *BZ* 2:134–38.

————. 1959. Review of *Un editto bilingue greco-aramaico di Aśoka*, by G. Pugliese-Carratelli et al. *VD* 37:369–77.

————. 1959a. Ad inscriptionem aramaicam Arpadensem (adnotationes criticae). *VD* 37:171–75.

————. 1959b. Review of *Un editto bilingue greco-aramaico di Aśoka*, by G. Pugliese-Carratelli, et al. *VD* 37:369–77.

————. 1960. Notula lexicalis ad $y^eba'\hat{o}n$, Dan 4,33. *VD* 38:35–37.

————. 1960a. De nuevo sobre el significado de āsparnā en Esdras. *EstBib* 19:111–12.

————. 1960b. Review of *Il semitico di nord-ovest*, by G. Garbini. *VD* 38:316–17.

————. 1961. Y'hûd (aram.) = Jerusalem(?). *VD* 39:110–13.

————. 1961a. Review of *A Grammar of Biblical Aramaic*, by F. Rosenthal. *Bib* 42:245–46.

Nöldeke, T. 1871. Die Namen der aramäischen Nation und Sprache. *ZDMG* 25:113–31.

————. 1879. Review of *Keilinschriften und Geschichtsforschung*, by E. Schrader. *ZDMG* 33:321–22.

————. 1884. Altaramäische Inschriften aus Teimâ (Arabien). *SPAW* 35:813–20.
Reviews: D. H. Müller 1884.

————. 1884a. Review of *Grammatik des Biblisch-Aramäischen*, by E. Kautzsch. *GGA* 136:1014–23.

————. 1886. Mene tekel upharsin. *ZA* 1:414–18.

————. 1892. Aramäische Inschrift aus Cilicien. *ZA* 7:350–53.

————. 1893. Bemerkungen zu den aramäischen Inschriften von Sendschirli. *ZDMG* 47:96–105.

————. 1899. *Die semitischen Sprachen: Eine Skizze*. 2nd ed. Leipzig: Tauchnitz.

————. 1907. Die aramäischen Papyri von Assuan. [Review article: A. H. Sayce and A. E. Cowley, *Aramaic Papyri Discovered at Assuan*.] *ZA* 20:130–50.

————. 1908. Neue jüdische Papyri. *ZA* 21:195–205.

————. 1908a. Aramäische Inschriften. *ZA* 21:375–88.

———. 1913. Untersuchungen zum Achiqar-Roman. *AbhKGWG* 14/4:1–63. Berlin: Weidmann.

———. 1913a. Zum Achiqar. *ZDMG* 67:766.

———. 1924. Zur Frage der Geschichtlichkeit der Urkunden im Esra-Buche. *DLZ* 45:1849–56.

Nöldeke, T., H. Lenzen, A. von Haller, and W. Göpner. 1936. Siebenter vorläufiger Bericht über die von der Deutschen Forschungsgemeinschaft in Uruk-Warka unternommenen Ausgrabungen. *Abh. d. preussischen Akad. d. Wissens.* 4:36–37, pls. 32b, 39b.

Nordio, M. 1980. *Lessico dei logogrami in Medio-Persiano.* Quaderni del seminario di iranistica dell'Università di Venezia 12. Venice: La Tipografica.

Norman, K. R. 1972. Notes on the Greek Version of Aśoka's Twelfth and Thirteenth Rock Edicts. *JRAS*: 111–18.

Norris, E. 1856. On the Assyrian and Babylonian Weights. *JRAS* 16:215–26.

Norris, H. T. 1951. Arslan Tash (Rock of the Lion). *PEQ* 83:168–74, pl. XVII + 3 figs. + 2 photos.

Noth, M. 1929. La'asch und Hazrak. *ZDPV* 52:124–41. Reprinted in *Aufsätze zur biblischen Landes- und Altertumskunde*, ed. H. W. Wolff, 135–47. Neukirchen-Vluyn: Neukirchener, 1971.

———. 1955. Die Heiligen des Höchsten. *Norsk Teologisk Tidsskrift* 56:146–61.

———. 1961. Der historische Hintergrund der Inschriften von Sefîre. *ZDPV* 77:118–72. Reprinted in *Aufsätze zur biblischen Landes- und Altertumskunde*, ed. H. W. Wolff, 161–210. Neukirchen-Vluyn: Neukirchener, 1971.

———. 1971. Das Reich von Hamath als Grenznachbar des Reiches Israel. In *Aufsätze zur biblischen Landes- und Altertumskunde*, ed. H. W. Wolff, 148–60. Neukirchen-Vluyn: Neukirchener.

Nyberg, H. 1931. Ein iranisches Wort im Buche Daniel. *Le Monde Oriental* 25:178–204.

Nylander, C. 1968. *Assyria grammata*: Remarks on the 21st "Letter of Themistocles." *Opuscula atheniensia* 8:119–36 + 3 figs.

O'Callaghan, R. T. 1948. *Aram Naharaim.* AnOr 26. Rome: Pontifical Biblical Institute.

O'Connor, M. 1977. The Rhetoric of the Kilamuwa Inscription. *BASOR* 226:15–29.

———. 1989. Semitic **mgn* and Its Supposed Sanskrit Origin. *JAOS* 109:25–32.

Oden, Jr., R. A. 1977. *Ba'al Šāmēm* and *'Ēl. CBQ* 39:457–73.

Oelsner, J. 1974. Review of *Development of the Aramaic Script*, by J. Naveh. *OLZ* 69:366–68.

———. 1975. Review of *Aramaic Ritual Texts from Persepolis*, by R. A. Bowman. *OLZ* 70:473–77.

———. 1976. Probleme der Entwicklung der aramäischen Schrift in Nordmesopotamien. *Philologia orientalis* 4:215–23.

———. 1976a. Zwischen Xerxes und Alexander: Babylonische Rechtsurkunden und Wirtschaftstexte aus der späten Achämenidenzeit. *WO* 8:310–18.

———. 1977. Review of *Eine weitere aramäo-iranische Inschrift der Periode des Aśoka aus Afghanistan*, by G. D. Davary and H. Humbach. *OLZ* 72:514–17.

————. 1980. Review of *The Akkadian Influences on Aramaic*, by S. A. Kaufman. *OLZ* 75:535–37.

————. 1980a. Review of *La langue de Ya'udi*, by P.-E. Dion. *OLZ* 75:553–56.

————. 1987. Aramäisches aus Babylonien–Notizen am Rande. In *Der Vordere Orient in Antike und Mittelalter: Festgabe für Heinrich Simon anlässlich seines 65. Geburtstages*, 38–46. Berlin: Humboldt-Universität zu Berlin.

————. 1987a. Review of *Early History of the Alphabet*, by J. Naveh. *OLZ* 82:467–70.

————. 1988. Review of *Aramaic Texts from North Saqqâra*, by J. B. Segal. *OLZ* 83:180–83.

————. 1989. Weitere Bemerkungen zu den Neirab-Urkunden. *Altorientalische Forschungen* 16:68–77.

Offord, J. 1900. Note on the Winged Figures on the Jar-Handles Discovered by Dr. Bliss. *PEFQS*: 279–80.

————. 1915. The Elephantine Papyri as Illustrative of the Old Testament. *PEFQS*: 72–80, 144–51.

Ohata, K. 1967. *Tel Zeror I: Preliminary Report of the Excavation, First Season 1964*. Tokyo: Univ. of Tokyo, The Society for Near Eastern Studies.

Ohnefalsch-Richter, M. 1893. *Kypros, die Bibel und Homer: Beiträge zur Cultur-, Kunst- und Religionsgeschichte des Orients im Alterthume*. Berlin: A. Asher.

Olmstead, A. T. 1931. *History of Palestine and Syria to the Macedonian Conquest*. New York: Scribner.

————. 1938. Darius and His Behistun Inscription. *AJSL* 55:392–416.

————. 1944. Tattenai, Governor of Across the River. *JNES* 3:46.

Oppert, M. J. 1874. L'Étalon des mesures assyriennes fixé par les textes cunéiformes. *JA* 7/4:417–86.

Oren, E. D. 1973. Tel Sera' (Tell esh-Shari'a). *RB* 80:401–5.

Osten, H. H. von der. 1928–29. Aghaya Kaleh. *AJSL* 45:275–78.

————. 1929. *Explorations in Hittite Asia Minor*. Oriental Institute Communications 6. Chicago: Univ. of Chicago.

————. 1957. *Altorientalische Siegelsteine der Sammlung Hans Silvius von Aulock*. Studia Ethnographica Upsaliensia 13. Uppsala: Almqvist & Wiksells.

Otzen, B. 1971. Review of *Archives from Elephantine*, by B. Porten. *DTT* 34:153–54.

————. 1988. Petitionary Formulae in the Aramaic Inscriptions from Hama. *ZAW Supplement* 100:233–43.

————. 1990. Appendix 2: The Aramaic Inscriptions. In *Hama: Fouilles et recherches de la Fondation Carlsberg 1931–1938 II 2. Les objets de la période dite syro-hittite (âge du fer)*, 267–318. Nationalmuseets Skrifter Større Beretninger XII. Copenhagen: National-museet.

Palache, J. L. 1939. *Over Beteckenisverandering der Woorden in het Hebreeuwsch (Semietisch) en andere Talen*. Amsterdam: Menno Hertzberger.

Palacios, L. 1953. *Grammatica aramaico-biblica*. 2nd ed. Rome: Desclée.

Paley, S. M. 1986. Inscribed Neo-Assyrian and Neo-Babylonian Cylinder Seals and Impressions. In *Insight through Images, Studies in Honor of Edith Porada*, ed. M. Kelly-Buccellati in collaboration with P. Matthiae and M. van Loon, 209–20. Bibliotheca Mesopotamica 21. Malibu: Undena.

Pande, B. M. See: M. C. Joshi.

Parayre, D. 1990. Les cachets ouest-sémitiques à travers l'image du disque solaire ailé (perspective iconographique). *Syria* 67:269–301; pls. I–XIII.

Pardee, D. 1977. Review of *The Akkadian Influences on Aramaic*, by S. A. Kaufman. *JNES* 36:318–19.

———. 1978. Review of *Textbook of Syrian Semitic Inscriptions, Vol. II*, by J. C. L. Gibson. *JNES* 37:195–97.

———. 1978a. Review of *Altaramäische Grammatik*, by S. Segert. *JNES* 37:197–99.

———. 1979. Review of *Aramaic Texts from Deir 'Alla*, by J. Hoftijzer et al. *JNES* 38:296–97.

———. 1991. The Linguistic Classification of the Deir 'Alla Text Written on Plaster. In *BTDAR*, 100–5.

Pardee, D., and R. D. Biggs. 1984. Review of *La statue de Tell Fekherye*, by A. Abou Assaf et al. *JNES* 43:253–57.

Parente, F. 1979. Ezra, 6.11: La pena comminata a chi altera l'editto di Dario. *Henoch* 1:189–200.

Parker, B. 1963. Economic Tablets from the Temple of Mamu at Balawat. *Iraq* 25:86–103, pls. xix–xxvi.

Parker, P. 1941. The Meaning of "Son of Man." *JBL* 60:151–57.

Parker, R. A. 1941. Persian and Egyptian Chronology. *AJSL* 58:285–301.

———. 1941a. Darius and His Egyptian Campaign. *AJSL* 58:373–77.

———. 1955. Some Considerations on the Nature of the Fifth-Century Jewish Calendar at Elephantine. *JNES* 14:271–74.

Parnas, M. 1975. עידות, עידות, עידוות במקרא על רקע תעודות חיצוניות. *Shnaton* 1:235–46, pl. xviii.

Parpola, S. 1974–79. The Alleged Middle/Neo-Assyrian Irregular Verb *naṣṣ and the Assyrian Sound Change š > s. *Assur* 1:1–10.

———. 1985. Si'gabbar of Nerab Resurrected. *OLP* 16:273–75.

———. 1987. Neo-Assyrian Treaties from the Royal Archives of Nineveh. *JCS* 39:161–89.

———. 1988. The Neo-Assyrian Word for "Queen". *SAAB* 2:73.

Parrot, A. 1939. *Malédictions et violations de tombes*. Paris: Geuthner.

———. 1961. *Nineveh and Babylon*. Transl. S. Gilbert and J. Emmons. London: Thames and Hudson.

Paul, S. 1983. Daniel 3: 29 — A Case Study of "Neglected" Blasphemy. *JNES* 42:291–94.

———. 1984. Dan 6, 8: An Aramaic Reflex of Assyrian Legal Terminology. *Bib* 65:106–10.

———. 1986. משא מלך שרים: Hosea 8:8–10 and Ancient Near Eastern Royal Epithets. In

Studies in Bible (Scripta Hierosolymitana XXXI), ed. S. Japhet, 193–204.

Peckham, B. 1971. Review of *The Development of the Aramaic Script*, by J. Naveh. *Or* 40:491–2.

Peiser, F. E. 1890. *Babylonische Verträge des Berliner Museums in Autographie, Transscription und Übersetzung*. Berlin: W. Peiser Verlag.

———. 1898. Aus dem kaiserlich-ottomanischen Museum in Constantinopel. *OLZ* 1:6–9.

Pennacchietti, F. 1968. *Studi sui pronomi determinativi semitici*. Pubblicazioni del Seminario di Semitistica: Ricerche IV. Naples: Istituto Orientale di Napoli.

———. 1981. Storia e massime di Achicar. In *Apocrifi dell'Antico Testamento*, ed. P. Sacchi, 51–95. Classici delle religioni, sez. 2a. Turin: UTET.

Pericoli Ridolfini, F. S. 1949–54. Elefantina. In *Enciclopedia Cattolica* 197–98. Vatican City: Ente per l'Enciclopedia Cattolica e per il Libro Cattolico.

Perles, F. 1911–12. Zu Sachaus "Aramäischen Papyrus und Ostraka." *OLZ* 14:497–503, 15:54–57.

———. 1926. Das Land Arzâph (IV Ezra 13, 45). *AfO* 3:120–21.

Perrot, G., and C. Chipiez. 1884. *A History of Art in Chaldaea and Assyria*. Transl. W. Armstrong. 2 volumes. London: Chapman and Hall.

Pestman, P. W. See: J. Hoftijzer.

Peters, J. P. 1884–85. Miscellaneous Notes. *Hebraica* 1:115–19.

———. 1896. Notes on the Old Testament. *JBL* 15:106–17.

Peters, N. 1907. Die jüdische Gemeinde zu Syene im fünften Jahrhundert vor dem Geburt v. Chr. nach den Papyri von Assuan. *Katholik* ser. 3, vol. 36:310–20, 369–77.

———. 1907a. Ein jüdischer Tempel in Ägypten im 6. und 7. Jahrh. v. Chr. *Wissenschaftliche Beilage zur Germania* 9:385.

Petit, T. 1988. L'Evolution sémantique des termes hébreux et araméens *phḥ* et *sgn* et accadiens *pāḫatu* et *šaknu*. *JBL* 107:53–67.

Petrie, W. M. F. 1888. *A Season in Egypt, 1887*. London: Field and Tuer.

Petschow, H. 1956. *Neubabylonisches Pfandrecht*. Abhand. d. säch. Akad. d. Wissen. zu Leipzig, Phil.-Hist. Kl. Bd. 48, Heft 1. Berlin: Akademie Verlag.
Reviews: G. Cardascia 1958.

Piattelli, D. 1984. Effetti giuridici dell'affrancazione degli schiavi alla luce dei documenti aramaici di Elefantina. In *Atti del xvii congresso internazionale di papirologia*, vol. 3, 1233–44. Naples: Centro Internazionale per lo Studio dei Papiri Ercolanesi.

Picard, C. 1959. Review of *Un editto bilingue greco-aramaico di Aśoka*, by G. Pugliese-Carratelli et al. *RArch* 1:102–6.

———. 1961. Le rite magique des εἴδολα de cire brûlés, attesté sur trois stèles araméennes de Sfiré (vers le milieu du VIIIᵉ s. av. notre ère). *RArch* 2:85–88.

Pigulevskaja, N. V. 1949. Novye aramejskie pamjatniki iz Germupol'a [New Aramaic monuments from Hermopolis]. *VDI* 28:267–68.

Pilcher, E. J. 1901. A Cylinder Seal Bearing the Name "Gehazi." *PSBA* 23:362.

———. 1912. The Assuan Papyri and the Grave-Goods of Gezer. *PEFQS*: 30–35.

Pilter, W. T. 1914. The Word אגורא and Its Cognate Forms. *OLZ* 17:66–68.

Pinches, T. G. 1890. *Babylonian and Assyrian Cylinder-Seals and Signets in the Collection of Sir Henry Peek*. London: Harrison and Sons.

———. 1900. The Collection of Babylonian Tablets Belonging to Joseph Offord, Esq. *PEFQS* 31:258–68.

———. 1910. *An Outline of Assyrian Grammar*. London: H. J. Glaisher.

Pitard, W. T. 1987. *Ancient Damascus: A Historical Study of the Syrian City-State from Earliest Times until Its Fall to the Assyrians in 732 B.C.E.* Winona Lake, Ind.: Eisenbrauns.
Reviews: J.-M. de Tarragon 1988: *RB* 95:607–8.

———. 1988. The Identity of the Bir Hadad of the Melqart Stela. *BASOR* 272:3–21.

Plöger, O. 1965. *Das Buch Daniel*. KAT 18. Gütersloh: G. Mohn.

Poebel, A. 1932. *Das appositionell bestimmte Pronomen der 1. Pers. Sing. in den westsemitischen Inschriften und im Alten Testament*. Oriental Institute of the University of Chicago, Assyriological Studies 3. Chicago: Univ. of Chicago Press.

———. 1938. Chronology of Darius' First Year of Reign. *AJSL* 55:142–65, 285–314.

Pognon, H. 1907–8. *Inscriptions sémitiques de la Syrie, de la Mésopotamie, et de la région de Mossoul*. Paris: Imprimerie Nationale/Gabalda.
Reviews: H. Grimme 1909; M. Lidzbarski 1908; S. Ronzevalle 1909; R. Savignac 1908.

———. 1911. Chronologie des papyrus araméens d'Éléphantine. *JA* 10/18:337–65.

Pohl, A. 1948. Neue aramäische Papyri von West-Hermopolis. *Or* 17:549–50.

———. 1949. Aramäisch als diplomatische Sprache im 7. Jahrhundert. *Or* 18:512.

———. 1954. Personalnachrichten. *Or* 23:83–4.

———. 1956. Personalnachrichten. *Or* 25:153–161.

———. 1958. Personalnachrichten. *Or* 27:288–91, 420.

———. 1959. Personalnachrichten. *Or* 28:215–6, 298.

Polotsky, H. J. 1932. Aramäisch prš und das "Huzvaresch." *Le Muséon* 45:273–83.

Polzin, R. 1976. *Late Biblical Hebrew: Toward an Historical Typology of Biblical Hebrew Prose*. HSM 12. Missoula, Mont.: Scholars Press.

Pope, M. H. 1961. Review of *Il semitico di nord-ovest*, by G. Garbini. *JBL* 80:290–91.

Porada, E., et al. 1948. *Corpus of Ancient Near Eastern Seals in North American Collections*. Bollingen Series 14. Washington: Bollingen Foundation, Pantheon.

Porten, B. 1961. The Structure and Orientation of the Jewish Temple at Elephantine — A Revised Plan of the Jewish District. *JAOS* 81:38–42.

———. 1963. שיבת ציון לאור כתבי יב. *BM* 16:66–79.

———. 1968. *Archives from Elephantine. The Life of an Ancient Jewish Military Colony*. Berkeley: Univ. of California Press.
Reviews: H. Bardtke 1971; R. A. Bowman 1970: *Or* 39:454–59; R. J. Coggins 1970: *SOTS Book List*: 80; B. Couroyer 1970; B. Couroyer 1970: *RB* 77:463–65; A.-M. Denis 1969: *Le Muséon* 82:531–32; G. Fohrer 1970: *ZAW* 82:167; M. A. Friedman: *Conservative Judaism* 24:64–68; C. H. Gordon 1969: *American Historical Review* 75:88; P. Grelot 1970a; R. W. Klein 1970: *Concordia Theological Monthly* 41:745–46; P. D. Miller 1970: *Interpretation* 24:385–86; G. Nahon 1971; B. Otzen 1971; M. H. Pope 1970: *JBL* 89:92–94; G. Rinaldi 1969: *BibOr* 11:214; J. J. Scullion 1970:

Australian Biblical Review *18:45; J. B. Segal 1971; J. J. Stamm 1970:* AfO 23:114–15; E. Stern 1970; J. Teixidor 1970: *JAOS* 90:543–44; W. White, Jr. 1969–70: *Westminster Theological Journal* 32:233–36; R. Yaron 1969: *Israel Law Review* 4:588–91; R. Yaron 1971.

———. 1969. The Religion of the Jews of Elephantine in Light of the Hermopolis Papyri. *JNES* 28:116–21.

———. 1971. The Restoration of Fragmentary Aramaic Marriage Contracts. In *Gratz College Anniversary Volume: On the Occasion of the Seventy-fifth Anniversary of the Founding of the College, 1895–1970,* ed. I. D. Passow and S. T. Lachs, 243–61. Philadelphia.

———. 1972. חוזה הנישואין הארמי של האמה תמת. In *Bible and Jewish History: Studies in Bible and Jewish History Dedicated to the Memory of Jacob Liver,* ed. B. Uffenheimer, 307–29. Tel Aviv: Tel Aviv Univ.

———. 1978. ארכיון ידניה בן גמריה מיב: מבנה האיגרות וסגנונן (א). *EI (Ginsberg Volume)* 14:165–77.

———. 1978–79. The Aramaic "Passover Papyrus": Physical Format and Textual Reconstruction. In *Actes du XVᵉ Congrès International de Papyrologie,* ed. J. Bingen and G. Nachtergael, 39–45. Papyrologica Bruxellensia 16–19. Brussels: Fondation Égyptologique Reine Élisabeth.

———. 1978–79a. המסמכים בספר עזרא ושליחותו של עזרא. *Shnaton* 3:174–96.

———. 1979. Aramaic Papyri and Parchments: A New Look. *BA* 42:74–104.

———. 1980. Aramaic Letters: A Study in Papyrological Reconstruction. *JARCE* 17:39–75.

———. 1981. Structure and Chiasm in Aramaic Contracts and Letters. In *Chiasm in Antiquity: Structure, Analysis, Interpretation,* ed. J. W. Welch, 169–82. Hildesheim: Olms.

———. 1981a. The Identity of King Adon. *BA* 44:36–52.

———. 1982. ארכיון ידניה בן גמריה מיב: מבנה האיגרות וסגנונן (ב). In *Irano-Judaica: Studies Relating to Jewish Contacts with Persian Culture throughout the Ages,* ed. S. Shaked, Hebrew Section, 11–24. Jerusalem: Ben-Zvi Institute.

———. 1983. Aramaic Papyri in the Egyptian Museum: The Missing Endorsements. In *The Word of the Lord Shall Go Forth: Essays in Honor of David Noel Freedman in Celebration of His Sixtieth Birthday,* ed. C. L. Meyers and M. O'Connor, 527–44. Winona Lake, Ind.: Eisenbrauns.

———. 1983a. Une lettre araméenne conservée à l'Académie des Inscriptions et Belles-Lettres (AI 5–7): Une nouvelle reconstruction. *Sem* 33:89–100.

———. 1983b. The Address Formulae in Aramaic Letters: A New Collation of Cowley 17. *RB* 90:396–415, pls. II–IV.

———. 1983c. An Aramaic Oath Contract: A New Interpretation (Cowley 45). *RB* 90:563–75, pls. VIII–IX.

———. 1983d. היהודים במצרים. In ימי שלטון פרס—שיבת ציון, ed. H. Tadmor et al., ההיסטוריה של עם ישראל, vol. 1:8. Jerusalem: Alexander Peli. 104–95.

———. 1984. The Jews in Egypt. In *The Cambridge History of Judaism I: Introduction: The Persian Period,* ed. W. D. Davies and L. Finkelstein, 372–400. Cambridge: Cambridge Univ. Press.

———. 1985. Aramaic Letters in Italian Museums. In *Studi in onore di Edda Bresciani,* ed. S. F. Bondi et al., 429–53. Pisa: Giardini.

——— . 1985a. Two Aramaic Contracts Without Dates: New Collations (C 11, 49). *BASOR* 258:41–52.

——— . 1986. *Select Papyri from Ancient Egypt.* Jerusalem: Institute for the Study of Aramaic Papyri.

——— . 1986a. Une autre lettre araméenne à l'Académie des Inscriptions (AI 2–4): Une nouvelle reconstruction. *Sem* 36:71–86.

——— . 1987. Seven Aramaic Lists of Names: A New Collation. In *La vie de la parole: De l'Ancien au Nouveau Testament: Etudes d'exégèse et d'herméneutique bibliques offertes à Pierre Grelot professeur à l'Institut Catholique de Paris*, 31–47. Paris: Desclée.

——— . 1987a. Cowley 7 Reconsidered. *Or* 56:89–92.

——— . 1988. Aramaic Papyrus Fragments in the Egyptian Museum of West Berlin. *Or* 57:14–54.

——— . 1989. Five Fragmentary Aramaic Marriage Documents: New Collations and Restorations. *AbrN* 27:80–105.

——— . 1989a. Fragmentary Aramaic Deeds of Obligation and Coveyance: New Collations and Restorations. *JNES* 48:161–83.

——— . 1990. The Calendar of Aramaic Texts from Achaemenid and Ptolemaic Egypt. In *Irano-Judaica II: Studies Relating to Jewish Contacts with Persian Culture Throughout the Ages*, ed. S. Shaked and A. Netzer, 13–32. Jerusalem: Ben-Zvi Institute.

Porten, B., and A. Yardeni. 1986. *Textbook of Aramaic Documents from Ancient Egypt Newly Copied, Edited and Translated into Hebrew and English: 1. Letters (Appendix: Aramaic Letters from the Bible.* Department of the History of the Jewish People. Texts and Studies for Students. Jerusalem: The Hebrew University. (Distributed by Eisenbrauns, Winona Lake, Indiana)
Reviews: P. Grelot 1988; S. A. Kaufman 1988: *JNES* 47:289–90; E. Lipiński 1988: *Or* 57:434–36; J. Oelsner 1990: *Archiv für Papyrusforschung* 36:93–94; H. G. M. Williamson 1987: *VT* 37:493.

——— . 1988. The Aramaic Boat Papyrus (P. Ber 23000): A New Collation. *Or* 57:76–81.

——— . 1989. *Textbook of Aramaic Documents from Ancient Egypt Newly Copied, Edited and Translated into Hebrew and English. 2: Contracts.* Department of the History of the Jewish People. Texts and Studies for Students. Jerusalem: The Hebrew University. (Distributed by Eisenbrauns, Winona Lake, Indiana)

Porten, B., and H. Z. Szubin. 1982. "Abandoned Property" in Elephantine: A New Interpretation of Kraeling 3. *JNES* 41:123–31.

——— . 1982a. Exchange of Inherited Property at Elephantine (Cowley 1). *JAOS* 102:651–54.

——— . 1985. Hereditary Leases in Aramaic Letters. *BO* 42:283–88.

——— . 1987. A Dowry Addendum (Kraeling 10). *JAOS* 107:231–38.

——— . 1987a. Litigants in the Elephantine Contracts: The Development of Legal Terminology. *Maarav* 4:45–67.

——— . 1987b. An Aramaic Deed of Bequest (Kraeling 9). In *Community and Culture: Essays in Jewish Studies in Honor of the Nineteeth Anniversary of the Founding of Gratz College*, ed. N. Waldman, 179–92. Philadelphia: Gratz College.

Porten, B., and J. C. Greenfield. 1968. The Aramaic Papyri from Hermopolis. *ZAW* 80:216–31.

––––––. 1969. The Guarantor at Elephantine-Syene. *JAOS* 89:153–57.

––––––. 1974. Hermopolis Letter 6. *IOS* 4:14–30.

Porten, B., in collaboration with J. C. Greenfield. 1974. *Jews of Elephantine and Arameans of Syene (Fifth Century B.C.E.): Fifty Aramaic Texts with Hebrew and English Translations.* Jerusalem: Academon.
Reviews: P. Grelot 1975; S. Segert 1976; P. Swiggers 1982.

Porten, B. See also: J. C. Greenfield, H. Z. Szubin.

Postgate, J. N. 1970. More "Assyrian Deeds and Documents." *Iraq* 32:129–64.

––––––. 1973. Assyrian Texts and Fragments. *Iraq* 35:13–36, pl. XII.

––––––. 1976. *Fifty Neo-Assyrian Legal Documents.* Warminster: Aris & Phillips.

Powell, H. H. 1907. *The Supposed Hebraisms in the Grammar of the Biblical Aramaic.* University of California Publications. Semitic Philology, vol. 1, no. 1. Berkeley: Univ. of California Press.

Poythress, V. S. 1976. The Holy Ones of the Most High in Daniel vii. *VT* 26:208–13.

Poznánski, S. 1921. Review of A. E. Cowley, *Jewish Documents of the Time of Ezra Translated from the Aramaic. OLZ* 24:303–5.

Prášek, J. V. 1895. Nálezy Sendžirliskév Berlínském musei [The discoveries from Zenjirli at the Berlin Museum]. *Zlatá Praha* 12:82–83, 91–93.

––––––. 1912. Review of *Chronological Notes from the Aramaic Papyri*, by M. Sprengling. *OLZ* 15:168–70.

Praetorius, F. 1881. Aegyptisch-Aramäisches. *ZDMG* 35:442–44.

Preiswerk, H. 1902. *Der Sprachenwechsel im Buche Daniel.* Bern: Berner Tagblatt.

Prideaux, W. F. 1876–77. On an Aramaean Seal. *Transactions of the Society of Biblical Archaeology* 5:456–58.

Prince, J. D. 1893. *Mene Mene Tekel Upharsin: An Historical Study of the Fifth Chapter of Daniel.* Baltimore: Author.

Pritchard, J. B. 1962. *Gibeon, Where the Sun Stood Still.* Princeton: Princeton University Press.

––––––. 1985. *Tell es-Sa'idiyeh: Excavations on the Tell, 1964–1966.* University Museum Monograph 60. Philadelphia: Univ. of Pennsylvania University Museum.

Pritsch, E. 1911. Bemerkungen zum oxforder ägyptisch-aramäischen Papyrus H. *ZA* 25:345–52.

––––––. 1912. Jüdische Rechtsurkunden aus Aegypten. *ZVR* 27:7–70.

––––––. 1957. Zum gegenwärtigen Stand der juristischen Papyrusforschung: Die aramäischen Urkunden. *ZVR* 60:99–117.

Procksch, O. 1927. Der Menschensohn als Gottessohn. *Christentum und Wissenschaft* 3:425–43.

Przeworski, S. 1928. Vier nordsyrisch-hethitische Denkmäler. *OLZ* 31:233–38.

Puech, E. 1971. Sur la racine 'ṢLḤ' en hébreu et en araméen. *Sem* 21:5–19.

———. 1975. Review of *Altaramäische Grammatik der Inschriften des 10.–8. Jh. v. Chr.*, by R. Degen. *RB* 82:614–15.

———. 1977. Review of *La langue de Ya'udi*, by P.-E. Dion. *RB* 84:446–47.

———. 1977a. Review of *La langue de Ya'udi*, by P.-E. Dion. *RA* 71:183–85.

———. 1978. Un ivoire de Bît-Guši (Arpad) à Nimrud. *Syria* 55:163–69.

———. 1981. L'ivoire inscrit d'Arslan-Tash et les rois de Damas. *RB* 88:544–62.

———. 1982. Les inscriptions araméennes I et III de Sfiré: Nouvelles lectures. *RB* 89:576–87 + 2 pls.

———. 1982a. Note sur la particule accusativale en phénicien. *Sem* 32:51–55.

———. 1982–84. La racine *ŠYT–Š'T* en araméen et en hébreu: A propos de Sfiré I A 24, 1 Q Hᵃ III, 30 et 36 (= XI, 31 et 37) et Ézéchiel. *RevQ* 11:367–78.

———. 1983. Review of *La statue de Tell Fekherye*, by A. Abou Assaf et al. *RB* 90:594–96.

———. 1985. L'inscription sur plâtre de Tell Deir 'Alla. *BAT*, 354–65.

———. 1985a. Review of *Aramaic Texts from Deir 'Alla*, by J. Hoftijzer et al. *RB* 85:114–17.

———. 1986. L'inscription de Deir Alla. *MDB* 46:36–37.

———. 1986a. Origine de l'alphabet: Documents en alphabet linéaire et cuneiforme du IIe millénaire. *RB* 93:161–213.

———. 1986b. Review of *The Balaam Text from Deir 'Alla*, by J. A. Hackett. *RB* 93:285–87.

———. 1987. Le texte "ammonite" de Deir 'Alla: Les admonitions de Balaam (première partie). In *La vie de la parole: De l'Ancien au Nouveau Testament: Etudes d'exégèse et d'herméneutique bibliques offertes à Pierre Grelot professeur à l'Institut Catholique de Paris* 13–30. Paris: Desclée.

———. 1988. Review of *The Aramaic Proverbs of Ahiqar*, by J. M. Lindenberger. *RB* 95:588–92.

———. 1991. Approches paléographiques de l'inscription sur plâtre de Deir 'Allā. In *BTDAR*, 221–38.

Pugliese-Carratelli, G. 1960. *Gli editti di Aśoka*. Filosofia e comunità mondiale, vol. 1. Florence: Nuova Italia.

Pugliese-Carratelli, G., and G. Garbini. 1964. *A Bilingual Graeco-Aramaic Edict by Aśoka: The First Greek Inscription Discovered in Afghanistan.* Serie Orientale Roma, vol. 29. Rome: Istituto italiano per il medio ed estremo oriente.

Pugliese-Carratelli, G., G. Tucci, G. Scerrato, and G. Levi della Vida. 1958. *Un editto bilingue greco-aramaico di Aśoka: La prima iscrizione greca scoperta in Afghanistan.* Serie orientale Roma, vol. 21. Rome: Istituto italiano per il medio ed estremo oriente.

Reviews: P. H. L. Eggermont 1959; P. Nober 1959; C. Picard 1959.

Qimron, E. 1981–82. המלות אשר, ש-, די בראש משפט עיקרי בעברית ובארמית. *Leš* 46:27–38.

———. 1987–88. קטלתוני and Related Forms in Hebrew. *JQR* 78:49–55.

Qohut, S. 1981–82. הכינוי היתר בלשון המקרא. *Leš* 46:9–26; 97–123.

Quinn, J. D. 1961. Alcaeus 48 (B 16) and the Fall of Ascalon (604 B. C.) *BASOR* 164:19–20.

Raabe, P. R. 1985. Daniel 7: Its Structure and Role in the Book. *Hebrew Annual Review* 9:267–75.

Rabinowitz, I. 1956. Aramaic Inscriptions of the Fifth Century B. C. E. from a North-Arab Shrine in Egypt. *JNES* 15:1–9.

———. 1959. Another Aramaic Record of the North-Arabian Goddess Han-'ilat. *JNES* 18:154–55, pls. I–III.

Rabinowitz, J. J. 1953. Marriage Contracts in Ancient Egypt in the Light of Jewish Sources. *HTR* 46:91–97.

———. 1955. A Legal Formula in the Susa Tablets, in an Egyptian Document of the Twelfth Dynasty, in the Aramaic Papyri, and in the Book of Daniel. *Bib* 36:74–77.

———. 1955a. The Meaning of the Phrase מחר או יום אחרן in the Aramaic Papyri. *JNES* 14:59–60.

———. 1956. *Jewish Law: Its Influence on the Development of Legal Institutions.* New York: Bloch.

———. 1956a. The Meaning of תתב על מוזנא in the Aramaic Papyri. *VT* 6:104.

———. 1957. The Aramaic Papyri, the Demotic Papyri from Gebelên and Talmudic Sources. *Bib* 38:269–74.

———. 1957a. Demotic Papyri of the Ptolemaic Period and Jewish Sources. *VT* 7:398–400.

———. 1957b. A Legal Formula in Egyptian, Egyptian-Aramaic and Murabba'at Documents. *BASOR* 145:33–34.

———. 1958. Ad inscriptionem aramaicam. *Bib* 39:401.

———. 1958a. Grecisms and Greek Terms in the Aramaic Papyri. *Bib* 39:77–82.

———. 1959. The "Great Sin" in Ancient Egyptian Marriage Contracts. *JNES* 18:73.

———. 1959a. An Additional Note on בראש. *VT* 9:209–10.

———. 1960. More on Grecisms in Aramaic Documents. *Bib* 41:72–74.

———. 1961. The Susa Tablets, the Bible and the Aramaic Papyri. *VT* 11:55–76.

Rahmani, L. Y. 1964. המטמון של מטבעות-אלכסנדר. *EI (L. A. Mayer Volume)* 7:33–38.

———. 1964a. Two Syrian Seals. *IEJ* 14:180–84 + 1 pl.

Rainey, A. F. 1965. Royal Weights and Measures. *BASOR* 179:34–36.

———. 1966. Private Seal Impressions: A Note on Semantics. *IEJ* 16:187–90.

———. 1969. The Satrapy Beyond the River. *AJBA* 1/2:51–78.

Rashid, S. A. 1974. Einige Denkmäler aus Tēmā und der babylonische Einfluss. *Baghdader Mitteilungen* 7:155–65 + 2 pls.

Rauschen, G. 1913. *Neues Licht aus dem alten Orient: Keilschrift- und Papyrusfunde aus dem jüdisch-christlichen Altertum—Ausgrabung der Menasstadt.* Bonn: P. Hanstein.

Rawlinson, H. C. 1865. Bilingual Readings. Cuneiform and Phoenician. Notes on Some Tablets in the British Museum, containing Bilingual Legends (Assyrian and Phoenician). *JRAS* 1:187–246.

————. 1870. *The Cuneiform Inscriptions of Western Asia.* 5 vols. London: British Museum, Department of Egyptian and Assyrian Antiquities.

Reed, W. L. See: F. A. Winnett.

Ray, J. D. 1988. Egypt 525–404 B.C.. In *The Cambridge Ancient History*, 2nd. ed., ed. J. Boardman et al., 254–86. Cambridge: Cambridge Univ. Press.

Reichardt, H. C. 1883. [Communication]. *PSBA*:16–17.

Reichelt, H. 1901. Aramäische Inschriften aus Kappadocien. *WZKM* 15:51–56.

Reider, J. 1953–54. Review of *The Brooklyn Museum Aramaic Papyri*, by E. G. Kraeling. *JQR* 44:337–40.

Reifenberg, A. 1938. Some Ancient Hebrew Seals. *PEQ*:113–16; pl. 6.

————. 1939. Ancient Jewish Stamps and Seals. *PEQ*:193–198; pls. 33–34.

————. 1942–43. Ancient Hebrew Seals III. *PEQ*:109–112; pl. 14.

————. 1950. *Ancient Hebrew Seals.* London: East and West Library.

Reinach, T. 1905. Note de la séance de 16 juin. *CRAIBL*: 332.

————. 1905a. Villes méconnues: III. Aranda. *REG* 18:159–64.

Reinhold, G. G. G. 1986. The Bir-Hadad Stele and the Biblical Kings of Aram. *AUSS* 24:115–26, pls. 1–3.

Reisner, G. A., C. S. Fisher, and D. G. Lyon. 1924. *Harvard Excavations at Samaria, 1908–10.* 2 vols. Cambridge, Mass.: Harvard Univ. Press.

Renan, E. 1856. Sur une inscription araméenne du Sérapéum de Memphis. *JA* 5/7:407–27.

————. 1884–85. Les inscriptions araméennes de Teimâ. *RA* 1:41–45.

Rendsburg, G. A. 1988. The Ammonite Phoneme /T/. *BASOR* 269:73–79.

————. 1988a. More on Hebrew *šibbōlet*. *JSS* 33:255–58.

Renger, J. 1971. Notes on the Goldsmiths, Jewelers and Carpenters of Neobabylonian Eanna. *JAOS* 91:494–503.

Revillout, E. 1910. Lettre à M. Clermont Ganneau de l'Institut sur les monnaies mentionnées dans les papyrus araméens d'Éléphantine. *Revue égyptologique* 13:158–63.

Reymond, P. 1980. Où en est "l'Hebräisches und aramäisches Lexikon zum Alten Testament" (HAL)? In *Unterwegs zur Einheit: Festschrift für Heinrich Stirnimann*, ed. J. Brantschen and P. Selvatico, 183–88. Fribourg: Presses universitaires; Vienna: Herder.

Ribera i Florit, J. 1983. Evolución morfológica y semántica de las partículas *k'n* y *'ry* en los diversos estadios del arameo. *AO* 1:227–33.

————. 1987. La partícula *bĕdyl*: Su origen y evolucioń en arameo. *AO* 5:306–9.

Ribera [i Florit], J. 1989. Evolución semántica y funcional del la partícula aramea "qbl". *AO* 7:263–68.

Ricci, S. de. 1906. Appendix II: Bibliography of Egyptian Aramaic Papyri. In A. E. Sayce and A. E. Cowley, *APA*, 25–34.

Ricciotti, G. 1929–39. Elefantina. In *Enciclopedia Italiana di scienze, lettere ed arti*, ed. G. Gentile et al., 13.626 + 1 pl. Milan: Istituto Giovanni Treccani.

Richardson, N. H. 1965. *A Practical Handbook for the Study of Biblical Aramaic.* Boston: Boston University Bookstore.

Ricke, H. 1960. *Die Tempel Nektanebos' II. in Elephantine und ihre Erweiterungen.* Beiträge zur ägyptischen Bauforschung und Altertumskunde 6. Cairo: Schweizerisches Institut für Ägyptische Bauforschung und Altertumskunde in Kairo.

Ricque, C. 1869. Note sur la XIIIe inscription phénicienne d'Égypte recueillie et copiée par M. Devéria. *JA* 6/13:382–83.

Ridder, A. de. 1911. *Collection De Clerq: Catalogue méthodique et raisonné. Tome VII,2: Les pierres gravées.* Paris: E. Leroux.

Rider, G. le. 1965. *Suse sous les Séleucides et les Parthes.* Paris: Geuthner.

Rigord, M. 1704. Lettre de Monsieur Rigord Commissaire de la Marine aux Journalistes de Trevoux sur une Ceinture de Toile trouvée en Egypte autour d'une Mumie. *Mémoires pour l'histoire des Sciences et les beaux Arts, Trevoux* 4:978–1000.

Rimalt, E. S. 1932. Wechselbeziehungen zwischen dem Aramäischen und dem Neubabylonischen. *WZKM* 39:100–22.

Rimbach, J. A. 1978. Bears or Bees? Sefire I A 31 and Daniel 7. *JBL* 97:565–66.

Rin, S. 1972. הארמית המקראית: Biblical Aramaic Transcribed in Hebrew and Interpreted. Jerusalem: Israel Society for Biblical Research.

Rinaldi, G. 1962. Review of *Il semitico di nord-ovest,* by G. Garbini. *BeO* 4:72.

———. 1965. Coppiere. *BeO* 7:68.

———. 1978. Balaam al suo paese. *BeO* 20:51–59.

Ringgren, H. 1977. Bileam och inskriften från Deir 'Alla [Balaam and the inscription from Deir 'Alla]. *Religion och Bibel* 36:85–89.

———. 1983. Balaam and the Deir 'Alla Inscription. In ספר יצחק אריה זליגמן: *Isac Leo Seeligmann Volume: Essays on the Bible and the Ancient World,* ed. Y. Zakovitch and A. Rofé, 93–98. Jerusalem: Rubinstein.

Rizack, M. A. 1984. A Coin with the Aramaic Legend *šrw,* a King-Governor of Liḥyân. *American Numismatic Society Museum Notes* 29:25–28.

Robert, J., and L. Robert. 1960. Bulletin épigraphique. *REG* 73:134–213.

Robert, L. See: A. Dupont-Sommer, J. Robert, D. Schlumberger.

Robinson, E. S. G. 1936. British Museum Acquisitions for the years 1933–34. *NC* 5/16:169–201.

———. 1958. The Beginning of the Achaemenid Coinage. *NC* 6/18:187–93.

Roca-Puig, R. 1976. Daniele: Due semifogli del codice 967: P. Barc. inv. nn. 42 e 43. *Aeg* 56:3–18.

Rödiger, E. 1828. Review of *Osservazioni sul basso-rilievo fenico-egizio che si conserva in Carpentrasso,* by M. Lanci. *Allgemeine Literatur-Zeitung* 3:265–74.

Rofé, A. 1979. *Book of Balaam.* Jerusalem: Simor.
Reviews: S. A. Kaufman 1986–87.

———. 1985. Response [to A. Lemaire]. In *BAT,* 365–66.

Rogers, E. 1914. *A Handy Guide in Jewish Coins.* London: Spink and Son.

Röllig, W. 1960. Griechische Eigennamen in Texten der babylonischen Spätzeit. *Or* 29:376–91.

———. 1962. Review of *Il semitico di nord-ovest*, by G. Garbini. *BO* 19:23–26.

———. 1974. Alte und neue Elfenbeininschriften. *NESE* 2:37–64.

———. 1977. Review of *The Akkadian Influences on Aramaic*, by S. A. Kaufman. *ZDMG* 127:453.

———. 1977a. Review of *La langue de Ya'udi*, by P.-E. Dion. *ZDMG* 127:449.

———. 1990. Zwei aramäische Inschriften vom Tall Šēḥ Ḥasan/Syrien. *Sem* 39:149–55.

———. See also: R. Degen, H. Donner, H. Kyrieleis.

Ronzevalle, S. 1907. Discovery of Aramaic Papyri in Egypt [in Arabic]. *Al-Mashriq* 10:673–83.

———. 1908. Kitâbah ārāmîyah li-Zakir ṣâḥib Ḥamâh wa-Laʿaš [An Aramaic inscription of Zakir, ruler of Hamath and Laʿaš]. *Al-Mashriq* 11:302–10.

———. 1909. La langue des inscriptions dites de Hadad et de Panammū. In *Florilegium ou recueil de travaux d'érudition dédiés à Monsieur le Marquis Melchior de Vogüé*, 519–28. Paris: Imprimerie Nationale.

———. 1909a. Review of *Inscriptions sémitiques de la Syrie, de la Mésopotamie, et de la région de Mossoul*, by H. Pognon. *MUSJ* 3/2:105–16.

———. 1914–21. Intailles orientales. *MUSJ* 7:181–87.

———. 1930–31. Fragments d'inscriptions araméennes des environs d'Alep. *MUSJ* 15:237–60.

———. 1932. Le prétendu «Char d'Astarté» et son «Bétyle» dans la numismatique de Sidon. *MUSJ* 16:51–63; pls. 1–11.

———. See also: A. Strazzulli.

Rosén, H. B. 1961. On the Use of the Tenses in the Aramaic of Daniel. *JSS* 6:183–203.

Rosenbaum, J. 1978. A Typology of Aramaic Lapidary Scripts from the Seventh to the Fourth Centuries B.C.E. Ph.D. diss., Harvard Univ.

Rosenthal, F. 1936. *Die Sprache der palmyrenischen Inschriften und ihre Stellung innerhalb des Aramäischen*. MVAG 41/1. Leipzig: J. C. Hinrichs.

———. 1939. *Die aramäistische Forschung seit Th. Nöldeke's Veröffentlichungen*. Leiden: Brill.

———. 1942. The Script of Ostracon No. 6043 from Ezion-geber. *BASOR* 85:8–9.

———. 1946. Aramaic Literature. In *Encyclopedia of Literature* 1:48–56. New York: The Philosophical Library.

———. 1949. Review of *Studies in Daniel*, by H. L. Ginsberg. *JAOS* 69:173–74.

———. 1953. Review of *Early Hebrew Orthography*, by F. M. Cross and D. N. Freedman. *JAOS* 73:46–47.

———. 1955. Canaanite and Aramaic Inscriptions. *ANET*, 499–505.

———. 1955a. Aram, Arameans, and the Aramaic Language. In *Twentieth Century Encyclopedia of Religious Knowledge*, 1:64–65. Grand Rapids, Mich.: Baker.

———. 1960. Notes on the Third Inscription from Sefîre-Sûjîn. *BASOR* 158:28–31.

———. 1961. *A Grammar of Biblical Aramaic*. Porta Linguarum Orientalium n.s. 5. Wiesbaden: Harrassowitz.

Reviews: W. Baumgartner 1962: *BO* 19:266; P. Boccaccio 1963; H. Donner 1963; G. Fohrer 1961: *ZAW* 73:340; G. Garbini 1961; H. L. Ginsberg 1961; P. Grelot 1962; H. Michaud 1961; P. Nober 1961: *Biblica* 42:245–46.

———. 1969. Canaanite and Aramaic Inscriptions. *ANESTP*, 655–57.

———. 1972. Review of *Lexicon linguae aramaicae Veteris Testamenti documentis antiquis illustratum*, by E. Vogt. *JBL* 91:552–53.

———. 1976. Review of *La langue de Ya'udi*, by P.-E. Dion. *JBL* 95:153–55.

———. 1978. The Second Laghmân Inscription. *EI (Ginsberg Volume)* 14:97*–99*.

———. 1978a. Aramaic Studies during the Past Thirty Years. *JNES* 37:81–92.

Rosenthal, F., ed. 1967. *An Aramaic Handbook*. 2 vols. in 4 parts. Porta Linguarum Orientalium n.s. 10. Wiesbaden: Harrassowitz.

    Reviews: H. Donner 1968a.

Rosenthal, F., J. Greenfield, and S. Shaked. 1986. Aramaic. In *Encyclopaedia Iranica II/3*, ed. E. Yarshater, 250–61. London: Routledge & Kegan Paul.

Ross, J. F. 1970. Prophecy in Hamath, Israel, and Mari. *HTR* 63:1–28.

Rössler, O. 1983. Aramäische Staatsverträge. In *Rechts- und Wirtschaftsurkunden; Historisch-chronologische Texte*, ed. O. Kaiser, 178–89. TUAT 1. Gütersloh: G. Mohn.

Rost, L. 1952–53. Neue Papyri aus Elephantine. *AfO* 16:378–79.

———. 1958. Zur Deutung des Menschensohnes in Dan 7. In *Gott und die Götter: Festschrift E. Fascher*, ed. G. Delling, 41–43. Berlin: Evangelische Verlaganstalt.

———. 1969. Bemerkungen zu Aḥiqar. *MIO* 15:308–11.

Rost, P. 1893. *Die Keilschrifttexte Tiglat-Pileser III*. 2 vols. Leipzig: E. Pfeiffer.

Rostovtzeff, M. 1932. *Seleucid Babylonia: Bullae and Seals of Clay with Greek Inscriptions*. Yale Classical Collections 3. New Haven: Yale Univ. Press.

Rothstein, J. W. 1913. Review of *Die Elephantiner Papyri und die Bücher Esra-Nehemja*, by G. Jahn. *ZDMG* 67:718–31.

Rouillard, H. 1985. *La péricope de Balaam (Nombres 22–24): La prose et les 'oracles'*. Études Bibliques 4. Paris: Gabalda.

Rowley, H. H. 1924. The Belshazzar of Daniel and of History. *Expositor* 9:182–95; 255–72.

———. 1928. The "Chaldeans" in the Book of Daniel. *ExpTim* 39:188–89.

———. 1929. *The Aramaic of the Old Testament*. London: Oxford Univ. Press.

———. 1930–31. The Historicity of the Fifth Chapter of Daniel. *JTS* 32:12–31.

———. 1932. The Bilingual Problem of Daniel. *ZAW* 9:256–68.

———. 1933. Early Aramaic Dialects and the Book of Daniel. *JRAS*: 777–805.

———. 1935. *Darius the Mede and the Four World Empires in the Book of Daniel: A Historical Study of Contemporary Theories*. Cardiff: University of Wales.

———. 1966. Review of "The Aramaic of Daniel," by K. A. Kitchen. *JSS* 11:112–16.

———. 1968–69. Review of *The Aramaic Inscriptions of Sefîre*, by J. A. Fitzmyer. *ExpTim* 80:182.

Rubensohn, O. 1907. *Elephantine-Papyri*. Ägyptische Urkunden aus den Kgl. Museen in Berlin: Griechische Urkunden — Sonderheft. Berlin: Weidmannsche Buchhandlung.

———. See also: W. Honroth.

Rüger, H. P. 1969. 'Das Tor des Königs' — der königliche Hof. *Bib* 50:247–50.

———. 1981. Die gestaffelten Zahlensprüche des Alten Testaments und aram. Achikar 92. *VT* 31:229–34.

Rundgren, F. 1953. Zum Lexikon des Alten Testaments. *AcOr* 21/4:301–45.

———. 1957. Elephantine-aramäisches *Mallaḥ di Mayyā* und altägyptisches *mw byn*. *Studia Linguistica* 11:57–60.

———. 1957a. Zur Bedeutung von ŠRŠW — Esra VII 26. *VT* 7:400–404.

———. 1958. Über einen juristischen Terminus bei Esra 6:6. *ZAW* 70:209–15.

———. 1965–66. Aramaica I. *OS* 14–15:75–88.

———. 1976–77. Aramaica III: An Iranian Loanword in Daniel. *OS* 25–26:45–55.

———. 1981. Aramaica IV: The Renaissance of Imperial Aramaic. *OS* 30:173–84.

———. 1982–83. Aramaica V: Biblical Aramaic *'adrazdā* and *šām bāl*. *OS* 31–32:143–46.

Ryckmans, G. 1965. Review of *La déesse de Hiérapolis Castabala (Cilicie)*, by A. Dupont-Sommer and L. Robert. *Le Muséon* 78:467–69.

Ryder, S. A. 1974. *The D-Stem in Western Semitic*. Janua Linguarum ser. practica, vol. 131. The Hague: Mouton.

Sacchi, P. 1959. Per una storia di Aram. *ParPass* 14:124–34.

———. 1960–61. Osservazioni sul problema degli Aramei. *Atti e memorie dell'Accademia Toscana di Scienze e Lettere "La Colombaria"* 25:83–142.

———. 1961. Osservazioni storiche alla prima iscrizione aramaica di Sfire. *Rendiconti delle sedute dell'Accademia Nazionale dei Lincei—Classe di Scienze morali, storiche e filologiche* ser. 8, vol. 16:175–91.

Sachau, E. 1887. Eine altaramäische Inschrift aus Lycien. *SKAWW* 114:3–7, pl. 1.

———. 1891. Inschrift, Corp. inscriptionum semiticarum II, 1 no. 75. *ZA* 6:432–36.

———. 1892. Zur historischen Geographie von Nordsyrien. *SPAW* 21:313–38.

———. 1893. Die Inschrift des Königs Panammû von Šam'al. In *Ausgrabungen in Sendschirli, I*, 55–84, pl. VIII. Mittheilungen aus den orientalischen Sammlungen Heft 11. Berlin: W. Spemann.

———. 1895. Baal-Harrân in einer altaramäischen Inschrift auf einem Relief des Königlichen Museums zu Berlin. *SPAW* 8:119–22.

———. 1896. Aramäische Inschriften. *SPAW* 41:1051–64.

———. 1907. *Drei aramäische Papyrusurkunden aus Elephantine*. Philosophische und historische Abhandlungen der königlich-preussischen Akademie der Wissenschaften, fasc. 1. Berlin: Verlag der königlichen Akademie der Wissenschaften. Reprint 1908.
Reviews: S. Fraenkel 1907; M. Lidzbarski 1907.

———. 1909. Ein altaramäischer Papyrus aus der Zeit des ägyptischen Königs Amyrtäus. In *Florilegium ou recueil de travaux d'érudition dédiés à Monsieur le Marquis Melchior de Vogüé à l'occasion du quatre-vingtième anniversaire de sa naissance*, 529–44. Paris: Imprimerie Nationale.

———. 1911. *Aramäische Papyrus und Ostraka aus einer jüdischen Militärkolonie zu Elephantine: Altorientalische Sprachdenkmäler des 5. Jahrhunderts vor Christus.* 2 vols. Leipzig: J. C. Hinrichs.
Reviews: M.-J. Lagrange 1912; F. Schwally 1912.

Sachs, A. 1952. The Answer to a Puzzle. *BA* 15:89.

Sachsse, E. 1927. 'Anî als Ehrenbezeichnung in inschriftlicher Beleuchtung. In *Sellin-Festschrift: Beiträge zur Religionsgeschichte und Archäologie Palästinas: Ernst Sellin zum 60. Geburtstage dargebracht*, 105–10. Leipzig: Deichert.

Sader, H. 1987. *Les états araméens de Syrie depuis leur fondation jusqu'à leur transformation en provinces assyriennes.* Beiruter Texte und Studien, 36. Beirut: Orient-Institut der Deutschen Morgenländischen Gesellschaft.

Saller, S. J. 1957. *Excavations at Bethany.* Jerusalem: Franciscan Press.

as-Samarra'i, I. 1959. Comparative Study of Duel [sic] [in Arabic]. *Sumer* 15:75–84.

———. 1960. A Comment on an Article [i.e. 'A. Fāḍil 1958, in Arabic]. *Sumer* 16:38–41.

Šanda, A. 1904. Zur Panammu-Inschrift Zeile 16. *BZ* 2:369.

San Nicolò, M. 1927. Vorderasiatisches Rechtsgut in den ägyptischen Eheverträgen der Perserzeit. *OLZ* 30:217–21.

San Nicolò, M., and A. Ungnad. 1935. *Neubabylonische Rechts- und Verwaltungsurkunden.* Leipzig: J. C. Hinrichs.

Sanders, B. G. 1955. The Burning Fiery Furnace. *Theology* 58:240–45.

Sapin, J. 1990. Essai sur les structures géographiques de la toponymie araméenne dans les Trouée de Homs (Liban-Syrie) et sur leur signification historique. *Transeuphratène* 2:73–107.

Sarauw, C. 1907. Zu den Inschriften von Sendschirli. *ZA* 20:59–67.

Sasson, J. M. 1983. Review of *La statue de Tell Fekherye*, by A. Abou Assaf et al. *Religious Studies Review* 9:67–68.

Sasson, V. 1985. Two Unrecognized Terms in the Plaster Texts from Deir 'Alla. *PEQ* 117:102–3.

———. 1985a. The Aramaic Text of the Tell Fakhriyah Assyrian-Aramaic Bilingual Inscription. *ZAW* 97:86–103.

———. 1986. The Book of Oracular Visions of Balaam from Deir 'Alla. *UF* 17:283–309.

———. 1986a. The Language of Rebellion in Psalm 2 and in the Plaster Texts from Deir 'Alla. *AUSS* 24:147–54.

Savignac, R. 1908. Review of *Inscriptions sémitiques de la Syrie, de la Mésopotamie, et de la région de Mossoul*, by H. Pognon. *RB* 5:596–600.

———. See also: A. J. Jaussen.

Sayce, A. H. 1886–87. New Phoenician & Israelitish Inscriptions. *Babylonian and Oriental Record* 1:193–94.

———. 1892. Note on an Aramaean Inscription from Egypt. *PEFQS*: 251.

———. 1893. The Aramaean Inscriptions of Sinjerli and the Name of the Jews. *The Academy* 44:16.

———. 1895. Gleanings from the Land of Egypt. *Recueil de travaux relatifs à la philologie et à l'archéologie égyptiennes et assyriennes* 17:160–64.

———. 1903. Note. *PSBA* 25:315–16.

———. 1904. Aramaic Inscriptions from Egypt. *PSBA* 26:207–8.

———. 1904a. Documents judéo-araméens d'Eléphantine. II: Ostraka. *RevSém* 12:55–66.

———. 1908. An Aramaic Ostracon from Elephantinê. *PSBA* 30:39–41.

———. 1909. The Aramaic Papyri of Assuan: a Rectification. *ZA* 22:210.

———. 1909a. An Aramaic Ostracon from Elephantinê. *PSBA* 31:154–55 + fig.

———. 1911. The Jewish Garrison and Temple in Elephantinê. *Expositor* 8/2:97–116.

———. 1911a. The Jews and Their Temple in Elephantinê. *Expositor* 8/2:417–34.

———. 1911b. An Aramaic Ostracon from Elephantinê. *PSBA* 33:183–84, pl. XXVII.

———. 1911–12. The Jewish Papyri of Elephantinê. *ExpTim* 23:92–93.

———. 1912. The Passover Ostrakon from Elephantiné. *PSBA* 34:212.

———. 1924. Unpublished Hebrew, Aramaic, and Babylonian Inscriptions from Egypt, Jerusalem, and Carchemish. *JEA* 10:16–17.

———. 1927. The Moscho-Hittite Inscriptions. *JRAS*: 699–715.

Sayce, A. H., and A. E. Cowley. 1906. *Aramaic Papyri Discovered at Assuan*. London: Alexander Moring.

Reviews: F. Schulthess 1907; E. Schürer 1907; U. Wilcken 1908.

———. 1907. An Aramaic Papyrus of the Ptolemaic Age from Egypt. *PSBA* 29:260–72 + 6 pls.

Saydon, P. P. 1951. The Interpretation of Daniel 5, 30–31. *Scripture* 4:362–63.

as-Sayrafi, F. 1960. The Excavations of Ein Dara [in Arabic]. *AASyr* 10:87–102, pls. 1–17.

Scerrato, G. See: G. Pugliese-Carratelli.

Scerrato, U. 1958. An Inscription of Aśoka Discovered in Afghanistan: The Bilingual Greek-Aramaic of Kandahar. *EAW* 9/1–2:4–6.

———. 1958a. Notizia sull'editto bilingue greco-aramaico di Asoka scoperto in Afghanistan. *Archeologia classica* 10:262–66.

———. 1958b. Attività del Museo di Kabul. *Ariana, Rivista della società storica Afghana* 1337 (April - May) 2:41–44.

Schaberg, J. 1982. Major Midrashic Traditions in Wisdom 1,1–6,25. *JSJ* 13:75–101.

Schaeder, H. H. 1929–30. Iranische Beiträge I. *Schriften der Königsberger gelehrten Gesellschaft, Geisteswiss. Kl.* 6/5:199–296. Halle (Saale): Niemeyer.

———. 1930a. *Esra der Schreiber*. Beiträge zur historischen Theologie 5. Tübingen: J. C. B. Mohr.

———. 1938. Eine verkannte aramäische Präposition. *OLZ* 41:593–99.

Schäfer, H. 1904. Die Auswanderung der Krieger unter Psammetich I. und der Söldneraufstand in Elephantine unter Apries. *Klio* 4:152–63 + 4 pls.

Scheftelowitz, I. 1923. *Die Bewertung der aramäischen Urkunden von Assuan und Elephantine für die jüdische und iranische Geschichte*. Scripta Universitatis atque Bibliothecae

Hierosolymitanarum — Orientalia et Judaica I/iv. Jerusalem.

Scheil, V. 1895. Notes d'épigraphie et d'archéologie assyriennes. *Recueil des travaux relatifs à la philogie et à l'archéologie égyptiennes et assyriennes* 17:78–84.

———. 1901. Empreintes achéménides. *RB* 10:567–70.

———. 1914. Contrat babylonien à légende araméenne. *RA* 11:183–87.

Schenkel, H. 1905. Eine griechische Inschrift aus Kleinasien. *Berliner philologische Wochenschrift* 25:814–16.

Schiffer, S. 1909. Der Gott אלור. *OLZ* 12:477–78.

———. 1911. *Die Aramäer: Historisch-geographische Untersuchungen.* Leipzig: J. C. Hinrichs.

———. 1913. Zu אלור = i-lu-mi-ir (OLZ 1913, Sp. 254). *OLZ* 16:471.

———. 1914. Review of *Epigraphes araméens*, by L. Delaporte. *OLZ* 17:115–16.

Schlottmann, K. 1878. Zur semitischen Epigraphik: 5. Metrum und Reim auf einer ägyptisch-aramäischen Inschrift. *ZDMG* 32:187–97.

———. 1879. Zur semitischen Epigraphik: 7. Persisch-aramäischen Inschrift auf der Silberschale von Moskau. *ZDMG* 33:292–93.

Schlumberger, D. 1964. Une nouvelle inscription grecque d'Açoka. *CRAIBL*: 126–40.

———. 1972. De la pensée grecque à la pensée bouddhique. *CRAIBL*: 188–89.

Schlumberger, D., L. Robert, A. Dupont-Sommer, and E. Benveniste. 1958. Une bilingue gréco-araméenne d'Asoka. *JA* 246:1–48.

Schmidt, E. F. 1939. *The Treasury of Persepolis and Other Discoveries in the Homeland of the Achaemenians.* Chicago: Univ. of Chicago Press.

———. 1953, 1957, 1970. *Persepolis.* 3 vols.. I. Structures, Reliefs, Inscriptions. II. Contents of the Treasury and other Discoveries. III. The Royal Tombs and Other Monuments. OIP 68–70. Chicago: Univ. of Chicago Press.
  Reviews: F. Altheim and R. Stiehl 1963, 1:17–21,79; E. Benveniste 1958; K. Erdmann 1960.

Schmitt, R. 1967. Griech. *maniakes*–ein iranisches Lehnwort. *Die Sprache* 13:61–4.

———. 1972. Ein iranischer Name aus Elephantine: 'SWRT. *Beiträge zur Namenforschung* 7:143–46.

———. 1975. Analecta Irano-aramaica. *Die Sprache* 21:178–84.

Schneider, N. 1949. Aram und Aramäer in der Ur III-Zeit. *Bib* 30:109–11.

Schober, L. 1981. *Untersuchungen zur Geschichte Babyloniens und der oberen Satrapien von 323–303 v. Chr.* Frankfurt: Lang.

Schollmeyer, A. 1912. Das Passahfest zu Elephantine. *ThGl* 4:314.

———. 1912a. Die Herkunft der Achikarsprüche. *ThGl* 4:660–61.

Schrader, E. 1878. *Keilinschriften und Geschichtsforschung: Ein Beitrag zur monumentalen Geographie, Geschichte und Chronologie der Assyrer.* Giessen: J. Ricker.
  Reviews: T. Nöldeke 1879.

Schröder, P. 1880. Phönicische Miscellen. *ZDMG* 34:675–84.

———. 1914. Vier Siegelsteine mit semitischen Legenden. *ZDPV* 37:172–79.

Schüler, E. von. 1965. *Die Kaškäer: Ein Beitrag zur Ethnographie des alten Kleinasien.* Untersuchungen zur Assyriologie und vorderasiatischen Archäologie 3. Berlin: De Gruyter.

Schürer, E. 1907. Der jüdische Kalendar nach den aramäischen Papyri von Assuan. *TLZ* 32:65–69.

———. 1907a. Review of *APA*, by A. H. Sayce and A. E. Cowley. *TLZ* 32:1–7.

Schulthess, F. 1907. Review of *APA*, by A. H. Sayce and A. E. Cowley. *GGA* 169:181–99.

Schuttermayr, G. 1970. *Rḥm* — Eine lexikalische Studie. *Bib* 51:499–532.

Schwally, F. 1904. Review of "Notice sur un papyrus égypto-araméen de la Bibliothèque Impériale de Strasbourg," by J. Euting. *Literarisches Zentralblatt für Deutschland* 55:1504.

———. 1912. Review of Aramäische Papyrus und Ostraka, by E. Sachau. *OLZ* 15:160–68.

Schwartz, G. M. 1989. The Origins of the Aramaeans in Syria and Northern Mespotamia: Research Problems and Potential Strategies. In *To the Euphrates and Beyond: Archaeological Studies in Honour of Maurits N. van Loon,* ed. O. Haex et al., 275–91. Rotterdam: Balkeme.

Schwertheim, E. See: F. Altheim.

Segal, J. B. 1957. An Aramaic Ostracon from Nimrud. *Iraq* 19:139–45.

———. 1969. Miscellaneous Fragments in Aramaic. *Iraq* 31:170–74 + 1 pl.

———. 1971. Review of *Archives from Elephantine,* by B. Porten. *BSOAS* 34:141–2.

———. 1975. The Aramaic Papyri. In *Proceedings of the XIV International Congress of Papyrologists: Oxford, 24–31 July, 1974* 252–55. London: Egyptian Exploration Society.

———. 1978. Review of *Aramaic Texts from Deir 'Alla,* by J. Hoftijzer et al. *PEQ* 110:69.

———. 1983. New Aramaic Texts from Saqqara: An Introduction. In *Arameans, Aramaic and the Aramaic Literary Tradition,* ed. M. Sokoloff, 23–29. Ramat-Gan: Bar-Ilan Univ. Press.

———. 1983a. *Aramaic Texts from North Saqqara with Some Fragments in Phoenician.* Texts from Excavations, Memoir 6. London: Egyptian Exploration Society.
Reviews: J. Blau 1984–85; S. P. Brock 1985; J. A. Fitzmyer 1986; F. Greenspahn 1988; A. Lemaire 1984; J. Naveh 1985; J. Oelsner 1988; S. Shaked 1987; J. Teixidor 1985; E. Ullendorff 1985; J. W. Wesselius 1984; H. Williamson 1987; R. Zadok 1985.

———. 1987. Five Ostraca Re-examined. *Maarav* 4:69–74 + 5 pls.

Segall, B. 1955. The Arts and King Nabonidus. *AJA* 59:315–18.

Segert, S. 1956. Neue aramäische Texte aus Ägypten. *ArOr* 24: 284–91.

———. 1956a. Aramäische Studien I. Die neuen Editionen von Brooklyn Papyri und Aršāms Briefe in ihrer Bedeutung für die Bibelwissenschaft. *ArOr* 24:383–403.

———. 1956b. Mluvnice aramejštiny [Aramaic Grammar]. In *Mluvnice hebrejštiny a aramejštiny,* by O. Klíma and S. Segert. Prague: Nakladatelství Československé akademie ved.

———. 1958. Aufgaben der biblisch-aramäischen Grammatik. *Communio Viatorum* 1:127–34.

————. 1958a. Aramäische Studien III. Zum Problem der altaramäischen Dialekte. *ArOr* 26:561–72.

————. 1958b. Aramäische Studien IV. Der Artikel in den ältesten aramäischen Texten. *ArOr* 26:578–84.

————. 1958c. Review of *Aramaic Documents of the Fifth Century B.C.*, by G. R. Driver. *ArOr* 26:670–72.

————. 1960. Considerations on Semitic Comparative Lexicography. *ArOr* 28:470–87.

————. 1962. Concerning the Methods of Aramaic Lexicography. *ArOr* 30:505–6.

————. 1963. Altaramäische Schrift und Anfänge des griechischen Alphabets. *Klio* 41:38–57.

————. 1964. Zur Schrift und Orthographie der altaramäischen Stelen von Sfire. *ArOr* 32:110–26.

————. 1965. Ugaritisch und Aramäisch. In *Studia Semitica philologica necnon philosophica Ioanni Bakoš terquinque lustra complectenti dicata*, ed. S. Segert, 215–26. Bratislava: VSAV.

————. 1965a. Kann das Ostrakon von Nimrud für aramäisch gehalten werden? *Asian and African Studies* 1:147–51.

————. 1967. Contributions of I. N. Vinnikov to Old Aramaic Lexicography. *ArOr* 35:463–66.

————. 1971. Zur Bezeichnung der Frauen in den aramäischen Verträgen von Elephantine. In *Studi in onore di Edoardo Volterra*, 619–21. Pubblicazioni della Facoltà di giurisprudenza dell'Università di Roma, vols. 40–45. Milan: Giuffrè.

————. 1975. *Altaramäische Grammatik mit Bibliographie, Chrestomathie und Glossar.* Leipzig: VEB Verlag Enzyklopädie.
Reviews: E. Clarke 1977; R. Degen 1979; G. Garbini 1977; P. Grelot 1977; S. A. Kaufman 1977; D. Pardee 1978.

————. 1975a. Review of *Documents araméens d'Égypte*, by P. Grelot. *WZKM* 67:273–75.

————. 1976. Review of *Jews of Elephantine and Arameans of Syene (Fifth Century B.C.E.)*, by B. Porten in collaboration with J. C. Greenfield. *WZKM* 68:216–17.

————. 1978. Vowel Letters in Early Aramaic. *JNES* 37:111–14.

————. 1980. Review of *Studies in Aramaic Inscriptions and Onomastics, I*, by E. Lipiński. *WZKM* 72:176–79.

————. 1980a. Review of *Aramaic Texts from Deir 'Alla*, by J. Hoftijzer et al. *WZKM* 72:182–89.

————. 1985. Review of *La statue de Tell Fekherye et son inscription bilingue assyro-araméenne*, by A. Abou Assaf et al. *AfO* 31:90–94.

————. 1986. Preliminary Notes on the Structure of the Aramaic Poems in the Papyrus Amherst 63. *UF* 18:271–99.

Seidel, M. 1912. Bemerkungen zu den aramäischen Papyrus und Ostraka aus Elephantine. *ZAW* 32:292–98.

Seidl, E. 1967. Juristische Papyruskunde: 16. Bericht. *Studia et Documenta Historiae et Iuris* 33:503–80.

————. 1968. *Ägyptische Rechtsgeschichte der Saiten- und Perserzeit*. 2. neubearbeitete Auflage. Glückstadt: J. J. Augustin.

Selle, F. 1890. *De Aramaismis Libri Ezechielis*. Halle (Saale): Formis Kaemmererianis.

Sellers, O. R. 1933. *The Citadel of Beth-Zur*. Philadelphia: Westminster.

Sellin, E. 1908. [Communication]. MDOG 39:38–40; figs. 17–18.

Sellin, E., and C. Watzinger. 1913. *Jericho*. Die Ergebnisse der Ausgrabungen. Wissenschaftliche Veröffentlichung der Deutschen Orientgesellschaft, vol. 22. Leipzig: J. C. Hinrichs.

Sellwood, D. G. 1962. The Parthian Coins of Gotarzes I, Orodes I, and Sinatruces. *NC* 7/2:73–89.

————. 1965. Wroth's Unknown Parthian King. *NC* 7/5:113–35 + 2 pls.

————. 1967. A Die-Engraver Sequence for Later Parthian Drachmas. *NC* 7/7:13–28 + 2 pls.

————. See also: M. T. Abgarians.

Senart, E. 1881–86. *Les inscriptions de Piyādasi*. 2 vols. Paris: Imprimerie Nationale.

Seton Williams, M. V. 1961. Preliminary Report on the Excavations at Tell Rifa'at. *Iraq* 23:68–87.

Seyrig, H. 1955. Antiquités syriennes [60. Quelques cylindres orientaux (5. Atarshamayn)]. *Syria* 32:29–48, pl. III/5.

Shaffer, A. 1965. Hurrian **kirezzi*, West-Semitic *krz*. *Or* 34:32–34.

Shaffer, A., and J. C. Greenfield. 1981–82. הערות לכתובת הדו-לשונית מתל פח'ריה. *Shnaton* 5–6:119–29.

Shaffer, A. See also: J. C. Greenfield.

Shaked, S. 1969. Notes on the New Aśoka Inscription from Kandahar. *JRAS*: 118–22.

————. 1987. Review of *Aramaic Texts from North Saqqâra*, by J. B. Segal. *Or* 56:407–13.

Shaked, S., and J. Naveh. 1986. Three Aramaic Seals of the Achaemenid Period. *JRAS*: 21–29.

Shaked, S. See also: E. Y. Kutscher, J. Naveh, F. Rosenthal.

Shea, W. H. 1976. Adon's Letter and the Babylonian Chronicle. *BASOR* 223:61–64.

————. 1978–79. The Kings of the Melqart Stela. *Maarav* 1:159–76.

————. 1981. The Carpentras Stela: A Funerary Poem. *JAOS* 101:215–17.

————. 1982. Daniel 3: Extra-Biblical Texts and the Convocation on the Plain of Dura. *AUSS* 20:29–52.

————. 1982a. Nabonidus, Belshazzar, and the Book of Daniel: An Update. *AUSS* 20:133–49.

————. 1982b. Darius the Mede: An Update. *AUSS* 20:229–47.

————. 1983. A Further Note on Daniel 6: Daniel as "Governor." *AUSS* 21:169–71.

————. 1985. Further Literary Structures in Daniel 2–7: An Analysis of Daniel 4. *AUSS* 23:193–202.

————. 1985a. Further Literary Structures in Daniel 2–7: An Analysis of Daniel 5, and the Broader Relationships within Chapters 2–7. *AUSS* 23:277–95.

―――. 1988. Bel(te)shazzar Meets Belshazzar. *AUSS* 26:67–81.

Sherman, M. E. 1966. Systems of Hebrew and Aramaic Orthography: An Epigraphic History of the Use of Matres Lectionis in Non-biblical Texts to circa A.D. 135. Ph.D. diss., Harvard Univ.

Shevoroshkin, V. See: P. Frei.

Shifman, I. Sh. See: V. A. Livshitz.

Shirun, H. 1975–86. Aramäische Texte aus Ägypten. In *Lexikon der Ägyptologie*, ed. W. Helck and E. Otto, 362–70. Wiesbaden: Harrassowitz.

Shunnar, Z. 1970. Ein neuer aramäischer Papyrus aus Elephantine. In *Geschichte Mittelasiens im Altertum*, ed. F. Altheim and R. Stiehl, 111–18, pls. 1–2. Berlin: De Gruyter.

―――. 1971, 1973. Zu einer 'revidierten' Lesung des aramäischen Papyrus Berol. 23000. In *Christentum am Roten Meer*, ed. F. Altheim, 277–89, 379–95. Berlin and New York: De Gruyter.

Sidersky, D. 1910. Le calendrier sémitique des papyri araméens d'Assouan. *JA* 10/16:587–92.

―――. 1926. Le comput des Juifs d'Égypte au temps des Achéménides. *REJ* 82:59–78.

Siegman, E. F. 1956. The Stone Hewn from the Mountain: Daniel 2. *CBQ* 18:364–79.

Silverman, M. H. 1969. Aramean Name-types in the Elephantine Documents. *JAOS* 89:691–709.

―――. 1969a. הערות לשמות שבטקסטים מאוסף מיכאלידיס. *Leš* 34:66–71.

―――. 1969b. Onomastic Notes to "Aramaica Dubiosa." *JNES* 28:192–96.

―――. 1970. Hebrew Name-Types in the Elephantine Documents. *Or* 39:465–91.

―――. 1973. Egyptian Aramaic Texts [Review article: P. Grelot, *Documents araméens d'Égypte.*] *CdE* 48:301–8.

―――. 1981. Servant ('ebed) Names in Aramaic and in Other Semitic Languages. *JAOS* 101:361–66.

―――. 1981a. Biblical Name-Lists and the Elephantine Onomasticon: A Comparison. *Or* 50:265–331.

―――. 1985. *Religious Values in the Jewish Proper Names at Elephantine*. AOAT 217. Neukirchen-Vluyn: Neukirchener.
Reviews: H. Williamson 1987.

Simonetta, A. M. 1966. Some Remarks on the Arsacid Coinage of the Period 90–57 B.C. *NC* 7/6:15–40 + 2 pls.

Simonetta, B. 1961. Notes on the Coinage of the Cappadocian Kings. *NC* 7/1:9–50.

―――. 1964. Remarks on Some Cappodocian Problems. *NC* 7/4:83–92.

―――. 1967. A Note on Vologeses V, Artabanus V and Artavasdes. *NC* 7/7:7–12.

―――. 1967a. Some Additional Remarks on the Royal Cappodocian Coinage. *NC* 7/7:7–12.

Simons, J. 1959. *The Geographical and Topographical Texts of the Old Testament*. Leiden: Brill.

Simpson, W. K. 1959. Historical and Lexical Notes on the New Series of Ḥammamat

Inscriptions. *JNES* 18:20–37.

Sims-Williams, N. 1981. The Final Paragraph of the Tomb Inscription of Darius I (DNb, 50–60): The Old Persian Text in the Light of an Aramaic Version. *BSOAS* 44:1–7.

Sjöberg, E. 1948. Människosonen och Israel i Dan 7 [The Son of Man and Israel in Dan 7]. *Religion och Bibel* 7:1–16.

———. 1950. Uttrycket "Människoson" i Gamla testamentet [The expression "Son of Man" in the Old Testament]. *Svensk TKv* 26:35–44.

———. 1950–51. בן אדם und בר אנש im Hebräischen und Aramäischen. *AcOr* 21:57–65, 91–107.

Skaist, A. 1978. A Note on the Bilingual Ostracon from Khirbet el-Kôm. *IEJ* 28:106–8.

———. 1983. The *Clasula* [sic] *Salvatoria* in the Elephantine and Neo-Assyrian Conveyance Documents. In *Arameans, Aramaic and the Aramaic Literary Tradition*, ed. M. Sokoloff, 31–41. Ramat-Gan: Bar-Ilan Univ. Press.

Smelik, K. A. D. 1983. Een aramese parallel voor psalm 20. *NedTT* 37:89–103.

———. 1985. The Origin of Psalm 20. *JSOT* 31:75–81.

Smend, R. 1907. Zu den von E. Sachau herausgegebenen aramäischen Papyrusurkunden aus Elephantine. *TLZ* 32:705–11.

———. 1908. Alter und Herkunft des Achikar-Romans und sein Verhältnis zu Aesop. *BZAW* 13:55–125.

Smirnov, Y. I. 1896. [no title]. *Zapisky Imperatorskoe Russkoe arkheologicheskoe obshchestvo* n.s. 8/3–4:444–46.

Smit, E. J. 1990. The Saqqara Letter: Historical Implications. *Journal for Semitics* 2:57–71.

Smith, G. 1876. *Assyrian Discoveries*. 6th ed. London: Sampson Low, Marston, Searle, & Rivington.

Smith, J. M. P. 1908. The Jewish Temple at Elephantine. *BW* 31:448–59.

———. 1916–17. Jewish Religion in the Fifth Century B.C. *AJSL* 33:322–33.

Smith, J. Z. 1971. Review of *Aramaic Ritual Texts from Persepolis*, by R. A. Bowman. *History of Religions* 11:239–40.

Smith, V. A. 1904. *The Early History of India*. Oxford: Clarendon.

Smitten, W. T. In der. 1971. Vordeuteronomischer Jahwismus in Elephantine? *BO* 28:173–74.

———. 1971a. Eine aramäische Inschrift in Pakistan aus dem 3. Jhdt. v. Chr. *BO* 28:309–11.

Smyly, J. G. 1909. An Examination of the Dates of the Assuan Aramaic Papyri. *Proceedings of the Royal Irish Academy* 27:Sect. C., 235–50.

Snell, D. C. 1976. Review of *La langue de Ya'udi*, by P.-E. Dion. *WZKM* 68:220–24.

———. 1980. Why is There Aramaic in the Bible? *JSOT* 18:32–51.

———. 1985. The Aramaeans. In *Ebla to Damascus: Art and Archaeology of Ancient Syria*, ed. H. Weiss, 326–29. Washington: Smithsonian Institution.

Snijders, L. A. 1954. The Meaning of זו in the Old Testament: An Exegetical Study. *OTS* 10:1–154.

Soden, W. von. 1935.   Eine babylonische Volksüberlieferung von Nabonid in den Danielerzählungen. *ZAW* 53 12:81–89.

———. 1936.   Die Unterweltsvision eines assyrischen Kronprinzen nebst einigen Beobachtungen zur Vorgeschichte des Aḥiqar-Romans. *ZA* 43:1–31 + 6 pls.

———. 1959–60.   Aramäisches *ḥ* erscheint im Spätbabylonischen vor *m* auch als *g*. *AfO* 19:149.

———. 1961.   Azitawadda = Mattî von Atunna; KTK und Kasku. *OLZ* 56:576–79.

———. 1963.   *izqātu, išqātu* "Kettenringe", ein aramäisches Lehnwort. *AfO* 20:155.

———. 1966–77.   Aramäische Wörter in neuassyrischen und neu- und spätbabylonischen Texten: Ein Vorbericht I, II, III. *Or* 35:1–20; 37:261–71; 46:183–97.

———. 1977.   Review of *The Akkadian Influences on Aramaic*, by S. A. Kaufman. *JSS* 22:81–86.

———. 1982.   Review of *La statue de Tell Fekherye*, by A. Abou Assaf et al. *ZA* 72:293–96.

———. 1985.   Das nordsyrische *KTK/Kiski* und der Turtan Šamši-ilu: Erwägungen zu einem neuen Buch. *Studi epigrafici e linguistici* 2:133–41.

———. 1989.   Die Nominalform *taqtûl* im Hebräischen und Aramäischen. *Zeitschrift für Althebraistik* 2:77–85.

Soden, W. von, and T. Fish. 1952.   Manchester Texts. *Manchester Cuneiform Studies* 2:16–20.

Soggin, J. A. 1965.   Tracce di antichi causativi in *š*- realizzati come radici autonome in ebraico biblico. *AION* 25:17–30. Reprinted as "Traces of Ancient Causatives in *š*- Realized as Autonomous Roots in Biblical Hebrew" in *Old Testament and Oriental Studies* (Rome: Pontifical Biblical Institute, 1975), 188–202.

———. 1968.   Review of *The Aramaic Inscriptions of Sefîre*, by J. A. Fitzmyer. *ZAW* 80:126–27.

Sokoloff, M. 1969–70. שתי פונימות בארמית מקראית /θ/–/t/. *Leš* 34:239.

———. 1976.   'ămar nĕqē', "Lamb's Wool" (Dan 7:9). *JBL* 95:277–79.

———. 1976a.   Review of *The Akkadian Influences on Aramaic*, by S. A. Kaufman. *Kiryat Sepher* 51:464–73.

———. 1989.   Review of *The Bisitun Inscription of Darius the Great: Aramaic Version*, by J. C. Greenfield and B. Porten. *JAOS* 109:685–86.

Sola-Solé, J. M. 1967.   Miscellanea punico-hispana IV. *Sefarad* 27:15.

Sommer, F. 1930.   Das lydische und etruskische F-Zeichen. *SBAW* heft 1:1–23.

——— . See also: P. Kahle.

Soyez, B. 1972.   Le bétyle dans le culte de l'Astarté phénicienne. *MUSJ* 47:147–69 + 6 pls.

Spadafora, F. 1951.   Hazael. In *Enciclopedia cattolica*, 6:1380. (12 vols. Vatican City: Ente per l'Enciclopedia cattolica, 1948–54).

Sparks, H. F. D. 1946.   On the Origin of 'Darius the Mede' at Daniel V. 31. *JTS* 47:41–46.

Speiser, E. A. 1934.   A Figurative Equivalent for Totality in Akkadian and West-Semitic. *JAOS* 54:200–203.

———. 1934a. Addendum on the Phrase מן חם ועד חוט. *JAOS* 54:299.

Speleers, L. 1943. *Catalogue des intailles et empreintes orientales des Musées Royaux d'Art et d'Histoire: Supplément.* Brussels: Vromant.

Sperling, D. 1968. The Akkadian Legal Term *dīnu u dabābu. JANES* 1:35–40.

———. 1969–70. The Informer and the Conniver. *JANES* 2:101–4.

Sperry, S. B. 1955. *The Aramaic Vocabulary of the Old Testament: Containing a Linear Translation of the Texts Together with Grammatical Notes for the Benefit of Beginners.* Provo, Utah: Brigham Young Univ.

Spiegelberg, W. 1904. Zu dem Strassburger aramäischen Papyrus. *OLZ* 7:10–11.

———. 1906. Ägyptisches Sprachgut in den aus Ägypten stammenden aramäischen Urkunden der Perserzeit. In *Orientalische Studien Theodor Nöldeke zum siebzigsten Geburtstag (2. März 1906) gewidmet,* vol. 2, ed. C. Bezold, 1093–1115. Giessen: Töpelmann.

———. 1912. Zu den ägyptischen Personennamen in den kürzlich veröffentlichten Urkunden von Elephantine. *OLZ* 15:1–10.

———. 1913. Die demotische Notiz in dem Papyrus 8 von Elephantine. *OLZ* 16:15–16.

———. 1913a. Zu den ägyptischen Personennamen der Urkunden von Elephantine. *OLZ* 16:346–47.

Spijkerman, A. 1961–62. Chronique du Musée de la Flagellation. *SBFLA* 12:323–33.

Spitaler, A. 1952–54. Zur Frage der Geminatendissimilation im Semitischen: Zugleich ein Beitrag zur Kenntnis der Orthographie des Reichsaramäischen. *Zeitschrift für indogermanische Forschungen* 61:257–66.

———. 1962. *Al-ḥamdu lillāhi lladī* und Verwandtes. *Oriens* 15:97–114.

———. 1968. Zum Problem der Segolisierung im Aramäischen. *Wissenschaftliche Zeitschrift der Martin-Luther-Universität, Halle* 17, vol. 2:193–99.

Spoer, H. H. 1907. Some Hebrew and Phoenician Inscriptions. *JAOS 28:355–59.*

Sprengling, M. 1910–11. Chronological Notes from the Aramaic Papyri. The Jewish Calendar. Dates of the Achaemenians (Cyrus-Darius II). *AJSL* 27:233–66.
Reviews: O. Holtzmann 1912; J. V. Prášhek 1912.

———. 1917. The Aramaic Papyri of Elephantine in English. *AJT* 21:411–52.

———. 1918. The Aramaic Papyri of Elephantine in English Continued. *AJT* 22:349–75.

———. 1928–29. The Epigraphic Material of Aghaya Kaleh. *AJSL* 45:279–80.

———. 1932. An Aramaic Seal Impression from Khorsabad. *AJSL* 49:53–55.

———. 1940. Kartīr, Founder of Sasanian Zoroastrianism. *AJSL* 57:197–228.

———. 1953. *Third Century Iran: Sapor and Kartir.* Chicago: Oriental Institute, Univ. of Chicago.

Spycket, A. 1981. *La statuaire du proche-orient ancien.* Handbuch der Orientalistik 7/1.2B. Leiden: Brill.
Reviews: A. Invernizzi 1982.

———. 1985. La statue bilingue de Tell Fekheriyé. *RA* 79:67–68.

Staerk, W. 1907. *Die jüdisch-aramäischen Papyri von Assuan sprachlich und sachlich erklärt.* KIT 22–23. Bonn: Marcus & Weber.

————. 1908. *Aramäische Urkunden zur Geschichte des Judentums im VI. und V. Jahrhundert vor Chr. sprachlich und sachlich erklärt.* KIT 32. Bonn: Marcus & Weber.

————. 1912. *Alte und neue aramäische Papyri übersetzt und erklärt.* KIT 94. Bonn: Marcus & Weber.

Stähelin, F. 1908. Elephantine und Leontopolis. *ZAW* 28:180–82.

Starcky, J. 1952. *Palmyre.* L'Orient ancien illustré 7. Paris: Maisonneuve.

————. 1960. Une tablette araméenne de l'an 34 de Nabuchodonosor (AO, 21.063). *Syria* 37:99–115.

Starcky, J., and A. Jamme. 1970. VIII — Aramaic Collection, in A. Jamme, "The Pre-Islamic Inscriptions of the Riyâdh Museum." *OrAnt* 9:115–39.

Starcky, J. See also: A. Dupont-Sommer.

Starkey, J. L. See: H. Torczyner.

Stec, D. M. 1987. The Use of *hēn* in Conditional Sentences. *VT* 37:478–86.

Stefanovic, Z. 1987. *Correlations between Old Aramaic Inscriptions and the Aramaic Section of Daniel.* Ph.D. diss., Andrews Univ.

Stein, W. 1927–30. Elephantine. In *Jüdisches Lexikon*, ed. G. Herlitz and B. Kirschner, 344–47. Berlin: Jüdischer Verlag.

Steindorff, G. 1894. Deutsche Ausgrabungen im Orient. *Deutsche Rundschau* 78:453–57.

————. 1905. Elephantine ('Ελεφαντίνη). In *Pauly-Wissowa*, vol. 5, 2321–24. Stuttgart: J. B. Metzler.

Steiner, R. C. 1980. *Yuqaṭṭil, Yaqaṭṭil* or *Yiqaṭṭil*: D-stem Prefix-Vowels and a Constraint on Reduction in Hebrew and Aramaic. *JAOS* 100:513–18.

————. 1987. *Lulav* versus **lu/law*: A Note on the Conditioning of **aw>ū* in Hebrew and Aramaic. *JAOS* 107:121–22.

Steiner, R. C., and C. F. Nims. 1984. You Can't Offer Your Sacrifice and Eat It Too: A Polemical Poem from the Aramaic Text in Demotic Script. *JNES* 43:89–114.

————. 1985. Ashurbanipal and Shamash-shum-ukin: A Tale of Two Brothers from the Aramaic Text in Demotic Script. *RB* 92:60–81 + 1 pl.

Steiner, R. C. See also: C. F. Nims.

Stern, E. 1970. Review of *Archives from Elephantine*, by B. Porten. *Qadmoniot* 3/4:145–6.

————. 1971. Seal-Impressions in the Achaemenid Style in the Province of Judah. *BASOR* 202:6–16.

————. 1982. *Material Culture of the Land of the Bible in the Persian Period 538–332 B.C.* Warminster: Aris & Phillips; Jerusalem: Israel Exploration Society.

Stern, E., and Y. Magen. 1982. A Persian Period Pottery Assemblage from Qadum in the Samaria Region [in Hebrew]. *EI* (Orlinsky Volume) 16:182–97.

————. 1984. A Pottery Group of the Persian Period from Qadum in Samaria. *BASOR* 253:9–27.

Steuernagel, C. 1909. Bemerkungen über die neuentdeckten jüdischen Bedeutung für das Alte Testament. *Theologische Studien und Kritiken* 105:1–12.

————. 1911. Zum Passa-Maṣṣothfest. *ZAW* 31:310.

————. 1912. Die jüdisch-aramäischen Papyri und Ostraka aus Elephantine und ihre Bedeutung für die Kenntnis palästinensischer Verhältnisse. *ZDPV* 35:85–104.

Stevenson, J. H. 1902. *Assyrian and Babylonian Contracts with Aramaic Reference Notes.* The Vanderbilt Oriental Series. New York: American Book Co.

Stevenson, W. B. 1924. *Grammar of Palestinian Jewish Aramaic.* Oxford: Clarendon. 2nd ed., with an appendix on the numerals by J. A. Emerton, 1962.

Reviews: G. Bergsträsser 1926: *OLZ* 29:495–500; G. Dalman 1925: *TLZ* 50:147–48; P. Dhorme 1926: *RB* 35:155; G. R. Driver 1924–25: *JTS* 26:210–12; I. Eitan 1935–36: "Aramaica,", *JQR* 26:165–72 esp. 167–69; M. Lambert 1924: *REJ* 79:213–14; S. A. B. Mercer 1924: *Anglican Theological Reveiw* 7:400; S. A. B. Mercer 1925: *Journal of the Society for Oriental Research* 9:186; A. van Hoonaker 1924: *Le Muséon* 37:306–7.

————. 1934–35. The Identification of the Four Kingdoms of the Book of Daniel. *Transact. Glasgow Univ. Or. Soc.* 7:4–8.

Stiehl, R. 1959–62. Wörterverzeichnis aramäischer Inschriften und anderer Urkunden aus parthischer Zeit. In *Geschichte der Hunnen*, ed. F. Altheim, 110–25. Berlin: De Gruyter.

————. 1964. Aramäisch als Weltsprache. In *Neue Beiträge zur Geschichte des Alten Welt*, vol. 1, 69–85. Berlin: Akademie Verlag.

————. See also: F. Altheim.

Stinespring, W. F. 1958. History and Present State of Aramaic Studies. *JBR* 26:298–303.

————. 1962. The Active Infinitive with Passive Meaning in Biblical Aramaic. *JBL* 81:391–94.

Stolper, M. W. 1976. A Note on Yahwistic Personal Names in the Murašû Texts. *BASOR* 222:25–28, p. 20 fig. 1.

————. 1985. *Entrepreneurs and Empire: The Murašû Archive, the Murašû Firm, and Persian Rule in Babylon.* Publications de l'Institut historique et archéologique néerlandais de Stamboul 54. Leiden: Nederlands Historisch-Archaeologisch Instituut te Istanbul.

————. 1989. The Governor of Babylon and Across-the-River in 486 B.C. *JNES* 48:283–85.

Stolz, F. 1970. *Strukturen und Figuren im Kult von Jerusalem.* BZAW 118. Berlin: De Gruyter.

Stone, M. E. 1971. Ahikar. *Encyclopaedia Judaica* 1:461–62.

Story, C. I. K. 1945. The Book of Proverbs and Northwest Semitic Literature. *JBL* 64:319–37.

Strack, H. L. 1896. Zum Kenntnis des älteren aramäisch. *Theologisches Literaturblatt* 17:153–58.

————. 1911. Review of *Aramäische Papyrus und Ostraka*, by E. Sachau. *ZDMG* 65:826–32.

————. 1911a. Review of *Aramäische Papyrus aus Elephantine*, by A. Ungnad. *ZDMG* 65:832–38.

————. 1921. *Grammatik des Biblisch-Aramäischen.* 6th ed. Munich: Beck.

Reviews: G. Bergsträsser 1912; C. Levias 1903.

Strazzulli, A., P. Bovier-Lapierre, and S. Ronzevalle. 1918–19. Rapport sur les fouilles à Éléphantine de l'Institut Biblique Pontifical en 1918. *ASAE* 18:1–7.

Struve, W. 1926. Zur Geschichte der jüdischen Kolonie von Elephantine. *Bulletin de l'Académie des Sciences de l'URSS* 6/20:445–54.

Stucky, R. A. 1985. Achämenidische Hölzer und Elfenbeine aus Ägypten und Vorderasien im Louvre. *Antike Kunst* 28:7–32 + 12 pls.

Stummer, F. 1914. *Der kritische Wert der altaramäischen Ahikartexte aus Elephantine.* Alttestamentliche Abhandlungen vol. 5, no. 5. Münster: Aschendorff.

———. 1914a. Zu den altaramäischen Achikarsentenzen. *OLZ* 17:252–54.

———. 1915. Zur Ursprache des Ahikarbuches. *OLZ* 18:103–5.

Sukenik, E. L. 1933. The 'Jerusalem' and 'The City' Stamps on Jar Handles. *JPOS* 13:226–31.

———. 1933a. Inscribed Hebrew and Aramaic Potsherds from Samaria. *PEFQS* 65:152–56.

———. 1934. Paralipomena Palaestinensia. *JPOS* 14:178–84 + 3 pls.

Sukenik, E. L., and J. [E. Y.] Kutscher. 1942. A Passover Ostracon from Elephantine [in Hebrew]. *Kedem* 1:32–36.

Sundermann, W. 1985. Schriftsysteme und Alphabete im alten Iran. *Altorientalische Forschungen* 12:101–13.

Swain, J. W. 1940. The Theory of the Four Monarchies: Opposition History under the Roman Empire. *Classical Philology* 35:1–21.

Swetnam, J. 1965. Some Observations on the Background of צדיק in Jeremias 23,5a. *Bib* 46:29–40.

Swiggers, P. 1980. Note sur un papyrus araméen d'el-Hibeh. *Aeg* 60:93–95.

———. 1981. Note sur le papyrus IV d'Hermoupolis. *Aeg* 61:65–68.

———. 1981a. Notes on the Hermopolis Papyri I and II. *AION* 41:144–46.

———. 1981b. A Syncretistic Anthroponym in the Aramaic Documents from Egypt. *Beiträge zur Namenforschung* 16:348–50.

———. 1981c. Review of *La langue de Ya'udi*, by P.-E. Dion. *Language* 57:505.

———. 1982. The Aramaic Inscription of Kilamuwa. *Or* 51:249–53.

———. 1982a. The Hermopolis Papyri III and IV. *AION* 42:135–40.

———. 1982b. Review of *Jews of Elephantine and Arameans from Syene*, by B. Porten and J. C. Greenfield. *Onoma* 26:327–29.

———. 1983. The Notation System of the Old Aramaic Inscriptions. *ArOr* 51:378–81.

———. 1983a. The Name *mspt* in the Aramaic Documents from Egypt. *Aeg* 63:177–79.

———. 1988. Possessives with Predicative Function in Official Aramaic. In *FUCUS: A Semitic/Afrasian Gathering in Remembrance of Albert Ehrman*, ed. Y. A. Arbeitman, 449–61. Amsterdam: Benjamins.

Sznycer, M. 1971. Trois fragments de papyri araméens d'Égypte d'époque perse. In *HomAD-S*, 161–76, pls. 1–2.

———. 1984. L'inscription araméenne sur un vase inscrit du Musée de Bahrain. *Syria* 61:108–18.

———. 1986. Une inscription araméenne de Tell Khazneh. In *Failaka: Fouilles françaises 1984–1985*, ed. Y. Calvet and J.-F. Salles, 273–80. Paris: n.p.

Szubin, H. Z., and B. Porten. 1982. "Ancestral Estates" in Aramaic Contracts: The Legal Significance of the Term *mhḥsn*. *JRAS*: 3–9.

———. 1983. Litigation Concerning Abandoned Property at Elephantine (Kraeling 1). *JNES* 42:279–84.

———. 1983a. Testamentary Succession at Elephantine. *BASOR* 252:35–46.

———. 1987. Royal Grants in Egypt: A New Interpretation of Driver 2. *JNES* 46:39–48.

———. 1988. A Life Estate of Usufruct: A New Interpretation of Kraeling 6. *BASOR* 269:29–45.

Szubin, H. Z. See also: B. Porten.

Türck, U. 1928. Die Stellung der Frau in Elephantine als Ergebnis persisch-babylonischen Rechtseinflusses. *ZAW* 46:166–69.

Tadmor, H. 1961. גבולה הדרומי של ארם-דמשק. *Yediot* 25:201–10. Reprinted as "The Southern Border of Aram" in *IEJ* 12 (1962): 114–22.

———. 1961a. Que and Muṣri. *IEJ* 11:143–50.

———. 1965. A Note on the Seal of Mannu-ki-Inurta. *IEJ* 15:233–34.

———. 1970. הערות לשורות הפתיחה של החוזה הארמי מספירה. In *Sepher Shmuel Yeivin*, ed. S. Abramski et al., 397–405. Jerusalem: Kirjath Sepher.

———. 1975. Assyria and the West: The Ninth Century and Its Aftermath. In *Unity and Diversity: Essays in the History, Literature, and Religion of the Ancient Near East*, ed. H. Goedicke and J. J. M. Roberts, 36–48. Baltimore: Johns Hopkins Univ. Press.

———. 1982. Treaty and Oath in the Ancient Near East: A Historian's Approach. In *Humanizing America's Iconic Book: Society of Biblical Literature Centennial Addresses 1980*, ed. G. M. Tucker and D. A. Knight, 127–52. Chico, Cal.: Scholars Press.

———. 1982a. The Aramaization of Assyria: Aspects of Western Impacts. In *Mesopotamien und seine Nachbarn: XXV. Rencontre assyriologique internationale, Berlin 1978*, Berliner Beiträge zum vorderen Orient I/2, 449–70. Berlin: Reimer.

———. 1989. על מקומה של הארמית בממלכת אשור: שלוש הערות על תבלית של סרגון. *EI (Yadin Volume)* 20:249–52.

———. See also: A. R. Millard, J. Naveh.

Talmon, S. 1958. Divergences in Calendar-Reckoning in Ephraim and Judah. *VT* 8:48–74.

Tawil, H. 1972. *Idioms in Old Aramaic Royal Inscriptions in the Light of Akkadian*. Ph.D. diss., Columbia Univ.

———. 1973. The End of the Hadad Inscription in the Light of Akkadian. *JNES* 32:477–82.

———. 1974. Some Literary Elements in the Opening Sections of the Hadad, Zākir, and the Nērab II Inscriptions in the Light of East and West Semitic Royal Inscriptions. *Or* 43:40–65.

———. 1977. A Curse concerning Crop-Consuming Insects in the Sefîre Treaty and in Akkadian: A New Interpretation. *BASOR* 225:59–62.

——. 1980. Two Notes on the Treaty Terminology of the Sefîre Inscriptions. *CBQ* 42:30–37.

Taylor, W. R. 1930. Recent Epigraphic Discoveries in Palestine. *JPOS* 10:16–22, pl. IIa.

Teixidor, J. 1964. Un nouveau papyrus araméen du règne de Darius II. *Syria* 41:285–90.

——. 1964a. Nota sobre un papiro arameo del año 417 antes de Cristo. *Sefarad* 24:325–26 + 1 pl.

——. 1967. Bulletin d'épigraphie sémitique. *Syria* 44:163–95.

——. 1968. Bulletin d'épigraphie sémitique. *Syria* 45:352–89.

——. 1969. Bulletin d'épigraphie sémitique. *Syria* 46:318–58.

——. 1970. Review of *Archives from Elephantine*, by B. Porten. *JAOS* 90:543–44.

——. 1970a. Bulletin d'épigraphie sémitique 1970. *Syria* 47:357–89.

——. 1971. Bulletin d'épigraphie sémitique. *Syria* 48:452–93.

——. 1972. On the Authenticity of the Madrid Papyrus. *JNES* 31:340–42.

——. 1972a. Bulletin d'épigraphie sémitique. *Syria* 49:412–49.

——. 1972b. Review of *The Development of the Aramaic Script*, by J. Naveh. *JAOS* 92:529–30.

——. 1973. Bulletin d'épigraphie sémitique. *Syria* 50:400–442.

——. 1974. Bulletin d'épigraphie sémitique. *Syria* 51:299–340.

——. 1975. Bulletin d'épigraphie sémitique. *Syria* 52:261–95.

——. 1976. Bulletin d'épigraphie sémitique. *Syria* 53:304–41.

——. 1976a. Review of *Documents araméens d'Égypte*, by P. Grelot. *JNES* 35:217–18.

——. 1977. Bulletin d'épigraphie sémitique. *Syria* 54:251–76.

——. 1978. The Aramaic Text in the Trilingual Stele from Xanthus. *JNES* 37:181–85.

——. 1979. Bulletin d'épigraphie sémitique. *Syria* 56:353–405.

——. 1984. Contexto epigráfico y literario de Esdras y Daniel. In *Simposio bíblico español (Salamanca, 1982)*, ed. M. Fernández Marcos et al., 129–40. Madrid: Universidad Complutense.

——. 1985. Review of *Aramaic Texts from North Saqqâra*, by J. B. Segal. *JAOS* 105:731–34.

——. 1986. *Bulletin d'épigraphie sémitique (1964–1980)*. Institut français d'archéologie du Proche Orient — Bibliothèque archeologique et historique 126. Paris: Geuthner.
Reviews: S. A. Kaufman 1990: *JAOS 110:162.*

——. See also: P. Bordreuil, J. Margueron, K. Yassine.

Temerev, A. N. 1979. The Problematical Character of Literal Interpretations of Military Terms in Aramaic Papyri of the Fifth Century B.C. from Upper Egypt [in Russian]. In *Problems in the History of the Countries of the Near and Middle East*, 111–22. Moscow: Nauka.

——. 1980. The Food-Supply System in Achaemenid Garrisons (according to Aramaic Texts from Upper Egypt and Arad) [in Russian]. *VDI* 151:124–31.

——. 1983. Social Organizations in Egyptian Military Settlements of the Sixth-Fourth

Centuries B.C.E: *dgl* and *m't*. In *The Word of the Lord Shall Go Forth: Essays in Honor of David Noel Freedman in Celebration of His Sixtieth Birthday*, ed. C. L. Meyers and M. O'Connor, 523–25. Winona Lake, Ind.: Eisenbrauns.

Termes, P. 1963–65. Ăḥīqār y el Libro de Tobías. In *Enciclopedia de la Biblia*, ed. A. Diez Macho and S. Bartina, 266–68. Barcelona: Garriga.

Testen, D. 1985. The Significance of Aramaic *r* < *n*. *JNES* 44:143–46.

Thapar, R. 1961. *Aśoka and the Decline of the Mauryas*. London: Oxford Univ. Press.

Thompson, J. A. 1965. Expansions of the *'d* Root. *JSS* 10:222–40.

Thomson, J. E. H. 1893. The Chaldee of Daniel compared with that of the Targums. *The Thinker* 4:486–93.

Thureau-Dangin, F. 1922. *Tablettes d'Uruk*. Musée orientale: Textes cunéiformes, vol. 6. Paris: Geuthner.

———. 1896. Anciens noms de mois chaldéens. *JA* 9/7:339–43.

Thureau-Dangin, F., A. Barrois, G. Dossin, and M. Durand. 1931. *Arslan Tash*. Bibliothèque archéologique et historique, vol. 16. Paris: Geuthner.
Reviews: R. Dussaud 1932.

Thureau-Dangin, F., and M. Dunand. 1936. *Til-Barsib*. Paris: Geuthner.

Tisdall, W. St. C. 1921. The Book of Daniel: Some Linguistic Evidence regarding its Date. *Journal of the Transactions of the Victoria Institute* 53:206–45.

———. 1921a. Egypt and the Book of Daniel. *Expositor* 22:340–57.

Tomback, R. S. 1984. An Unrecognized Maltese West-Semitic Isogloss. *JNSL* 12:121–23.

Toorn, K. van der. 1986. Ḥerem-Bethel and Elephantine Oath Procedure. *ZAW* 98:282–85.

Torczyner, H. 1912. Anmerkungen zu den Papyrusurkunden von Elephantine. *OLZ* 15:397–403.

———. 1916. Wissenschaftlicher Jahresbericht über die morgenländischen Studien Im Jahre 1915: Das Semitische 1913–1915, mit Ausschluss der Assyriologie, des Sabaeo-Mināischen und der abbesinischen Dialekte sowie der alttestamentlichen Studien. *ZDMG* 70:274–91.

Torczyner, H., L. Harding, A. Lewis, and J. L. Starkey. 1938. *Lachish I: The Lachish Letters*. The Wellcome Archaeological Research Expedition to the Near East: Publications, vol. 1. London: Oxford Univ. Press.

Torres, C. 1944. Dan 5,30s en relación con la historia de Caldea. *Boletín de la Univ. de Santiago de Compostela* 43:15–59.

Torrey, C. C. 1908. The Aramaic Portions of Ezra. *AJSL* 24:209–81.

———. 1909. Notes on the Aramaic Part of Daniel. *Transact. of the Connect. Acad. of Arts and Sciences* 15:239–82.

———. 1910. *Ezra Studies*. Chicago: Univ. of Chicago Press. Reprint, with a Prolegomenon by W. F. Stinespring. New York: Ktav, 1970.

———. 1912. New Notes on Some Old Inscriptions. *ZA* 26:77–92.

———. 1915. The Zakar and Kalamu Inscriptions. *JAOS* 35:353–69.

———. 1915a. An Aramaic Inscription from Cilicia, in the Museum of Yale University. *JAOS* 35:370–74.

———. 1917–18. The Bilingual Inscription from Sardis. *AJSL* 34:185–98.

———. 1921–22. A Few Ancient Seals. In AASOR 2–3:103–8.

———. 1923. Stray Notes on the Aramaic of Daniel and Ezra. *JAOS* 43:229–38.

———. 1926. A Specimen of Old Aramaic Verse. *JAOS* 46:241–47.

———. 1935. Hebrew and Aramaic from Beth Shemesh. *JAOS* 55:307–10.

———. 1937. *Aramaic Graffiti on Coins of Demanhur.* Numismatic Notes and Monographs 77. New York: American Numismatic Society.

———. 1938. Notes on the Aramaic Contract Published by Bauer and Meissner. *JAOS* 58:394–98.

———. 1939. The Two Persian Officers Named Bagoas. *AJSL* 56:300–301.

———. 1940. The Letters Prefixed to Second Maccabees. *JAOS* 60:119–150.

———. 1941. On the Ostraca from Elath (Bulletin No. 80). *BASOR* 82:15–16.

———. 1941a. A Synagogue at Elath? *BASOR* 84:4–5.

———. 1946. Medes and Persians. *JAOS* 66:1–15.

———. 1952. Ein griechisch transkribiertes und interpretiertes hebräisch-aramäisches Verzeichnis der Bücher des Alten Testaments aus dem 1. Jahrhundert n. Chr. *TLZ* 77:249–54.

———. 1954. More Elephantine Papyri [Review article: E. G. Kraeling, *The Brooklyn Museum Aramaic Papyri.*] *JNES* 13:149–53.

Tournay, R. 1957. Le nom du 'buisson ardent'. *VT* 7:410–13.

Trever, J. C. 1985. The Book of Daniel. *BA* 48:89–102.

Troickiy, J. G. 1895. [no title]. *Christianskoye Čtenie* 75:422–30.

Tsereteli, K. 1980. Zur Frage der Spirantisation der Verschlusslaute in den semitischen Sprachen. *ZDMG* 130:207–16.

Tsevat, M. 1959. The Neo-Assyrian and Neo-Babylonian Vassal Oaths and the Prophet Ezekiel. *JBL* 78:199–204.

———. 1960. A Chapter in Old West Semitic Orthography. In *The Joshua Bloch Memorial Volume: Studies in Booklore and History*, ed. A. Berger, L. Marwick, and I. Meyer, 82–91. New York: New York Public Library.

Tucci, G. See: G. Pugliese-Carratelli.

Tuland, C. G. 1958. Hanani—Hananiah. *JBL* 77:157–61.

———. 1958a. 'Uššayyā' and 'Uššarnā: a Clarification of Terms, Date, and Text. *JNES* 17:269–75.

Tur-Sinai (Torczyner), N. H. 1960. ארמית בנבואת ירמיהו. In *Sepher Z. Karl*, ed. A. Weiser and B. Z. Luria, 112–114. Scripta assoc. investigandae S. Scripturae in Israel, vol. 10. Jerusalem: Kiryat Sepher.

Tvedtnes, J. A. 1981. The Origin of the Name 'Syria'. *JNES* 40:139–40.

Tychsen, O. G. 1815. De linguae phoeniciae et hebraicae mutua aequalitate commentatio. *Nova acta regiae societatis scientiarum Upsaliensis* ser. 2, vol. 7:87–103.

Tzaferis, V. See: A. Biran.

Uffenheimer, B. 1965–66. מונה פולחני עתיק מן המזרח הקדמון – "המעוררין". *Leš* 30:163–74.

———. 1977. אל עליון קונה שמים וארץ. *Shnaton* 2:20–26.

Ullendorff, E. 1985. Review of *Aramaic Texts from North Saqqâra*, by J. B. Segal. *JRAS*: 68–70.

Unger, E. 1931. *Babylon, Die Heilige Stadt.* Berlin: De Gruyter.

Unger, M. 1957. *Israel and the Aramaeans of Damascus.* London: Clarke.

Ungnad, A. 1911. *Aramäische Papyrus aus Elephantine: Kleine Ausgabe unter Zugrundelegung von Eduard Sachau's Erstausgabe.* Leipzig: J. C. Hinrichs.
Reviews: H. L. Strack 1911.

———. See also: M. San Nicolò.

Unvala, J. M. 1935. [Communication]. Revue numismatique 38:160–61.

Vaccari, A. 1953. Due documenti contemporanei di Geremia. *RivB* 1:136–43.

Van Rooy, H. F. 1989. The Structure of the Aramaic Treaties of Sefire. *Journal for Semitics* 1:133–39.

van Selms, A. 1974. The Name Nebuchadnezzar. In *Travels in the World of the Old Testament: Studies Presented to Professor M. A. Beek on the Occasion of His 65th Birthday,* ed. M. S. H. G. Heerma van Voss et al., 223–29. Assen: Van Gorcum.

Vasholz, R. I. 1978. Qumran and the Dating of Daniel. *JETS* 21:315–21.

———. 1979–81. Two Notes on 11 Q tg Job and Biblical Aramaic. *RevQ* 10:93–94.

———. 1979–81a. A Further Note on the Problem of Nasalization in Biblical Aramaic, 11 Q tg Job, and 1 Q Genesis Apocryphon. *RevQ* 10:95–96.

Vattioni, F. 1958. Dan 3.8; 6.25 e i testi di Mari. *RivB* 6:371.

———. 1963. La III iscrizione de Sfiré A 2 e Proverbi 1, 23. *AION* 23:279–86.

———. 1965. La prima menzione aramaica di "figlio dell'uomo." In *Biblos Press*, vol.6, 6–7. Rome: S. Maxia.

———. 1965a. Il dio Resheph. *AION* 25:39–74.

———. 1965b. Un papiro aramaico del 417 a. C. *Aeg* 45:190–93.

———. 1966. A propos du nom propre syriaque Gusai. *Sem* 16:39–41.

———. 1966a. Il papiro di Saqqarah. *Studia papyrologica* 5:101–17.

———. 1967. Recenti studi sull'alleanza nella Bibbia e nell'antico oriente. *AION* 27:181–226.

———. 1969. Frustula epigraphica. *Aug* 9:366–69.

———. 1969a. Preliminari alle iscrizioni aramaiche. *Aug* 9:305–61.

———. 1969b. I sigilli ebraici. *Bib* 50:357–88.

———. 1970. Epigrafia aramaica. *Aug* 10:493–532.

———. 1971. Epigrafia aramaica. *Aug* 11:18–190.

———. 1971a. I sigilli, le monete e gli avori aramaici. *Aug* 11:47–87.

———. 1978. Saggio di bibliografia semitica 1976–1978. *AION* 38:465–500.

———. 1978a. Sigilli ebraici. III. *AION* 38:227–54.

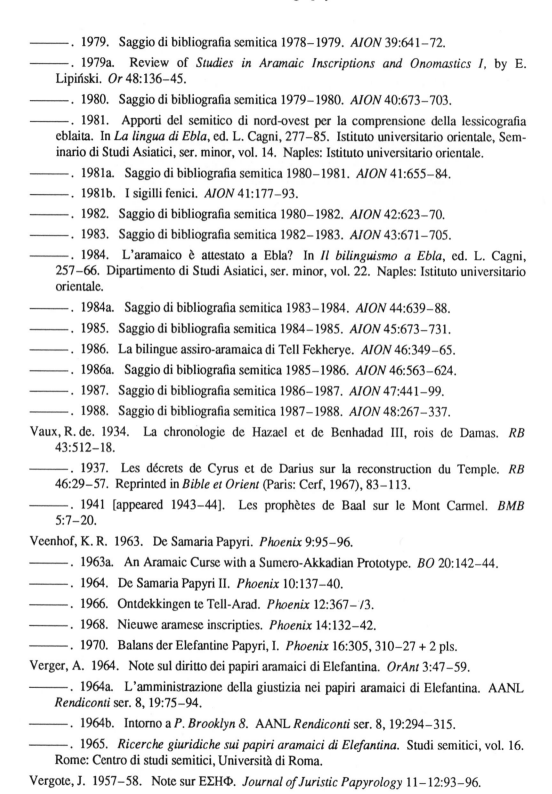

———. 1979. Saggio di bibliografia semitica 1978–1979. *AION* 39:641–72.

———. 1979a. Review of *Studies in Aramaic Inscriptions and Onomastics I*, by E. Lipiński. *Or* 48:136–45.

———. 1980. Saggio di bibliografia semitica 1979–1980. *AION* 40:673–703.

———. 1981. Apporti del semitico di nord-ovest per la comprensione della lessicografia eblaita. In *La lingua di Ebla*, ed. L. Cagni, 277–85. Istituto universitario orientale, Seminario di Studi Asiatici, ser. minor, vol. 14. Naples: Istituto universitario orientale.

———. 1981a. Saggio di bibliografia semitica 1980–1981. *AION* 41:655–84.

———. 1981b. I sigilli fenici. *AION* 41:177–93.

———. 1982. Saggio di bibliografia semitica 1980–1982. *AION* 42:623–70.

———. 1983. Saggio di bibliografia semitica 1982–1983. *AION* 43:671–705.

———. 1984. L'aramaico è attestato a Ebla? In *Il bilinguismo a Ebla*, ed. L. Cagni, 257–66. Dipartimento di Studi Asiatici, ser. minor, vol. 22. Naples: Istituto universitario orientale.

———. 1984a. Saggio di bibliografia semitica 1983–1984. *AION* 44:639–88.

———. 1985. Saggio di bibliografia semitica 1984–1985. *AION* 45:673–731.

———. 1986. La bilingue assiro-aramaica di Tell Fekherye. *AION* 46:349–65.

———. 1986a. Saggio di bibliografia semitica 1985–1986. *AION* 46:563–624.

———. 1987. Saggio di bibliografia semitica 1986–1987. *AION* 47:441–99.

———. 1988. Saggio di bibliografia semitica 1987–1988. *AION* 48:267–337.

Vaux, R. de. 1934. La chronologie de Hazael et de Benhadad III, rois de Damas. *RB* 43:512–18.

———. 1937. Les décrets de Cyrus et de Darius sur la reconstruction du Temple. *RB* 46:29–57. Reprinted in *Bible et Orient* (Paris: Cerf, 1967), 83–113.

———. 1941 [appeared 1943–44]. Les prophètes de Baal sur le Mont Carmel. *BMB* 5:7–20.

Veenhof, K. R. 1963. De Samaria Papyri. *Phoenix* 9:95–96.

———. 1963a. An Aramaic Curse with a Sumero-Akkadian Prototype. *BO* 20:142–44.

———. 1964. De Samaria Papyri II. *Phoenix* 10:137–40.

———. 1966. Ontdekkingen te Tell-Arad. *Phoenix* 12:367–73.

———. 1968. Nieuwe aramese inscripties. *Phoenix* 14:132–42.

———. 1970. Balans der Elefantine Papyri, I. *Phoenix* 16:305, 310–27 + 2 pls.

Verger, A. 1964. Note sul diritto dei papiri aramaici di Elefantina. *OrAnt* 3:47–59.

———. 1964a. L'amministrazione della giustizia nei papiri aramaici di Elefantina. AANL *Rendiconti* ser. 8, 19:75–94.

———. 1964b. Intorno a *P. Brooklyn 8*. AANL *Rendiconti* ser. 8, 19:294–315.

———. 1965. *Ricerche giuridiche sui papiri aramaici di Elefantina*. Studi semitici, vol. 16. Rome: Centro di studi semitici, Università di Roma.

Vergote, J. 1957–58. Note sur ΕΣΗΦ. *Journal of Juristic Papyrology* 11–12:93–96.

Vincent, A. 1937. *La religion des judéo-araméens d'Éléphantine*. Paris: Geuthner.

——. 1957. Les papyrus araméens d'Éléphantine. *BVC* 17:105–15.

Vincent, L.-H. 1910. Une nouvelle estampille judéo-araméenne. *RB* 7:578.

——. 1910a. Les fouilles allemandes à Jéricho. *RB* 7:404–20.

——. 1923. La date des épigraphes d''Arâq el-émîr. *JPOS* 3:55–68.

——. 1949. Les épigraphes judéo-araméennes postexiliques. *RB* 56:274–94.

Vinnikov, I. N. 1955. Novaja interpretacija nadpisi Zakara, carja Chamat i Luaša [A new interpretation of the inscriptions of Zakara, ruler of Hamat in Luaša]. *Epigrafika Vostoka* 10:84–94.

——. 1958–65. Dictionary of Aramaic Inscriptions [in Russian]. *PalSb* 3:171–216; 4:196–240; 7:192–237; 9:140–58; 11:189–232; 13:217–62.

Vittmann, G. 1989. Zu den ägyptischen Entsprechungen aramäisch überlieferter Personnamen. *Or* 58:213–29.

Vivian, A. 1981. *Studi di sintassi contrastiva: Dialetti aramaici*. Quaderni di semitistica 12/1. Florence: Istituto di Linguistica e di Lingue Orientali.
Reviews: T. Muraoka 1983: *JSS* 28:176–77.

Vleeming, S. P. 1981. Een lang uitgestelde benoeming. *Phoenix* 27:82–91.

Vleeming, S. P., and J. W. Wesselius. 1982. An Aramaic Hymn from the Fourth Century B.C. *BO* 39:501–9.

——. 1983–84. Betel the Saviour. *JEOL* 28:110–40.

——. 1985. *Studies in Papyrus Amherst 63: Essays on the Aramaic Texts in Aramaic/Demotic: Papyrus Amherst 63, 1*. Amsterdam: Juda Palache.

——. 1985a. Bijbelse parallellen in een aramees/demotische papyrus uit de vierde eeuw v. Chr. In *Vreemdeling in het land van Pharao*, ed. P. W. Pestman, 14–26. Zutphen: Terra.

Vogüé, C. J. M. de. 1862. Notice sur un talent de bronze trouvé à Abydos. *RArch* 3/5:30–39.

——. 1868. *Syrie centrale: inscriptions sémitiques*. Paris: J. Baudry.

——. 1868a. Intailles à légendes sémitiques. In *Mélanges d'archéologie orientale* 105–40. Paris: Imprimerie Impériale.

——. 1868b. Le Lion d'Abydos. In *Mélanges d'archéologie orientale* 179–96. Paris: Imprimerie Nationale.

——. 1886. Note sur quelques intailles sémitiques. *CRAIBL* 4/14:187–93.

——. 1902. [No title]. *CRAIBL*: 247–48.

——. 1902a. [No title.]. *CRAIBL*: 49–50.

——. 1903. Inscription araméenne trouvée en Egypte. *CRAIBL*: 269–76, with photo, pl. opp. p. 270.

——. 1906. Papyrus araméens d'Égypte. *CRAIBL*: 499–508.

——. 1908. Nouvelles de la mission de M. Clermont-Ganneau en Égypte. *CRAIBL*: 100, 127.

Vogelsang, W. 1986. Four Short Notes on the Bisitun Text and Monument. *Iranica antiqua* 21:121–40.

Vogelstein, M. 1942. Bakshish for Bagoas? *JQR* 33:89–92.

Vogt, E. 1953. Novae papyri aramaicae Elephantinae. *Bib* 34:265–67.

———. 1954. Ex novis documentis aramaicis. *Bib* 35:266–68.

———. 1957. Die neubabylonische Chronik über die Schlacht bei Karkemisch und die Einnahme von Jerusalem. In *Volume du congrès: Strasbourg 1956*, 67–96. VTSup 4. Leiden: Brill.

———. 1958. Nova inscriptio aramaica saec. 8 a. C. *Bib* 39:269–74.

———. 1958a. Nomina hebraica-phoenicia in Assyria. *Bib* 39:114–15.

———. 1971. *Lexicon linguae aramaicae Veteris Testamenti documentis antiquis illustratum*. Rome: Pontifical Biblical Institute.
Reviews: K. Beyer 1979; J. A. Fitzmyer 1973; P. Grelot 1972; D. J. Harrington 1972; S. A. Kaufman 1978; J. Körner 1985: *OLZ* 80:39–40; F. Rosenthal 1972.

———. 1975. Review of *Studies in the Aramaic Legal Papyri from Elephantine*, by Y. Muffs. *Or* 44:129–31.

Voigt, R. M. 1987. The Classification of Central Semitic. *JSS* 32:1–21.

Voigtlander, E. N. von. 1978. *The Bisitun Inscription of Darius the Great: Babylonian Version*. Corpus Inscriptionum Iranicarum I/2. London: Lund Humphries.
Reviews: R. Zadok 1981.

Volkwein, B. 1969. Masoretisches *'ēdūt, 'ēdwōt, 'ēdōt*: "Zeugnis" oder "Bundesbestimmungen"? *BZ* 13:18–40.

Vollenweider, M.-L. 1967–83. Catalogue raisonné des sceaux, cylindres et intailles. 3 vols. Geneva: Musée d'Art et d'Histoire.

Vollenweider, M.-L., F. Brüschweiler, and R. Stucky. 1966. *Trésors de l'ancien Iran; Musée Rath-Genève, 8 juin–25 september 1966*. Geneva: Musée d'Art et d'Histoire.

Volterra, E. 1956. Osservazioni sul divorzio nei documenti aramaici. In *Studi orientalistici in onore de Giorgio Levi della Vida*, vol. 2, 586–600. Pubblicazioni dell'Istituto per l'Oriente 52. Rome: Giovanni Bardi.

———. 1957. Le affrancazioni di schiavi nei documenti aramaici del V secolo a. C. *RSO* 32:675–96.

———. 1963. *Yhwdy* e *'rmy* nei papiri aramaici del V secolo provenienti dall'Egitto. AANL *Rendiconti* 18:131–73.

———. 1964. Intorno a AP. 13 lin. 17–18. In *Mélanges Eugène Tisserant*, vol. 1, 443–48. Studi e testi, vol. 231. Vatican City: Biblioteca Apostolica Vaticana.

———. 1964a. Osservazioni alla nota del Prof. R. Yaron. *Iura* 15:173–80.

Volz, P. 1912. Ein Beitrag aus den Papyri von Elephantine zu Hiob Kap. 31. *ZAW* 32:126–27.

Vriezen, T. C. 1963. Das Hiphil von *'āmar* in Deut. 26, 17.18. *JEOL* 17:207–10.

Wagenaar, C. G. 1928. *De joodsche Kolonie van Jeb-Syene in de 5de eeuw voor Christus*. Groningen/The Hague: J. B. Wolters.

Wagner, M. 1966. *Die lexikalischen und grammatikalischen Aramaismen im alttestamentlichen Hebräisch*. BZAW 96. Berlin: Töpelmann.
Reviews: K. Beyer 1970; R. Degen 1968–69; A. Hurvitz 1969; O. Klíma 1973: *ArOr* 41:78.

———. 1967. Beiträge zur Aramaismenfrage im alttestamentlichen Hebräisch. In *Hebräische Wortforschung, Festschrift zum 80. Geburtstag von Walter Baumgartner*, ed. B. Hartmann et al., 355–71. VTSup 16.

Wagner, S. 1984. Review of *Textbook of Syrian Semitic Inscriptions I-II*, by J. C. L. Gibson. *OLZ* 79:356–59.

Waldman, N. M. 1974. Notes on the Aramaic Lexicon. *JANES* 6:125–32.

Wallis, G. 1978. Review of *Aramaic Texts from Deir ʿAlla*, by J. Hoftijzer et al. *BO* 35:316–17.

Waltke, B. K. 1976. The Date of the Book of Daniel. *BSac* 133:319–30.

Ward, W. H. 1886. Two Seals with Phoenician Inscriptions. *AJA* 2:155–56.

———. 1910. *The Seal Cylinders of Western Asia*. Washington: Carnegie Institution.

———. 1920. *Cylinders and Other Ancient Oriental Seals in the Library of J. Pierpont Morgan*. New Haven: Yale Univ. Press.

Watanabe, K. 1987. *Die adê-Vereidigung anlässlich der Thronfolgeregelung Asarhaddons*. Baghdader Mitteilungen 3. Berlin: Gebr. Mann.

Waterman, L. 1946. A Gloss on Darius the Mede in Daniel 7, 5. *JBL* 65:59–61.

Watson, W. G. E. 1984. The Ahiqar Sayings: Some Marginal Comments. *AO* 2:253–61.

Watzinger C. See: E. Sellin.

Weber, O. 1920. *Altorientalische Siegelbilder*. Der alte Orient, vols. 17–18. Leipzig: J.C. Hinrichs.

Wehr, H. 1964. Das "Tor des Königs" im Buche Esther und verwandte Ausdrücke. *Islam* 39:247–60.

Weidner, E. F. 1932–33. Der Staatsvertrag, Aššurnirâris VI. von Assyrien mit Matiʾilu von Bît-Agusi. *AfO* 8:17–34.

———. 1952–53. Das Reich Sargons von Akkad. *AfO* 16:1–24.

———. 1939. Jojachim, König von Juda, in babylonischen Keilschrifttexten. In *Mélanges syriens offerts à M. René Dussaud*, 923–35. Bibliothèque archéologique des antiquités, vol. 30. Paris: Geuthner.

Weill, R. 1913. Un document araméen de la moyenne-Egypte. *REJ* 65:166–23.

Weinfeld, M. 1965. Traces of Assyrian Treaty Formulae in Deuteronomy. *Bib* 46:417–27.

———. 1970. The Covenant of Grant in the Old Testament and in the Ancient Near East. *JAOS* 90:184–203.

———. 1971–72. הברית והחסד — המונחים וגלגולי התפתחותם בישראל ובעולם העתיק. *Leš* 36:85–105.

———. 1972. *Deuteronomy and the Deuteronomic School*. Oxford: Clarendon.

———. 1973. Covenant Terminology in the Ancient Near East and Its Influence on the West. *JAOS* 93:190–99.

———. 1973–74. לעניין מונחי ברית ביונית וברומית. *Leš* 38:231–37.

———. 1975. שבועת אמונים לאסרחדון אופייה ומקבילותיה בעולם המזרח הקדום. *Shnaton* 1:51–88. Reprinted as "The Loyalty Oath in the Ancient Near East," *UF* 8 (1976):379–414.

——— . 1981–2. נבואת בלעם בכתובת מדיר עלא (סוכות). *Shnaton* 5–6:141–47.

——— . 1982. The Counsel of the "Elders" to Rehoboam and Its Implications. *Maarav* 3:27–53.

——— . 1985. [Section VI: Discussion]. *BAT*, 367.

Weippert, H., and M. Weippert. 1982. Die "Bileam"-Inschrift von Tell *Dēr Allā*. *ZDPV* 98:77–103.

Weippert, M. 1964. Archäologischer Jahresbericht. *ZDPV* 80:150–93.

——— . 1966. Archäologischer Jahresbericht. *ZDPV* 82:274–330.

——— . 1975. Zum Präskript der hebräischen Briefe von Arad. *VT* 25:202–12.

——— . 1981. Der Beitrag ausserbiblischer Prophetentexte zum Verständnis der Prosareden des Jeremiabuches. In *Le Livre de Jérémie: Le prophète et son milieu, les oracles et leur transmission*, ed. P. M. Bogaert, 83–104. Bibliotheca ephemeridum theologicarum lovaniensium, vol. 54. Louvain: Peeters.

——— . 1991. The Balaam Text from Deir 'Allā and the Study of the Old Testament. In *BTDAR*, 151–84.

——— . See also: H. Weippert.

Weisberg, D. B. 1967. *Guild Structure and Political Allegiance in Early Achaemenid Mesopotamia*. Yale Near Eastern Researches 1. New Haven: Yale Univ. Press.

Weissbach, F. H. 1911. *Die Keilinschriften der Achämeniden*. Vorderasiatische Bibliothek 3. Leipzig: J. C. Hinrichs.

Welles, C. B. 1949. Manumission and Adoption. *RIDA* 3:507–20.

Wellhausen, J. 1899. Review of *A Glossary of the Aramaic Inscriptions*, by S. Cook. *GGA*:244–46.

——— . 1899a. Review of *Handbuch der Nordsemitischen Epigraphik*, by M. Lidzbarski. *GGA*:602–8.

Wensinck, A. J. 1909. *Het oudste Arameesch*. Utrecht: A. Oosthoek.

——— . 1912. Zu den Achikarsprüchen der Papyri aus Elephantine. *OLZ* 15:49–54.

——— . 1931. *The Article of Determination in Arabic*. Mededeel. Kon. Akad. v. Wetensch., afd. Letterk., deel 71, serie A, no. 3. Amsterdam: Noordhollandsche Uitgeversmij.

Wesedonk, O. G. von. 1932. Über die Verwendung des Aramäischen im Achaemenidenreich. *Litterae orientales* 49 (Jan.):1–10.

Wesselius, J. W. 1980. Reste einer Kasusflektion in einigen früharamäischen Dialekten. *AION* 40:265–68.

——— . 1982. Notes on Aramaic Magical Texts. I: The Incantation in Cuneiform Script. *BO* 39:249–51.

——— . 1983. Het standbeeld van de arameese vorst Hada-yit͞ʿī. In *Schrijvend verleden: Documenten uit het oude Nabije Oosten vertaald en toegelicht*, ed. K. R. Veenhof, 55–59. Leiden: Ex Oriente Lux.

——— . 1983a. Review of *La statue de Tell Fekherye*, by A. Abou Assaf et al. *BO* 40:181–82.

——— . 1984. A New Reading in Sfire III, 18. *BO* 41:589–91.

————. 1984a. Official Aramaic *l'brt* = 'area'. *OLP* 15:77–80.

————. 1984b. Review of *Aramaic Texts from North Saqqâra*, by J. B. Segal. *BO* 41:700–7.

————. 1984c. Review of *The Bisitun Inscription of Darius the Great, Aramaic Version*, by J. C. Greenfield and B. Porten. *BO* 41:440–45.

————. 1985. A Document Concerning the Sustenance of a Mother by Her Sons. *AION* 45:506–8.

————. 1985a. Official Aramaic *rḥh wmršh* = 'Mill and Mortar' (Kraeling 9, 14). *AION* 45:503–5.

————. 1986. The Restoration of Hermopolis Letter 6 and the Ransom of Prisoners. In *Tradition and Reinterpretation in Jewish and Early Christian Literature: Essays in Honour of Jürgen C. H. Lebram*, ed. J. W. van Henten et al., 7–18. SPB 36. Leiden: Brill.

————. 1987. Thoughts about Balaam: The Historical Background of the Deir Alla Inscription on Plaster. *BO* 44:589–99.

————. 1988. Language and Style in Biblical Aramaic: Observations on the Unity of Daniel ii-vi. *VT* 38:194–209.

————. See also: S. P. Vleeming.

Westberg, F. 1910. *Die Biblische Chronologie nach Flavius Josephus*. Leipzig: Deichert.

Whitehead, J. D. 1974. Early Aramaic Epistolography: The Arsames Correspondence. Ph.D. diss., Univ. of Chicago.

————. 1978. Some Distinctive Features of the Language of the Aramaic Arsames Correspondence. *JNES* 37:119–40.

Whitehouse, O. C. 1908. Some Problems Suggested by the Recent Discoveries of Aramaic Papyri at Syene (Assuān). In *Transactions of the Third International Congress for the History of Religions*, 280–84. Oxford: Clarendon.

————. 1908–9. Some Problems Suggested by the Recent Discoveries of Aramaic Papyri at Syene (Assouan). *ExpTim* 20:200–205.

Whiting, R. M. 1988. A Late Middle Assyrian Tablet from North Syria. *SAAB* 2:99–101.

Wikander, S. 1974. Aramäisch *sprb*, Sanskrit *śvabhra*. In *Ksiega pamiatkowa ku czci Eugeniusza Sluszkiewicza*, ed. J. Reychmana, 271–72. Warsaw: Wydaunictwa Uniwersytetu.

Wilcken, U. 1908. Review of *Aramaic Papyri Discovered at Assuan*, by A. H. Sayce and A. E. Cowley. *Archiv für Papyrusforschung* 4:228–30.

————. 1913. Papyrus-Urkunden. *Archiv für Papyrusforschung* 5:198–300.

Will, E. 1987. Qu'est-ce qu'une *Baris*? *Syria* 64:253–59.

Williamson, H. 1983. The Composition of Ezra i-vi. *JTS* n. s. 34:1–30.

————. 1987. Review of *Religious Values in the Jewish Proper Names at Elephantine*, by M. H. Silverman. *SOTS Book List*: 124–25.

————. 1987a. Review of *Aramaic Texts from North Saqqâra*, by J. B. Segal. *JEA* 73:265–69.

Wilson, G. H. 1979. An Index to the Biblical Passages Cited in Franz Rosenthal, *A Grammar of Biblical Aramaic. JSS* 24:21–24.

———. 1985. Wisdom in Daniel and the Origin of Apocalyptic. *Hebrew Annual Review* 9:373–81.

Wilson, J. V. K. 1957. Two Medical Texts from Nimrud (continued). *Iraq* 19:40–49.

Wilson, R. D. 1912. The Aramaic of Daniel. In *Biblical and Theological Studies by the Members of the Faculty of Princeton Theological Seminary*, 261–306. New York: Scribner.

———. 1917–38. *Studies in the Book of Daniel*. 2 vols. Reprint: Baker, 1979 (one volume).

Winckler, H. 1893. Das syrische Land Jaudi und der angebliche Azarja von Juda. In *AF*, vol. 1, 1–23. Leipzig: Pfeiffer.

———. 1893a. Zu den Inschriften aus Sendschirli-Gerdschin. In *AF*, vol. 1, 105–7. Leipzig: Pfeiffer.

———. 1894. Bemerkungen zu semitischen Inschriften. In *AF*, vol. 2, 183–84. Leipzig: Pfeiffer.

———. 1896. Die Bauinschrift Bar-rekub's aus Sendschirli. *MVAG* 1:198–202.

———. 1898. Zur Inschrift von Teima. In *AF*, Zweite Reihe, vol. 2, 76–77. Leipzig: Pfeiffer.

Winnett, F. A., and W. L. Reed. 1970. *Ancient Records from North Arabia*. Near & Middle East Series, vol. 6. Toronto: Univ. of Toronto.

Winter, I. J. 1981. Is There a South Syrian Style of Ivory Carving in the Early First Millennium B.C.? *Iraq* 43:101–30.

———. 1989. North Syrian Ivories and Tell Halaf Reliefs: The Impact of Luxury Goods upon "Major" Arts. In *Essays in Ancient Civilization Presented to Helene J. Kantor*, ed. Albert Leonard, Jr. and Bruce Beyer Williams, 321–32. Studies in Ancient Oriental Civilization, vol. 47, Chicago: The Oriental Institute of the University of Chicago.

Winton Thomas, D. 1950. The Age of Jeremiah in the Light of Recent Archaeological Discovery. *PEQ*:1–15.

———. 1960. Review of *Les inscriptions araméennes de Sfiré*, by A. Dupont-Sommer and J. Starcky. *JSS* 5:281–84.

Winton Thomas, D., ed. 1958. *Documents from Old Testament Times, Translated with Introductions and Notes by Members of the Society for Old Testament Study*. London: Nelson; New York: Harper.

Wise, M. O. 1990. A Calque from Aramaic in Qoheleth 6:12, 7;12; and 8:13. *JBL* 109:249–57.

Wiseman, D. J. 1958. The Vassal-Treaties of Esarhaddon. *Iraq* 20:1–99 + 65 pls.
Reviews: I. J. Gelb 1962.

———. 1978. They Lived in Tents. In *Biblical and Near Eastern Studies: Essays in Honor of William Sanford LaSor*, ed. G. A. Tuttle, 195–200. Grand Rapids, Mich.: Eerdmans.

———. n.d. *Cylinder Seals of Western Asia*. London: Batchworth Press.

Witakowski, W. 1976. Aramejskie papirusy z Elefantyny i ich znaczenie historyczne. *Przegld orientalistyczny* 1:57–67.

———. 1978–79. The Origins of the Jewish Colony at Elephantine. *OS* 27–28:34–41.

Wittstruck, T. 1978. The Influence of Treaty Curse Imagery on the Beast Imagery of Daniel 7. *JBL* 97:100–102.

Witzel, T. 1909. Documenti aramaici del secolo V avanti Cristo trovati nell'Egitto superiore. *Rivista storico-critica delle scienze teologiche* 5:680–90, 737–52.

———. 1909a. Urkundenfunde in Oberägypten (aus dem 5. Jahrh. v. Chr.) *Pastor Bonus* 21:371–79, 437–42, 481–87.

Wolters, A. 1988. The Balaamites of Deir 'Alla as Aramean Deportees. *HUCA* 59:101–13.

———. 1991. Aspects of the Literary Structure of Combination I. In *BTDAR*, 294–304.

Woolley, L. 1962. *The Neo-Babylonian and Persian Periods*. Ur Excavations, vol. 9. London: British Museum.

Woolley, L., and R. D. Barnett. 1952. *Carchemish. Part III: The Excavations in the Inner Town. The Hittite Inscriptions*. London.

Wood, L. H. See: S. H. Horn.

Woude, A. S. van der. 1986. Erwägungen zur Doppelsprachigkeit des Buches Daniel. In *Scripta signa vocis: Studies about Scripts, Scriptures, Scribes and Languages in the Near East, Presented to J. H. Hospers*, ed. H. L. J. Vanstiphout et al., 305–16. Groningen: Forsten.

Wright, Ch. H. H. 1908. *Light from Egyptian Papyri on Jewish History before Christ*. London: Williams and Norgate.

Wright, W. 1883. [Communication]. *PSBA*:100–101.

Wright, W., ed. 1875–83. *The Paleographical Society: Facsimiles of Manuscripts and Inscriptions (Oriental Series)*. London: W. Clowes and Sons.

Wroth, W. 1899. *Catalogue of the Greek Coins of Galatia, Cappodocia, and Syria*. A Catalogue of the Greek Coins in the British Museum, vol. 20. London: British Museum, Dept. of Coins and Medals. Reprint. Bologna: Arnaldo Forni, 1964.

———. 1903. *Catalogue of the Coins of Parthia*. A Catalogue of the Greek Coins in the British Museum, vol. 23. London: British Museum, Dept. of Coins and Medals. Reprint. Bologna: Arnaldo Forni, 1964.

Görg, M. 1984. Ein Keilschrift-Fragment des Berichtes vom dritten Feldzug des Senaherib mit dem Namen des Hiskija. *BN* 24:16–17.

Yadin, Y. 1957. Note. *IEJ* 7:153.

———. 1961. The Fourfold Division of Judah. *BASOR* 163:6–12.

———. 1967. A Note on the Nimrud Bronze Bowls. *EI (Sukenik Volume)* 8: 6.

———. 1967a. ‏על סמלי האלים בשמאל (זינגירלי, בקארתאגו ובחצור‎. *Yediot* 31:29–63.

———. 1970. Symbols of Dieties at Zinjirli, Carthage and Hazor. In *Essays in Honor of Nelson Glueck: Near Eastern Archaeology in the Twentieth Century*, ed. J. A. Sanders, 199–231. Garden City, N.Y.: Doubleday.

Yalon, H. 1931. Assimilation of ‏ת"ו‎ in Hebrew and Aramaic [in Hebrew]. *Tarbiz* 3:99–106.

———. 1935. ‏פלל‎ and ‏פלפל‎ in Hebrew and Aramaic [in Hebrew]. *Tarbiz* 6:223–29.

Yamauchi, E. M. 1970. The Greek Words in Daniel in the Light of Greek Influence in the Near East. In *New Perspectives on the Old Testament*, ed. J. B. Payne, 170–200. Waco,

Texas: Word.

———. 1980. Hermeneutical Issues in the Book of Daniel. *JETS* 23:13–21.

Yardeni, A. See: B. Porten.

Yaron, R. 1957.   Two Greek Words in the Brooklyn Museum Aramaic Papyri. *HUCA* 28:49–51.

———. 1957a. The Schema of the Aramaic Legal Documents. *JSS* 2:33–61.

———. 1958. Identities in the Brooklyn Museum Aramaic Papyri. *Bib* 39:344–54.

———. 1958a. On Defension Clauses of Some Oriental Deeds of Sale and Lease from Mesopotamia and Egypt. *BO* 15:15–22.

———. 1958b. Aramaic Marriage Contracts from Elephantine. *JSS* 3:1–39.

———. 1958c. Notes on Aramaic Papyri. *RIDA* ser. 3, 5:299–310.

———. 1959. Redemption of Persons in the Ancient Near East. *RIDA* ser. 3, 6:155–76.

———. 1960. Aramaic Marriage Contracts: Corrigenda et Addenda. *JSS* 5:66–70.

———. 1960a. Aramaic Deeds of Conveyance. *Bib* 41:248–74, 379–94.

———. 1961. המשפט של מסמכי יב. Jerusalem: Hebrew Univ.

———. 1961a. *Introduction to the Law of the Aramaic Papyri.* Oxford: Clarendon.

———. 1961b. Notes on Aramaic Papyri II. *JNES* 20:127–30.

———. 1964. Who Is Who at Elephantine. *Iura* 15:167–72.

———. 1967. "כסף זוז בתעודות יב". *Leš* 31:287–88.

———. 1968. Minutiae Aramaicae. *JSS* 13:202–11 + 1 pl.

———. 1970. Aramaica recentia. In *Proceedings of the 12th International Congress of Papyrology*, ed. D. H. Samuel, 537–44. Toronto: Hakkert.

———. 1971. Review of *Archives from Elephantine*, by B. Porten. *JSS* 16:240–44.

Yassine, K., and P. Bordreuil. 1982. Deux cachets ouest sémitiques inscrits decouverts a Tell Mazar. In *Studies in the History and Archaeology of Jordan*, vol. 1, ed. A. Hadidi, 192–94. Amman: Department of Antiquities.

———. 1984. Two West Semitic Inscribed Stamp Seals. In *Tell el Mazar I, Cemetery A*, ed. K. Yassine, 132–34. Amman: The University of Jordan.

Yassine, K., and J. Teixidor. 1986. Ammonite and Aramaic Inscriptions from Tell El-Mazār in Jordan. *BASOR* 264:45–51.

Yelin, A. 1937. ספר אחיקר החכם. 2nd ed. Jerusalem: HaMaarav.

Young, E. J. 1958. *Daniel's Vision of the Son of Man.* London: Tyndale.

Young, R. S. See: M. Mellink.

Younger, K. L., Jr. 1986. Panammuwa and Bar-Rakib: Two Structural Analyses. *JANES* 18:91–103.

Zadok, R. 1976. On Five Iranian Names in the Old Testament. *VT* 26:246–47.

———. 1976a. Review of *Studies in Aramaic Inscriptions and Onomastics I*, by E. Lipiński. *BO* 33:227–31.

———. 1977. *On West Semites in Babylonia during the Chaldean and Achaemenian Periods: An Onomastic Study.* Jerusalem: Wanaarta and Tel-Aviv Univ.

————. 1977a. Historical and Onomastic Notes. *WO* 9:35–56.

————. 1979. New Documents from the Chaldean and Achaemenian Periods. *OLP* 15:65–75.

————. 1980. Notes on the Biblical and Extra-Biblical Onomasticon. *JQR* 71:107–17.

————. 1981. Review of *The Bisitun Inscription of Darius the Great: Babylonian Version*, by E. N. von Voigtlander. *BO* 38:657–65.

————. 1981–82. Iranian and Babylonian Notes. *AfO* 28:135–39.

————. 1982. Remarks on the Inscription of *HDYS'Y* from Tell Fakhariya. *Tel Aviv* 9:117–29.

————. 1982a. Three Non-Akkadian Words in Late Babylonian Documents. *JAOS* 102:115–17.

————. 1984. On the Historical Background of the Sefire Treaty. *AION* 44:529–38.

————. 1984a. Assyrians and Chaldeans in Achaemenian Babylonia. *Assur* 4:1–28.

————. 1984b. Review of *Les inscriptions araméennes de Sfiré et l'Assyrie de Shamshi-ilu*, by A. Lemaire and J.-M. Durand. *WO* 15:210–12.

————. 1985. Some Problems in Early Aramean History. In *XXII. Deutscher Orientalistentag vom 21. bis 25. März 1983 in Tübingen: Ausgewählte Vorträge*, ed. W. Röllig, 81–85. ZDMG, Supplement 6. Stuttgart: F. Steiner.

————. 1985a. Suteans and Other West Semites during the Latter Half of the Second Millennium B.C. *OLP* 16:59–70.

————. 1985b. Samarian Notes. *BO* 42:567–72.

————. 1985c. Review of *Aramaic Texts from North Saqqâra*, by J. B. Segal. *WO* 16:173–76.

————. 1986. On Some Iranian Names in Aramaic Documents from Egypt. *Indo-Iranian Journal* 29:41–44.

————. 1986a. In *Cuneiform Archives and Libraries*, ed. K. R. Veenhof, 278–88. Publications de l'Institut historique-archéologique néerlandais de Stamboul, 57. Leiden: Nederlands Instituut voor het Nabije Oosten.

Zahdi, B. 1958–59. Mamlakat Dimašq al Aramiyya [The Aramean kingdom of Damascus]. *AASyr* 8–9:75–102 + 6 pls.

Zakharov, A. A. 1931. Material for the Corpus Sigillorum Asiae Anterioris Antiquae. *ArOr* 3:508–12 + 2 pls.

Zaki Saad, E. 1945. Saqqarah: Fouilles royales (1942). *CdE* 20:80–82.

Zauzich, K. T. 1976. Demotische Fragmente zum Ahikar-Roman. In *Folia rara: Wolfgang Voigt LXV diem natalem celebranti*. 180–85. Wiesbaden: F. Steiner.

————. 1985. Ägyptologische Bemerkungen zu den neuen aramäischen Papyri aus Saqqara. *Enchoria* 13:115–18.

————. 1985a. Der Gott des aramäisch-demotischen Papyrus Amherst 63. *Göttinger Miszellen* 85:89–90.

Zevit, Z. 1984. The Khirbet el-Qôm Inscription Mentioning a Goddess. *BASOR* 255:39–47.

————. 1990. The Common Origin of the Aramaicized Prayer to Horus and of Psalm 20. *JAOS* 110:213–28.

Zimmermann, F. 1938. The Aramaic Original of Daniel 8–12. *JBL* 57:255–72.

———. 1939. Some Verses in Daniel in Light of a Translation Hypothesis. *JBL* 58:349–54.

———. 1961. Hebrew Translation in Daniel. *JQR* 51:198–208.

———. 1964–65. The Writing on the Wall (Dan. 5:25f.) *JQR* 55:201–7.

———. 1975. *Biblical Books Translated from the Aramaic*. New York: Ktav.
    Reviews: J. D. Whitehead 1978.

Zivie, P. 1978. Review of *Documents araméens d'Égypte*, by P. Grelot. *Revue d'Égyptologie* 30:178–83.

Zobel, H.-J. 1971. Das Gebet um Abwendung der Not und seine Erhöhung in den Klageliedern des Alten Testaments und in der Inschrift des Königs Zakir von Hamath. *VT* 21:91–99.

Zotenberg, H. 1868. Nouvelles inscriptions phéniciennes d'Égypte. *JA* 6/11:431–50, 2 pls.

Zucker, F. 1959. Mitteilung über eine kürzlich gefundene griechisch-aramäische Bilingue des Königs Aśoka. AAASH 7:103–6.

Zucker, F. See: W. Honroth.

Zuckerman, B. 1983. "For Your Sake...": A Case Study in Aramaic Semantics. *JANES* 15:119–29.

———. 1987. *Puzzling Out the Past: Making Sense of Ancient Inscriptions from Biblical Times*. Los Angeles: West Semitic Research Project.

APPENDIX A: ARAMAICA?

Ap.1   Ördek-Burnu Stele (Zinjirli, 9th c.)   OrdBurn
Limestone stela with a mostly illegible 10-line inscription. Istanbul Museum.

Ed. Pr.   F. E. Peiser 1898.

EASY ACCESS
  Editions: *AC* 6 • *ESE* 3.192–206, pls. 13, 15.

LITERATURE
  A. H. Sayce 1927, esp. pp. 713–14 • S. Przeworski 1928 • J. Friedrich 1932, esp. pp. 38–39 • H. T. Norris 1951.

Ap.2   Khorsabad Maces (?)   KhorsabadMace
Bronze mace heads (3.01 cm. ht.) Iraq Museum, Louvre.

לאסרסרצר

Ed. Pr.   Louvre) *CIS* 50; Iraq) K. 'Abada 1974, esp. pp. 333–34.

LITERATURE
  A. Lemaire 1987.

Ap.3   Clay Tube (Nineveh, 8th–7th c.?)   NinCTu
Baked clay fragmentary tube (lamp?).

בלטסו

Ed. Pr.   R. Campbell Thompson and R. W. Hamilton 1932

Ap.4   Calah (Nimrud) Ostracon (725–675)   CalahOstr
Ostracon containing personal names, probably Ammonite.

Ed. Pr.   J. B. Segal 1957.

LITERATURE
  G. Garbini 1956a, esp. pp. 270–72 • W. F. Albright 1958 • E. Vogt 1958a • S. Segert 1965a • G. Garbini 1967a, esp. pp. 94–95 • J. Naveh 1971c, esp. p. 14 • P. Bordreuil 1979 • J. Naveh 1979–80 • J. Naveh 1982, pl. 13B • K. P. Jackson 1983a, esp. pp. 63–67 • B. Becking 1988.

Ap.5   Nimrud Ivory Inscriptions (7th c.)   NimrIv

Six inscriptions on ivory furniture adornments, four possibly in Aramaic, but only one (no. 3) certainly so. London.
1) Ivory label (9.2 x 6.5 cm.) (ND 10151).
2) Triangular plaque (ND 10359).
3) Fragment of dedication on strip of ivory (ND 8184a).
4) Fragment of plaque (3 x 1.5 cm.) (ND 8184b).

חמת (1
לעש (2
[...] זי הקרב [...] (3
[...]בא[..] (4

Ed. Pr.   A. R. Millard 1962.

LITERATURE

R. D. Barnett 1935 ● R. D. Barnett 1939 ● P. Amandry 1958 ● R. D. Barnett 1957, esp. p. 161, pl. 132 ● R. Giveon 1958 ● B. L. Goff 1960 ● R. D. Barnett 1963 ● J. Naveh 1964–65, esp. pp. 183–84 ● J. Naveh 1966, esp. pp. 20–21 ● W. Röllig 1974 ● E. Puech 1978.

Ap.6   Nimrud Bronzes (7th c.)   NimrBr

16 inscriptions on bronze bowls, tripods, and scepters. British Museum.

Ed. Pr.   1) A. H. Layard 1853.
2–4) P. Berger 1884.
5–16) R. D. Barnett 1967.

EASY ACCESS
Editions: 1) *CIS* II 49.
2) *CIS* II 47.
3) *CIS* II 48.
4) *CIS* II 46.

LITERATURE
J. Euting 1883, nos. 7,8 ● Y. Yadin 1967 ● M. Heltzer 1978 ● M. Heltzer 1982.

Ap.7   Amman Statue (7th c.[?])   AmmStat

Limestone statue (45 cm. ht.).   Archaeological Museum, Amman.

[...]שׁ[..] ירחעזר 1
[...]כר בר שנב

Ed. Pr.   G. L. Harding 1950.

LITERATURE
  W. Aufrecht 1989.

Ap.8   Heshbon Ostracon II (late 6th c.)   HeshOstr

Broken sherd with administrative (?) text (3.25 x 4.2 cm.) Archaeological Museum, Amman.

1 [...] נ[...]
... סכת פד]ן [...]
תמכאל]...[
בני גבל.]...[
5 [...]מ א[...]

Ed. Pr.   F. M. Cross 1973, pl. 16A.

LITERATURE
  W. Aufrecht, 1989.

Ap.9   Endir-kach Graffito (Kurdistan, 500)   EndirKGr

Graffito on the wall of a rock tomb. In situ.

זרתו]...[

Ed. Pr.   J. de Morgan 1896.

LITERATURE   E. Herzfeld 1947, esp. p. 53.

Ap.10   Jericho Ostracon (Elephantine?!, 5th c.)   JerichoOstr

Sherd with list of 14 non-Semitic names. Louvre (AO 25431).

Ed. Pr.   A. Lemaire 1975.

LITERATURE
  J. Teixidor 1976, esp. pp. 332–33.

Ap.11   Lachish Altar (5th–4th c.)   Lach

Stone altar (15 x 10 cm.) Rockefeller Museum, Jerusalem.

1 לבנת אי
ש בן מח
ליה מל]כ]ש[

Ed. Pr.   A. Dupont-Sommer 1953.

EASY ACCESS

Translations: *RTAT* 267 ● *NERTOT* 250–51.

LITERATURE
W. F. Albright 1953a ● A. Dupont-Sommer 1953b ● J. T. Milik 1958–59, esp. p. 334, n. 4 ● Anon. 1960 ● J. T. Milik 1960a ● M. Dahood 1960b, esp. pp. 407–8 ● B. Porten 1968, esp. p. 292, n.27 ● Y. Aharoni 1968, esp. pp. 163–64 ● F. M. Cross 1969c, esp. pp. 21–24 ● Y. Aharoni 1970–71 ● J. Teixidor 1970a, esp. pp. 374–75 ● N. Glueck 1971a ● R. Degen 1972 ● J. Teixidor 1973, esp. pp. 429–30 ● A. Lemaire 1974 ● J. Teixidor 1975, esp. p. 285 ● E. Lipiński 1975, esp. p. 267 ● E. Lipiński 1975a, esp. pp. 143–45 ● E. Lipiński 1978a, esp. p. 250–51 ● A. Lemaire 1989a, esp. p. 101.

Ap.12　　Gibeon Jar Fragment (Persian period)　　　　　　Gibeon
Part of a name (4 x 4 cm.). Israel Department of Antiquities.

פניה[צ]

Ed. Pr.　　　　J. Naveh 1985a, p. 120, pl. 20.

LITERATURE
J. Naveh 1971, esp. p. 31 n. 25.

Ap.13　　Araq el Emir (5th c.?)　　　　　　　　　　　Araq
Personal name on a tomb entrance. In situ.

טוביה

Ed. Pr.　　　　E. Littmann 1907, pp. 1–7.

LITERATURE
J. Derenbourg 1867 ● K. Budde 1918 ● G. Dalman 1920 ● L.-H. Vincent 1923 ● W. F. Albright 1932, esp. pp. 171, 222 ● B. Mazar (Maisler) 1940–41 ● R. A. Bowman 1948, esp. p. 82, n. 99 ● B. Mazar 1957 ● C. C. McCown 1957.

Ap.14　　Graffiti on Coins of Demanhur (318)　　　　　DemanGr
Ten Alexander tetradrachms with incised inscriptions. One is Demotic, the rest are names or letters in Aramaic square script.

Ed. Pr.　　　　C. C. Torrey 1937.

Ap.15   Naqsh i-Rustam Inscription (early 3d c.)   **Naqsh**

Portion of an Old Persian inscription in Aramaic script. In situ.

Ed. Pr.   E. Herzfeld 1926, esp. p. 244 + drawing.

LITERATURE

H. H. Schaeder 1929–30, esp. p. 268 • E. Herzfeld 1935, esp. p. 48 • G. Messina 1936 • E. Herzfeld 1937 • E. Herzfeld 1938, esp. pp. 12–13, pl. 4 • F. Altheim 1947–48, esp. pp. 36–39 • F. Altheim 1947a, esp. pp. 1:36–39 • F. Altheim 1948–50, esp. p. 2:186 • R. G. Kent 1953, esp. p. 109 • J. Friedrich 1957, esp. pp. 40–41 • W. B. Henning 1958, esp. pp. 24–25 • F. Altheim and R. Stiehl 1963, esp. pp. 10–13 • F. Altheim and R. Stiehl 1964–69, esp. pp. 2:368–69; 4:214 • F. Altheim and R. Stiehl 1970, esp. pp. 334–38.

Ap.16   Tell el-Mazār Jar Fragments   **Mazar**

Two pottery fragments with possible Aramaic inscriptions.

יהויה (1

בלל יֹין / [...]שׁ בֹר עגל (2

Ed. Pr.   Kh. Yassine and J. Teixidor 1986 + photos.

LITERATURE

M. Heltzer 1989.

APPENDIX B: TEXTUAL CONCORDANCES

I. CAL SIGLA

CAL Siglum	Biblio. No.	Title
ABCOstr	B.3.c.26	ABC Ostracon
AECT.1–42	B.2.5	Tablets from Nineveh and Environs
AECT.43–44	B.2.6	Nimrud Labels
AECT.45	B.2.7	Nimrud Bullae (ND 2348 and 2349)
AECT.46–51	B.2.8	Assur Tablets
AECT.52	B.2.9	Freydank Assur Tablet
AECT.5357	B.2.10	Tell Halaf Tablets
AECT.58	B.2.11	A Judicial Settlement
AECT.59	B.2.12	AECT 59
AECT.60	B.2.14	Loan Settlement
AECT.61	B.2.15	Copenhagen Conveyance
AGironOstr.1	B.3.c.27	Aimé-Giron Ostracon 1
AGironOstr.2	B.3.c.28	Aimé-Giron Ostracon 2
AP.50	B.3.c.14	AP 50
AP.57	B.3.c.6	Elephantine: Miscellaneous Letters
AP.58	B.3.c.6	Elephantine: Miscellaneous Letters
AP.64	B.3.c.14	AP 64
AP.68	B.3.c.14	AP 68
AP.79	B.3.c.15	Inventory
AP.82	B.3.c.13	Legal Document
APE.91	B.3.c.36	Uriah Ostracon
APE.92	B.3.c.37	Cucumber Ostracon
APE.94	B.3.c.38	Ismun-Seho Ostracon
APE.96	B.3.c.39	Golenischeff Ostracon I
APE.97	B.3.c.40	Golenischeff Ostracon II
APO76.1	B.3.c.22	Ostracon to Uriah and Ahutab
APO76.2	B.3.c.41	HWNY Ostracon
APO77.1	B.3.c.42	Mahseiah Ostracon
APO77.2	B.3.c.21	Passover Ostracon 2
APO78.2	B.3.c.23	Ahutab Ostracon
APO84.7	B.3.c.43	Meshullak Ostracon
AbuPapFrag.12	B.3.f.6	Abusir Papyri
AbydI	B.3.f.23	Abydos Inscriptions
AbydLiW	B.5.3	Abydos Lion Weight
AbydPap	B.3.f.14	Abydos Papyrus
AgacaKale	B.5.15	Agaca Kale Bilingual
AlexNecr	B.3.f.39	Alexandrian Necropolis Texts
AmmStat	Ap.7	Amman Statue
AradOstr	B.1.36	Tell Arad Ostraca
Araq	Ap.13	Araq el Emir
Arebsun	B.5.9	Arebsun Stelae
ArslanTash	B.1.4	Hazael Ivory Inlays

AshdodOstr	B.1.31	Ashdod Ostracon
Asok.1	B.6.6	Asoka I
Asok.2	B.6.7	Asoka II
Asok.3	B.6.8	Asoka III
Asok.4	B.6.9	Asoka IV
Asok.5	B.6.10	Asoka V
Asok.6	B.6.11	Asoka VI
AssOstr	B.2.13	Assur Ostracon
AswSarc	B.3.f.4	Aswan Sarcophagi
AswStel	B.3.f.3	Aswan Stele
BMAP 16	B.3.c.14	BMAP 16
BMDoc	B.2.19	Babylonian Dockets in the British Museum
BabBrick	B.2.21	Bricks from Babylon
BabDoc	B.2.20	Late Babylonian Contracts from Babylon
Bahad	B.5.10	Bahadirli Inscriptions
BahrVase	B.4.27	Bahrain Vase Inscription
BakFrag	B.3.f.9	Bakenrenef Fragment
BarH	B.1.1	Bar-Hadad Stele
BarRak	B.1.14	Bar-Rakkab Inscriptions
BeershebaOstr.54	B.1.38	Tell Beer-Sheba Jar
BeershebaOstr	B.1.37	Tell Beer-Sheba Ostraca
BelStat	B.3.a.1	Bel-shar-uṣur Statuette
BilTab	B.2.17	Bilingual Tablet
BodOstr.1	B.3.c.29	Bodleian Ostracon
BrusTab	B.2.18	Brussels Tablets
CairoOstr.1	B.3.c.30	Cairo Ostracon 1
CairoOstr.2	B.3.c.31	Cairo Ostracon 2
CairoOstr.3	B.3.c.32	Cairo Ostracon 3
CalahOstr	Ap.4	Calah (Nimrud) Ostracon
Carp	B.3.f.18	Carpentras Stele
CaucSilBo	B.5.1	Caucasus Silver Bowl
ClGan	B.3.c.33	Clermont-Ganneau Elephantine Ostraca
Coins	B.7.2	Coins
CowleyOstr	B.3.c.34	Cowley Ostracon 1
DA	B.1.19	Deir 'Alla Plaster Text
DAEpig	B.1.20	Deir 'Alla Epigraphs
DahshurGr	B.3.f.36	Dahshur Graffiti
Daskyleion	B.5.5	Daskyleion Funerary Stele
Decree	B.1.23	Beirut Decree
DegenPapFrag	B.3.c.55	Degen Papyrus Fragments
DemanGr	Ap.14	Graffiti on Coins of Demanhur
DreamOstr	B.3.c.47	Dream Ostracon
EdfuOstr	B.3.f.33	Edfu Ostraca
EdfuTomb	B.3.f.41	Edfu Tomb Inscriptions
EgAramStat	B.3.f.31	Egyptian Aramaic Statuette
EinGedi	B.1.34	Ein Gedi Ostraca
EinGev	B.1.2	Ein Gev Jar
ElJarI	B.3.c.49	Elephantine Jar Inscriptions
ElMumLab	B.3.c.52	Elephantine Mummy Label

ElSt.1	B.3.c.50	Elephantine Stone 1
ElSt.2	B.3.c.51	Elephantine Stone 2
ElWoStamp	B.3.c.53	Elephantine Wooden Stamp
ElWoStrip	B.3.c.54	Elephantine Wooden Strip
ElathOstr	B.1.25	Elath Ostraca
EmarSt	B.1.13	Emar Stone
EndirKGr	Ap.9	Endir-kach Graffito
Fakh	B.2.2	Tell Fakhariyeh Bilingual Statue
Gaza	B.1.48	Gaza Ostracon
Gibeon	Ap.12	Gibeon Jar Fragment
GizGr	B.3.f.19	Gizeh Graffito
GozBdSt	B.5.7	Gözneh Boundary Stone
Had	B.1.9	Hadad
HalAlph	B.2.3	Tell Halaf Alphabet
HalAlt	B.2.1	Tell Halaf "Altar"
HamAl	B.3.f.10	Wâdi Hammamath Alphabet
HamGr	B.1.5	Hamath Graffiti
HamWt	B.1.12	Hamath Weight
HazBrid	B.1.17	Hazael Bridles
Hem	B.5.11	Hemite Inscription
HeshOstr	Ap.8	Heshbon Ostracon II
HilprDock	B.2.24	Hilprecht Dockets
HorvDor	B.1.41	Ḥorvat Dorban Jar Fragment
Information	B.3.c.1	Elephantine Texts: General
Information	B.6.5	Asoka Inscriptions General
Ira	B.1.49	Tel 'Ira Ostracon
IranSilLab	B.6.4	Silver Label
JarH	B.1.40	Jar Handle Stamps and Inscriptions
Jemmeh	B.1.21	Tell Jemmeh Ostracon
JerichoOstr	Ap.10	Jericho Ostracon
JerusOstr	B.1.51	Jerusalem Ostracon
Kerak	B.1.44	Kerak Altar Fragment
Kesecek	B.5.4	Kesëcëk Köyü Votive
KetefYer	B.1.35	Ketef Yeriḥo Papyrus
KhElKom	B.1.50	Khirbet el-Kom Ostraca
KhShJar	B.1.32	Khan Sheikhoun Jar
KhorsabadMace	Ap.2	Khorsabad Maces
Kil	B.1.8	Kilamuwa Scepter
Lach	Ap.11	Lachish Altar
LarOstr	B.2.25	Larsa Ostracon
LimBil	B.5.12	Limyra Bilingual
LouvPal	B.3.f.35	Louvre Palette
LouvTab	B.1.24	Louvre (Starcky) Tablet
LurBr	B.6.1	Luristan Bronze Vessels
LuxorOstr	B.3.f.32	Luxor Ostracon
LydBil	B.5.13	Lydian (Sardis) Bilingual
Masarah	B.3.f.37	Ma'sârah Quarry Inscription
Maskh	B.3.f.12	Maskhûṭa Bowls
Mazar	Ap.16	Tell el-Mazār Jar Fragments

MelMWr	B.3.f.11	Mellawi Mummy Wrapper
MemLibAlt	B.3.e.8	Memphis Libation Altar
MemOJar	B.3.e.7	Memphis Ointment Jar
MemPap.3	B.3.e.4	Memphis Papyrus 3
MemPap.4	B.3.e.5	Memphis Papyrus 4
MemPlaque	B.3.e.11	Memphis Plaque
MemStel	B.3.e.9	Ptah Stele
MemWoJar	B.3.e.10	Memphis Wooden Jar
MemWoTab	B.3.e.12	Memphis Wooden Tablet
Meyd	B.5.2	Meydancikkale Inscriptions
MiscBab	B.2.23	Miscellaneous Babylonian Tablets and Dockets
MiscPapFrags	B.3.c.55	Papyrus Fragments
MousBowl	B.1.28	Moussaief Bowl
MunichOstr.1	B.3.c.24	Munich Ostracon 1
MunichOstr.2	B.3.c.25	Munich Ostracon 2
MurDoc	B.2.22	Murashû Dockets
NSaqOstr	B.3.e.25	North Saqqara Ostraca
NSaqPap	B.3.e.24	North Saqqara Papyri
Naqsh	Ap.15	Naqsh i-Rustam Inscription
NebYun	B.1.45	Nebī Yūnis Ostracon
NerTab	B.1.27	Nerab Tablets
Nerab	B.1.16	Nerab Stelae
NimJar	B.2.16	Nimrud Jar Inscriptions
NimrBr	Ap.6	Nimrud Bronzes
NimrIv	Ap.5	Nimrud Ivory Inscriptions
NinCTu	Ap.3	Clay Tube
NinLiW	B.2.4	Nineveh Lion Weights
NipOstr	B.2.26	Nippur Ostracon
Olymp	B.1.22	Olympian Bowl
OrdBurn	Ap.1	Ördek-Burnu Stele
PIBPap	B.3.f.8	Pontifical Biblical Institute Papyrus
Pad.3	B.3.c.5	Padua Papyrus Letter III
Pad	B.3.c.5	Padua Letters
Pan	B.1.10	Panamuwa
PapAmherst	B.3.f.27	Amherst Demotic Papyrus
PassOst	B.3.c.20	Passover Ostracon
Persep	B.6.3	Persepolis Inscriptions
PersepTab	B.6.2	Persepolis Tablets
PhilBil	B.1.53	Philotas Bilingual
Qadum	B.1.30	Qadum Bowl
RosPh	B.3.f.38	Rosette Phialê
Rub	B.3.f.34	Fayum Wooden Panel
SaidOstr	B.1.26	Tell es-Saidiyeh Ostraca
SaltSt	B.3.f.17	Salt Stele
SamPap	B.1.39	Samaria Papyri
SamSh	B.1.29	Samaria Sherds
SaqBaalStel	B.3.e.2	Saqqarah Baal Stele
SaqMumLab	B.3.e.23	Saqqarah Mummy Labels
SaqOstr	B.3.e.1	Saqqarah Ostracon

SaqPapFrag.4	B.3.e.17	Saqqarah Papyrus Fragment 4
SaqPapFrag.5	B.3.e.18	Saqqarah Papyrus Fragment 5
SaqPtahTomb	B.3.e.19	Saqqarah Ptah Tomb Papyrus
SaqSarcI	B.3.e.27	Saqqarah Sarcophagi
SaqPlt	B.3.e.20	Saqqarah Plate
SaqSteleFrag	B.3.e.28	Saqqarah Stele Fragment
SaqStel	B.3.e.22	Saqqarah Funerary Stele
SaqWoodFrag	B.3.e.21	Saqqarah Wooden Fragment
SarGr	B.5.8	Saraidin Graffito
Seals	B.7.1	Seals
SegalOstr	B.3.c.35	Segal Ostracon
SerapiumPap	B.3.f.7	Serapium Papyrus
Sf	B.1.11	Sefire Treaty
ShFTl	B.3.f.2	Sheikh Fadl Tomb
ShHasOst	B.1.43	Tell Sheikh Ḥasan Ostracon
StrasbourgOstr.1	B.3.c.44	Strasbourg Ostracon 1
StrasbourgOstr.2	B.3.c.45	Strasbourg Ostracon 2
StrasbourgOstr.3	B.3.c.46	Strasbourg Ostracon 3
SultStel	B.5.6	Sultaniye Köy Stele
TA.86bis	B.3.f.26	An Endorsement
TA.914	B.3.f.1	Graffiti
TA	B.3.f.21	Aimé-Giron Papyrus Fragments
TADA1.1	B.3.a.5	Adon Letter
TADA2	B.3.b.1	Hermopolis Letters
TADA3.1	B.3.c.6	Elephantine: Miscellaneous Letters
TADA3.2	B.3.c.6	Elephantine: Miscellaneous Letters
TADA3.3	B.3.c.5	Padua Papyrus Letter I
TADA3.4	B.3.c.5	Padua Papyrus Letter II
TADA3.5	B.3.c.6	Elephantine: Miscellaneous Letters
TADA3.6	B.3.c.6	Elephantine: Miscellaneous Letters
TADA3.7	B.3.c.6	Elephantine: Miscellaneous Letters
TADA3.8	B.3.c.6	Elephantine: Miscellaneous Letters
TADA3.9	B.3.c.6	Elephantine: Miscellaneous Letters
TADA3.10	B.3.c.6	Elephantine: Miscellaneous Letters
TADA3.11	B.3.f.24	El-Hibeh Papyrus Letter
TADA4	B.3.c.4	The Yedaniah Archive
TADA5.1	B.3.e.16	Saqqarah Papyrus Letter
TADA5.2	B.3.c.6	Elephantine: Miscellaneous Letters
TADA5.3	B.3.f.15	Turin Papyrus
TADA5.4	B.3.f.16	Fragmentary Letter
TADA5.5	B.3.c.6	Elephantine: Miscellaneous Letters
TADA6	B.3.d.1	The Arsames Letters
TADB1.1	B.3.a.4	Bauer-Meissner Land Lease
TADB2	B.3.c.7	The Mibtaḥiah Archive
TADB3	B.3.c.8	The Anani Archive
TADB4	B.3.c.9	Elephantine: Miscellaneous Contracts
TADB4.7	B.3.e.24	North Saqqarah Papyus 35
TADB5	B.3.c.10	Elephantine: Conveyances
TADB5.6	B.3.e.24	Sale of Slaves

TADB6	B.3.c.11	Elephantine: Marriage Contracts
TADB7	B.3.c.12	Elephantine: Affidavits and Legal Records
TADB8.1	B.3.e.24	North Saqqarah Papyus 29
TADB8.2	B.3.e.24	North Saqqarah Papyus 10+44
TADB8.3	B.3.e.24	North Saqqarah Papyus 5
TADB8.4	B.3.e.24	North Saqqarah Papyus 28+30+61
TADB8.5	B.3.c.14	Lepsius Fragments
TADB8.6	B.3.e.24	North Saqqarah Papyus 9
TADB8.7	B.3.e.24	North Saqqarah Papyus 4
TADB8.8	B.3.e.24	North Saqqarah Papyus 1
TADB8.9	B.3.e.24	North Saqqarah Papyus 2
TADB8.10	B.3.e.24	North Saqqarah Papyus 3+16
TADB8.11	B.3.e.24	North Saqqarah Papyus 21
TADB8.12	B.3.e.24	North Saqqarah Papyus 6
TADC1.1	B.3.c.3	Aḥiqar
TADC1.2	B.3.e.26	Bar Pawenesh
TADC2.1	B.3.c.2	Bisitūn Inscription
TADC3.1	B.3.a.2	RES 1791
TADC3.2	B.3.a.3	Göttingen Papyrus
TADC3.3	B.3.c.15	List of Names
TADC3.4	B.3.c.55	Berlin 23103
TADC3.5	B.3.e.15	Papyrus Fragment 2
TADC3.6	B.3.e.24	North Saqqarah Papyus 47
TADC3.7	B.3.e.6	Memphis Shipyard Journal
TADC3.8	B.3.e.24	North Saqqarah Papyus 20+19
TADC3.9	B.3.c.15	Aḥiqar Palimpsest
TADC3.10	B.3.e.13	Family List
TADC3.11	B.3.f.13	Cairo Papyrus 3484
TADC3.12	B.3.c.16	Papyrus Luparensis
TADC3.13	B.3.c.15	List
TADC3.14	B.3.c.15	Account
TADC3.15	B.3.c.15	Donor List
TADC3.16	B.3.c.15	Fragmentary Account
TADC3.17	B.3.f.22	Fragmentary Account of Grain
TADC3.18	B.3.e.24	North Saqqarah Papyus 45
TADC3.19	B.3.f.25	Vatican Papyrus
TADC3.20	B.3.e.24	North Saqqarah Papyus 57
TADC3.21	B.3.f.5	Mariette Papyrus Fragments
TADC3.22	B.3.e.24	North Saqqarah Papyus 48
TADC3.23	B.3.e.24	North Saqqarah Papyus 87
TADC3.24	B.3.e.24	North Saqqarah Papyus 106
TADC3.25	B.3.c.15	de Vogüé Papyrus Fragments
TADC3.26	B.3.f.30	Jequier Papyrus
TADC3.27	B.3.c.18	Harrow School Papyrus
TADC3.28	B.3.c.17	Account
TADC3.29	B.3.f.42	Levi della Vida Papyrus
TADC4.1	B.3.e.14	Papyrus Fragment 1
TADC4.2	B.3.e.24	North Saqqarah Papyus 53
TADC4.3	B.3.e.3	Memphis Name List

TADC4.4	B.3.c.15	List of Names
TADC4.5	B.3.c.15	List of Names
TADC4.6	B.3.c.15	List of Names
TADC4.7	B.3.c.15	List of Names
TADC4.8	B.3.c.15	List of Names
TADC4.9	B.3.c.15	List of Names
TAbuZeitun	B.1.42	Tell Abu Zeitun Ostracon
TDan	B.1.3	Tell Dan Bowl
TDanBil	B.1.52	Tell Dan Bilingual
TFara	B.1.46	Tell el-Fara' Ostraca
TSifr	B.1.15	Tell Sifr Stele
TZerB	B.1.18	Tell Zeror Ostracon
Teima.1	B.4.4	Teima Stele I
Teima.2	B.4.21	Teima Votive II
Teima.2a	B.4.22	Teima Votive II Draft
Teima.3	B.4.23	Teima Funerary Stele III
Teima.4	B.4.24	Teima Funerary Stele IV
Teima.5	B.4.5	Teima Inscription V
Teima.6	B.4.6	Teima Funerary Stele VI
Teima.7	B.4.2	Teima Funerary Stele VII
Teima.8	B.4.3	Teima Funerary Stele VIII
Teima.9	B.4.7	Teima Plaque
Teima.10	B.4.25	Teima Funerary Stele X
Teima.11	B.4.30	Teima Stone Basin
Teima.12	B.4.8	Khubu el-Gharbi Funerary Stele
Teima.13	B.4.9	Jebel ed-Dighš Funerary Stele
Teima.14	B.4.28	Wâdi Madhbah Grave Marker
Teima.15	B.4.10	Hejra Grave Marker
Teima.16	B.4.11	Engraver's Block
Teima.17	B.4.12	Teima Ostracon XVII
Teima.18	B.4.13	El-'Ula Stele
Teima.19	B.4.29	El-'Ula Stele
Teima.20	B.4.14	Teima Stele XX
Teima.21	B.4.15	Teima Funerary Stele XXI
Teima.22	B.4.16	Teima Funerary Stele XXII
Teima.23	B.4.17	Teima Funerary Stele XXIII
Teima.24	B.4.18	Teima Funerary Stele XXIV
Teima.25	B.4.19	Teima Funerary Stele XXV
Teima.26	B.4.26	Teima Ostracon XXVI
Teima.27	B.4.20	Teima Stele XXVII
TelBr	B.2.27	Tello Bricks
TumStel	B.3.e.29	Tumma Stele
UrukBr	B.2.28	Uruk Bricks
UrukInc	B.2.29	Uruk Cuneiform Incantation
VatFunStel	B.3.f.28	Vatican Funerary Stele
ViennaOstr.1	B.3.c.19	Vienna Ostracon I
ViennaOstr.24	B.3.f.40	Vienna Ostraca
WHudiGr	B.3.f.20	Wâdi El-Hudi Horus Stele Graffiti
WaSabRigGr	B.3.a.6	Wâdi es-Saba' Riggaleh Graffiti

WaSh	B.3.f.29	Wâdi Sheikh Sheikhun Graffito
Xanthos	B.5.14	Xanthos Inscriptions
Yatta	B.1.47	Yatta Ostracon
Yoqneam	B.1.33	Yoqneam Ostracon
Zak	B.1.6	Zakur Stele

II. MAJOR COLLECTIONS

AC

Texts found in J. J. Koopmans, *Aramäische Chrestomathie*.

AC	CAL Siglum	AC	CAL Siglum
1	[Phoenician]	31	TADC1.1
2	Kil	32	TADC2.1
3	HalAlt	33A	ClGan.152
4	BarH	33B	ClGan.186
5	ArslanTash.1	34	CairoOstr.1
6	Ord	35	CairoOstr.2
7	HamGr	36	APO76.1
8	Zak	37	StrasbourgOstr.1
9	Had	38	NipOstr
10	Sf	39	LarOstr
11	Pan	40	AbydI
12	BarRak.1	42	GozBdSt
13	NinLiW	43	HamAl
14	AssOstr	44A	Maskh.1
15	ShFTI	44B	Maskh.2
16	TADA1.1	44C	Maskh.3
17	Nerab.1	45	Teima.1
18	Nerab.2	46	LydBil
19	TADB1.1	47	SarGr
20	AbydLiW	48	Kesecek
21	SaqStel	49	Carp
22	AswStel	50	Teima.2
23	TADB3.1	51	DreamOstr
24	TADB3.2	52	TADA5.3
25	TADB3.6	53A	Asok.2
26	TADB3.9	53B	Asok.3
27	TADB2.11	54	Asok.1
28	TADA4.7	55	PapAmherst
29	TADA4.9	56	UrukInc
30	TADA6.11		

AP

Texts found in A. Cowley, *Aramaic Papyri of the Fifth Century B.C.*

AP	CAL Siglum	AP	CAL Siglum	AP	CAL Siglum
1	TADB5.1	31	TADA4.8	61	TADC3.9
2	TADB4.4	32	TADA4.9	62	TADC3.13
3	TADB4.3	33	TADA4.10	63	TADC3.13
4	AP.4	34	TADA4.4	64	AP.64
5	TADB2.1	35	TADB4.6	65+67	TADB5.2
6	TADB2.2	36	TADB6.2	66	TADA4.6
7	TADB7.2	37	TADA4.2	68	AP.68
8	TADB2.3	38	TADA4.3	68/12	TADA4.6
9	TADB2.4	39	TADA3.7	69	TADB8.5
10	TADB3.1	40	TADA3.6	70	TADA5.3
11	TADB4.2	41	TADA3.5	71	TADC1.2
12	TADC4.4	42	TADA3.8	72	TADC3.12
13	TADB2.7	43	TADB5.5	73	TADC3.19
14	TADB2.8	44	TADB7.3	74	TADC4.9
15	TADB2.6	45	TADB7.1	75	TADC3.21
16	TADA5.2	46	TADB6.3	76	TADA5.4
17	TADA6.1	47	TADB5.3	77	SerapiumPap
18	TADB6.4	48	TADB2.5	78	TADC3.25
19	TADC4.5	49	TADB4.1	79	AP.79
20	TADB2.9	50	AP.50	80	TADA5.5
21	TADA4.1	51	TADC4.7	81	TADC3.28
22	TADC3.15	52	TADC3.16	82	AP.82
23	TADC4.6	53	TADC4.8	83	TADC3.27
24	TADC3.14	54	TADA3.1	App. A.	TADC4.1
25	TADB2.10	55	TADA3.2	App. B-C.	TADC3.5
26	TADA6.2	56	TADA4.4	pp. 204-48	TADC1.1
27	TADA4.5	57	AP.57	pp. 248-71.	TADC2.1
28	TADB2.11	58	AP.58		
29	TADB4.5	59	TADB7.4		
30	TADA4.7	60	[Greek]		

CIS

Texts found in *Corpus Inscriptionarum Semiticarum* II.

CIS II	CAL Siglum	*CIS II*	CAL Siglum	*CIS II*	CAL Siglum
1-14	NinLiW	44-45	NimJar.1-2	120	Teima.14
15	AECT.30	46-49	NimrBr.1-4	121	Teima.19
16	AECT.1	50	KhorsabadMace	122	SaqStel
17	AECT.5	51-52	Seals	123	MemLibAlt
18	AECT.24	53-60	BabBrick	124	Seals
19	AECT.17	61	BMDoc.3	125-133	AbydI
20	AECT.28	62	BMDoc.1	134	WaSh
21	AECT.33	63	BMDoc.2	135	WaSabRigGr.1
22	AECT.27	64	BMDoc.4	136	WaSabRigGr.2
23	AECT.31	65	BMDoc.18	137	DreamOstr
24	AECT.32	66	Seals	138	APE.94
25	AECT.8	67	BMDoc.7	139	APE.95
26	BMDoc.17	68	BMDoc.15	140	Seals
27	AECT.10	69	MiscBab.1	141	Carp
28	AECT.23	70	BMDoc.21	142	VatFunStel
29	AECT.19	71	BMDoc.20	143	SaltSt
30	AECT.21	72	TelBr	144	TADA5.3
31	AECT.16	73-107	Seals	145	TADC1.2
32	AECT.2	108	AbydLiW	146	TADC3.12
33	AECT.20	109	LimBil	147	TADC3.19
34	BilTab	110	CaucSilBo	148	TADC4.9
35	AECT.11	111	SenKaleh	149	TADB8.5
36	AECT.26	112	Olymp	150	TADC3.21
37	AECT.35	113	Teima.1	151	TADA5.4
38	AECT.3	114	Teima.2	152	SerapiumPap
39	AECT.9	115	Teima.3	153	TADC3.25
40	AECT.6	116	Teima.4	154	APE.97
41	AECT.7	117	Teima.15	155	APE.96
42	AECT.15	118	Teima.17		
43	AECT.13	119	Teima.18		

KAI/TSSI

Texts found in H. Donner and W. Röllig, *Kanaanäische und Aramäische Inschriften*, 3d ed., and J. C. L. Gibson, *Textbook of Syrian Semitic Inscriptions*, Vol. 2.

KAI	CAL Siglum	*TSSI*	CAL Siglum
25	Kil	1	BarH
201	BarH	2	ArslanTash
202	Zak	3	EinGev
203-13	HamGr	4	TDan
214	Had	5	Zak
215	Pan	6	HamGr
216	BarRak.1	7	Sf.1
217	BarRak.8	8	Sf.2
218	BarRak.2	9	Sf.3
219	BarRak.3	10	HalAlt
220	BarRak.4	11	LurBr.1
221	BarRak.5	12	LurBr.2
222	Sf.1	13	Had
223	Sf.2	14	Pan
224	Sf.3	15	BarRak.1
225	Nerab.1	16	BarRak.8
226	Nerab.2	17	BarRak.2
227	LouvTab	18	Nerab.1
228	Teima.1	19	Nerab.2
229	Teima.2	20	AssOstr
230	Teima.3	21	TADA1.1
231	HalAlt	22	LouvTab
232	ArslanTash.1	23	SaqStel
233	AssOstr	24	Carp
234	AECT.47	25	Maskh.3
235	AECT.48	26	DreamOstr
236	AECT.49	27	TADA2
258	Kesecek	28	Pad.1
259	GozBdSt	29	AbydPap
260	LydBil	30	Teima.1
261	SarGr	31	AradOstr.38
262	LimBil	32	NebYun
263	AbydLiW	33	Kesecek
264	Arebsun	34	GozBdSt
266	TADA1.1	35	SarGr
267	SaqStel	36	Bahad
268	MemLibAlt	37	Dask
269	Carp		
270	DreamOstr		
271	APE.94		
272	VatFunStel		
273	Asok.1		
278	Bahad		
279	Asok.3		